HOSPITAL DEPARTMENTS DEMYSTIFIED

A Practical Guide Volume-I

Dr. Arun K. Agarwal

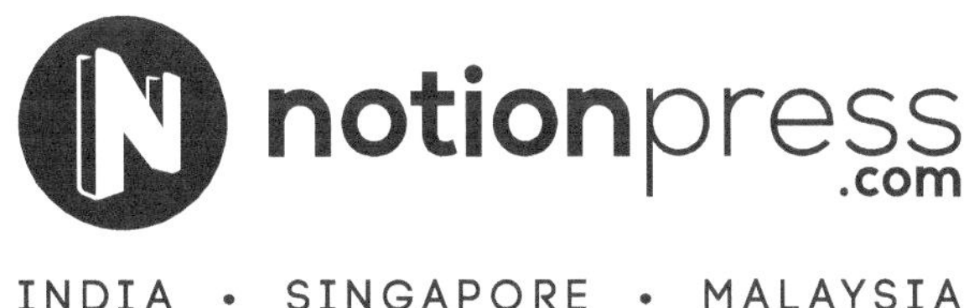

INDIA • SINGAPORE • MALAYSIA

ISBN 979-8-89026-946-1

Disclaimer

The information provided in this book, "Hospital Departments Demystified: A Practical Guide," is intended for educational and informational purposes only. While every effort has been made to ensure the accuracy and completeness of the content, the authors and publishers do not guarantee or warrant the reliability, suitability, or applicability of the information for any specific purpose.

The content of this book is based on research, professional experience, and the authors' understanding of the subject matter up to the date of publication. However, healthcare practices, guidelines, and regulations are constantly evolving, and the information in this book may become outdated or subject to change. Readers are advised to consult current medical literature, authoritative sources, and healthcare professionals for the most up-to-date and accurate information.

The authors and publishers disclaim any liability, loss, or risk incurred as a direct or indirect consequence of the use, application, or interpretation of the information presented in this book.

The authors and publishers are not responsible for any errors or omissions or for any consequences arising from the use of the information contained in this book.

Furthermore, the views and opinions expressed in this book are those of the authors and do not necessarily reflect the official policy or position of any institution or organization they may be affiliated with.

Readers are encouraged to independently verify any information provided in this book and exercise their own judgment and discretion in applying it to their specific circumstances.

By reading this book, the reader acknowledges and accepts the above disclaimer and agrees to release the authors and publishers from any and all liability arising from the use or reliance upon the information presented herein.

Dr. Arun K. Agarwal

CONTENTS

ACKNOWLEDGEMENT

Writing a book is a collaborative effort that would not be possible without the support, guidance, and contributions of numerous individuals. We would like to express our deepest gratitude to all those who have played a part in the creation of "Hospital Departments Demystified: A Practical Guide." Their unwavering support and valuable input have been invaluable throughout this journey.

First and foremost, we would like to thank the healthcare professionals who graciously shared their expertise, insights, and real-life experiences with us. Their willingness to impart their knowledge has enriched the content of this book and made it more relevant and meaningful.

We extend our heartfelt appreciation to the medical professionals, administrators, and staff from various hospital departments who provided us with valuable information, answered our queries, and gave us a glimpse into the inner workings of their respective departments. Their dedication to patient care and their commitment to excellence have inspired us in our endeavour to demystify the complexities of hospital departments.

Lastly, we are indebted to the readers of this book. Your curiosity, enthusiasm, and commitment to learning have driven us to create a resource that we hope will enrich your understanding of hospital departments and contribute to improved healthcare outcomes.

To everyone who has contributed, directly or indirectly, to the creation of this book, we extend our heartfelt thanks. Your support and involvement have been instrumental in making this project a reality.

Dr. Arun K. Agarwal
drarunghaziabad@yahoo.co.in

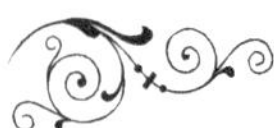

PREFACE

Welcome to "Hospital Departments Demystified: A Practical Guide." - Volume -1.

In this book, we aim to unravel the intricacies of hospital departments, shedding light on their planning, roles, functions, key performance indicator, checklists, duties of staff and interdependencies within the healthcare ecosystem. Whether you are a healthcare professional, a student, or simply an inquisitive reader, we hope this guide will provide you with valuable insights into the inner workings of hospitals.

The healthcare landscape can be overwhelming, with its myriad of departments and specialised areas. Understanding how these departments operate and collaborate is crucial for anyone involved in healthcare delivery, management, or even patient advocacy. This book endeavours to simplify and demystify the complexity of hospital departments, helping you navigate the healthcare system with confidence and clarity.

Through the pages of this guide, we will take you on a comprehensive tour of the most common hospital departments, exploring their unique functions, key personnel, and the essential services they provide. Each chapter will delve into the specific nuances of these departments, presenting a holistic view of their significance within the healthcare continuum.

We sincerely hope that this guide will empower you with a deeper appreciation of the collaborative efforts that drive hospital operations, ultimately leading to improved patient outcomes. Our goal is to equip you with the knowledge necessary to engage effectively with healthcare professionals, fostering meaningful partnerships and enhancing the overall patient experience.

We would like to express our gratitude to all the healthcare professionals who tirelessly work in various hospital departments, dedicating their lives to patient care. Their commitment and expertise have been instrumental in shaping the content of this book.

Lastly, we encourage you to embark on this enlightening journey through the fascinating world of hospital departments. By the end of this guide, we hope you will have gained valuable insights and a newfound appreciation for the intricate web of healthcare services that operate behind the scenes in hospitals.

As the subject is very wide, the complete information has been compiled in three volumes.

Wishing you an informative and enriching reading experience!

Dr. Arun K. Agarwal
drarunghaziabad@yahoo.co.in

INTRODUCTION

Welcome to "Hospital Departments Demystified: A Practical Guide," a comprehensive resource designed to unravel the intricacies of hospital departments and provide a practical understanding of their roles within the healthcare system. This three-volume series aims to provide a holistic view of the diverse departments that make up a hospital, offering insights into their functions, interdependencies, and the vital services they provide.

"Hospital Departments Demystified" is a comprehensive guide for doctors and hospitals on department Planning, Infrastructure required, Standard Operating Procedures (SOPs), Checklists, Key Performance Indicators, Duties of its staff and more. I have has also included suggested stationary formats used in these departments.

Volume I:

The departments covered in this volume are: Alternate Medicine, Ambulance, Anaesthesia, Biomedical Engineering, Cardiology, Cath lab, Dental, Dietetics, Emergency, Emergency Codes, Endocrinology, ENT, Gastroenterology, Materials Management (Store), Mortuary, Nephro – Dialysis, Nephrology, Ophthalmology, Urology.

Volume II:

The departments covered in this volume are: ICU, Radiology + Ultrasound, MRD, Neurology, Obs & Gynae, OPD, Orthopaedics, Paediatrics & Neonatology, Microbiology, Pathology, Physiotherapy, Plastic Surgery, Psychiatry, Pulmonology, Skin & VD, Surgery.

Volume III:

The departments covered in this volume are: Medicine, Code of Ethics, Nursing, and Code of Nurses Ethics, CSSD, Infection Control, HRD, Laundry, Front Office, Blood Bank, and Maintenance

We explore the critical aspects of all departments. We shed light on the unique responsibilities of each department and the dedicated professionals who work tirelessly to ensure the well-being of patients. By understanding the intricacies of departments, readers will gain a comprehensive view of the clinical care landscape within hospitals.

Ancillary and support departments focus on the ancillary and support departments those are vital to the smooth functioning of a hospital. These departments, often operating behind the scenes, play an integral role in supporting patient care. We delve into departments such as laboratory services, and nutrition, among others. By exploring these crucial components, readers will gain an appreciation for the comprehensive nature of hospital operations and the collaborative efforts required to provide high-quality care.

Administrative and Management Departments take readers into the administrative and management departments that oversee the strategic and operational aspects of a hospital. Understanding the administrative and management aspects of a hospital is crucial for healthcare professionals, administrators, and anyone interested in the efficient and effective operation of healthcare organizations.

Throughout this three-volume series, we aim to demystify the complexity of hospital departments, providing readers with a practical guide to navigate the healthcare system with confidence. Each volume is designed to stand alone, allowing readers to focus on specific areas of interest or explore the entire series for a comprehensive understanding of hospital departments.

Dr. Arun K. Agarwal

Chapter – 1

DEPARTMENT OF ALTERNATE MEDICINE

INDEX

INTRODUCTION:

The history of medicine indicates that almost every major civilisation and culture had developed their own system for curing diseases, though the approaches varied. From the very beginning of the human civilization, there has been on interest in controlling diseases, ensuring good health und prolonging life. (*Chandrakant Lahariya*)

ALTERNATIVE MEDICINE refers to a broad range of healing philosophies, approaches and therapies that exist largely outside the modern medical centres. Some people also refer to it as "Integrative" or "Complementary" medicine.

Complementary and alternative medicine (CAM) is defined as a group of diverse medical and health-care systems, practices, and products that are not generally considered part of conventional modern medicine or Western medicine.

According to one definition alternative medicine is a broad domain of healing resources that encompasses all health systems, modalities, practices and their accompanying theories and beliefs.

Alternative medicine refers to unproven or disproven methods used instead of standard medical treatments to prevent, diagnose, or treat numerous diseased. These methods have never been scientifically proven to be effective. Clinical trials are also lacking.

Alternative medicine includes dietary supplements, vitamins, natural products, herbal recipes, massage therapy, magnet therapy, and spiritual healing.

Alternative Medicine is an increasing feature of health-care practice, but still confusion exists on types of disciplines that are included in it.

In India, diverse systems of medicine are official and professionalized as to their service in education, treatment and research.

Alternative medicine is different from COMPLEMENTARY THERAPIES. Complementary methods are those that are used along with and support standard treatments (Allopathic).

Some people describe Alternative Medicine as unconventional, non-conventional, and non-traditional methods.

The renewed public interest has revitalized due to the lack of curative treatment for several emerging and chronic diseases, high cost of modern drugs, time constrain from patients and healthcare providers, microbial resistance and side effects of modern medicine.

"The Judicious use of Alternative Systems of Medicine is found cost effective and having lesser or no side effects. India stays in rural setup, where medicines from alternative systems can play very big role in curing the primary healthcare problems."

India is in process of integrating AYUSH system of medicine with the existing health system in the country, at all levels of health care so that preventive, promotive and rehabilitative health care services can be offered to all sections of society.

TYPES OF ALTERNATIVE MEDICINE:

Complementary and Alternative Medicine is a very brad department and there are too many types of therapies which constitute Alternative Medicine.

In India it is called AYUSH medicine and includes;

1. Ayurveda,
2. Yoga and Naturopathy,

3. Unani,
4. Siddha,
5. Homeopathy

Other types of therapeutic methods included in this group are;

1. Acupuncture
2. Acupressure
3. Chiropractic/Naprapathy
4. Anthroposophic Medicine
5. Electromagnetic Therapy (Magneto Therapy)
6. Reiki
7. Therapeutic (Healing) Touch
8. Apitherapy
9. Applied Kinesiology
10. Aqua Therapy
11. Aromatherapy
12. Aromatherapy
13. Bach Flower Remedy
14. Bach Flower Therapy
15. Balneotherapy
16. Bioresonance Therapy
17. Body Work OR Massage Therapy
18. Chelation Therapy
19. Colour Therapy/Light Therapy
20. Cupping Therapy
21. Dietary Supplements
22. Dowsing
23. Eclectic Psychotherapy
24. Feng Shui
25. Flower Essence Therapy
26. Gua Sha
27. Hatha Yoga
28. Hijama (Wet Cup Therapy)
29. Home Remedies
30. Hypnosis/Hypnotherapy
31. Laughter Therapy
32. Manipulative Therapy
33. Meditation
34. Moxibustion
35. Pranic Healing
36. Recreational Therapy
37. Reflexology
38. Reiki
39. T'ai Chi Ch'uan

40. Tea Therapy (Tea Leaves, Plant, Tree, Roots, Green Tea)
41. Tibetan Medicine
42. Urine Therapy/Uropathy
43. And many more.

AYURVEDA

One of the most ancient healing systems known to man, ayurveda is composed of two Sanskrit worlds, Ayus, and Veda, which means knowledge of life and how to live that life free from stress and with physical and mental wellbeing. It incorporates all aspects of life whether physical, psychological, spiritual or social. What is beneficial and what is harmful to life, what is happy life and what is sorrowful life; all these four questions and life span allied issues are elaborately and emphatically discussed in ayurveda.

Ayurveda is considered a form of medical care, equal to conventional allopathic medicine.

Ayurveda is the science of longevity and living. It is propounded that the knowledge of ayurveda came straight from BRAHMA and that makes it the medical science of highest order.

Ayurvedic medicine is a traditional medicine of India. Ayurveda believes in the existence of three elemental substances, the doshas (called vata, pitta and kapha), and states that a balance of the doshas results in health, while imbalance results in disease.

a. If "vata' gets out of balance, for instance, it leads to overactive mind, poor circulation, poor nerve conduction, loss of memory, irregular elimination & uncomfortable menses etc - all things related to movement.
b. If "Pitta" is out of balance, we can get excessive digestive fire, resulting in heartburn, excess stomach acid, hot temper & inflammations etc -all things related to heat and digestion.
c. If "Kapha" gets out of balance, it can lead to chronic congestion, weight gain, cellulite, cholesterol build-up, acne & oily skin etc - all things related to structure and lubrication.

Such disease-inducing imbalances can be adjusted and balanced using traditional herbs, minerals and heavy metals. Ayurveda stresses the use of plant-based medicines and treatments, with some animal products, and added minerals, including sulphur, arsenic, lead, copper sulphate.

Ayurveda is one of the world's oldest medical systems. It started in India more than 3,000 years ago and is still widely used today.

Health is not only the state of disease-free body but - 'Ayu' that is 'Life' which incorporates four components, namely;

1. Sharir: (physical body)
2. Indriya
3. Cognitive sense organs
4. Satva: (mind) & aatma (soul)

A healthy and disease-free existence of all four of the above components constitutes a healthy life.

Branches of Ayurveda: (courtesy: Planet Ayurveda)

Ayurveda is categorised into eight different branches and collectively it is known as Ashtang Ayurveda. Ashtang means eight parts or limbs. The basic mode of treatment of all these is same.

1. Kaaya Chikitsa (Internal medicine)
2. Baala Chikitsa (Paediatrics treatment)

3. Graha Chikitsa or Bhoot Vidya (Psychiatry)
4. Urdhyaanga Chikitsa (Treatment of eyes, nose, throat, head related diseases)
5. Shalyaroga Chikitsa (Surgery)
6. Damstra Chikitsa - Agad Tantra (Toxicology)
7. Jara Chikitsa - Rasayana (Geriatrics)
8. Vrishya Chikitsa or Vajjikarana (Aphrodisiac therapy)

STRENGTHS OF AYURVEDA:

It is helpful in many incurables, non-life-threatening conditions that may be chronic.

It improves the immune system.

Oil Massage Therapy or Kerala Ayurveda (*Dhara*)

Oil massage therapy or *Dhara* traces its roots back to 3000 years. This therapy is generally practiced by the Kerala's people. Many centres are established in Kerala these days, which provide this therapy. Basically, this therapy is a cure for a variety of physical and mental diseases, strains and tensions, arthritis, spondylitis, paralysis, obesity, sinusitis, migraine, rheumatism, etc.

The treatment called Panchkarma is based on the principal of Tridosha (three faults), which are Vata, Pita and Kapha. Through this five-fold purification therapy healers revive the disturbed equilibrium of these three doshas.

Panchkarma therapy has three main stages: poorvakarma, pradhanakarma and paschatkarma.

Poorvakarma is the first stage that comprises essential preliminary procedures preparing the body to unload stored toxins.

Pradhanakarma is the second stage and main cleaning therapies.

Paschatkarma is the final stage and describes the measures employed after the main treatment.

YOGA AND NATUROPATHY

Yoga is a group of physical, mental, and spiritual practices or disciplines which originated in ancient India and aim to control and still the mind, recognising a detached witness-consciousness untouched by the mind and mundane suffering.

Yoga is a comprehensive term comprising yogasanas, breath control, meditation, etc. The main aim of yoga is to build physical and mental powers in a human body. Yogasanas or asanas form only a part of yoga and are meant to keep the body in good health. Recent scientific research and experiments have proved beyond doubt the efficacy of yoga in controlling and curing many serious diseases like blood pressure, heart diseases, hypertension, nervous disorders, etc.

Yoga is now being adapted to correct lifestyle by cultivating a rational, positive and spiritual attitude towards all life situations.

Yoga is classified as per its style:

A. Ashtanga Yoga

Astanga or Ashtanga (aṣṭāṅga) is a Sanskrit compound translating to "having eight limbs or components".

B. Ashtanga Vinyasa Yoga

Ashtanga Vinyasa Yoga is a style of yoga as exercise created by K. Pattabhi Jois during the 20th century, often promoted as a modern-day form of classical Indian yoga. The style is energetic, synchronising breath with movements. The individual poses (asanas) are linked by flowing movements (vinyasas).

C. Bikram yoga

Bikram Yoga is a proprietary system of hot yoga as exercise devised by Bikram Choudhury; it became popular in the early 1970s. Classes consist of a fixed sequence of 26 postures, practised in a room heated to 105 °F (41 °C) with a humidity of 40%, intended to replicate the climate of India. The room is fitted with carpets and the walls are covered in mirrors; the instructor does not adjust the students, who are expected to adjust themselves.

What does YOGA do?

1. It lowers stress
2. It improves sleep
3. It improves balance
4. It manages anxiety or depression
5. It reduces neck and lower back pain
6. It can manage weight
7. It alleviates the symptoms of menopause
8. It reduces the symptoms of chronic conditions

Naturopathic medicine is based on a belief that the body heals itself using a supernatural vital energy that guides bodily processes, a view in conflict with the paradigm of evidence-based medicine.

Naturopathy or the naturopathic medicine is a drugless, non- invasive system of medicine imparting treatments with natural elements based on the theories of vitality, toxaemia and the self-healing capacity of the body, as well as the principles of healthy living.

Naturopathic practice aims at treating the underlying disease & disorders & restoring the natural body functions by encouraging the body's own healing capacities. It assist's the body's healing powers by using safe & effective non-pharmaceutical approaches.

Naturopathy is an integrating division by combining traditional practices and health care approaches. This medication system provides a unique way of treating patients, which maintains the homeostatic principle of the body identifies the source as well as treats the diseases. Naturopathic practitioners tend to employ the self-healing process by maintaining healthier lifestyles, diet and nutrition. Popular naturopathic therapies include physical treatments (light therapy, ultrasound and electric currents), dietary supplements, homeopathy, medical counselling.

Naturopathic practitioners use many different treatment approaches. Examples include:

1. Dietary and lifestyle changes
2. Stress reduction
3. Natural Herbal therapy - Herbs and other dietary supplements
4. Manipulative therapies
5. Exercise therapy
6. Natural Spa therapy
7. Natural Mud & Clay therapy

8. Practitioner-guided detoxification
9. Psychotherapy and counselling

UNANI MEDICINE

Unani medicine, also called Unani tibb, Arabian medicine, or Islamic medicine, a traditional system of healing and health maintenance observed in South Asia. The origins of Unani medicine are found in the doctrines of the ancient Greek physicians Hippocrates and Galen.

Unani medicine treats a patient with diet, pharmacotherapy, exercise, massages and surgery.

At present it is popular in the states of Andhra Pradesh, Karnataka, Tamil Nadu, Bihar, Madhya Pradesh, Maharashtra, Uttar Pradesh, Delhi and Rajasthan.

SIDDHA

The Siddha system of medicine is mainly practised in the Southern part of India. It is one of the earliest traditional medicine systems in the world which treats not only the body but also the mind and the soul. The word Siddha has its origin in the Tamil word Siddhi which means "an object to be attained" or "perfection" or "heavenly bliss". India being the birth place of many traditional philosophies also gave birth to Siddha. The roots of this system are intertwined with the culture of ancient Tamil civilization.

Siddha practitioners believe that five basic elements– earth, water, fire, air, sky – are in food, "humours" of the human body, and herbal, animal or inorganic chemical compounds, such as sulphur and mercury, used as therapies for treating diseases.

It takes into account the patient, his surroundings, age, sex, race, habitat, diet, appetite, physical condition etc. to arrive at the diagnosis. Siddha System uses minerals, metals and alloys and drugs and inorganic compounds to treat the patients.

Homeopathy

Homeopathy comes from the Greek word in which homoios means 'similar' and pathos indicates 'suffering'. Homeopathic drugs treat diseases by triggering the body's natural defences instead of fighting against them.

Homeopathy is a system developed in a belief that a substance that causes the symptoms of a disease in healthy people will cure similar symptoms in sick people; this doctrine is called similia similibus curentur, or "like cures like".

This medicine industry solely depends on a "minimum dose law," in which dosage concentrations are inversely related to the active potency. Many homeopathic medicines contain active substances overly diluted and minimal amounts of active substances throughout the resulting dosages.

The concept of disease in homoeopathy is that disease is a total affection of mind and body, the disturbance of the whole organism. Individual organs are not the cause of illness but disturbance at the inner level (disturbance of the life force, the vital energy of the body) is the cause of illness.

Homoeopathy treats the patient as a whole and not just the disease.

Issues with Homeopathy:

It was developed before knowledge of atoms and molecules, or of basic chemistry, which shows that repeated dilution as practiced in homeopathy produces only water, and that homeopathy is not scientifically valid.

ACUPUNCTURE

It is a traditional Chinese Medicine technique. Here special needles are used to stimulate specific points in the body of a patient. These sterile needles are introduced at specific points in the body, which leads to the release of certain Neurohumoral transmitters and endorphins that relive pain. In some cases, Acupuncture needles dipped in certain homeopathic medicines are also used. This methodology can also be used in conjugation with modern medical treatments.

In acupuncture, it is believed that a supernatural energy called Qi (the life-force, vitality, or energy that makes us alive) flows through the universe and through the body, and helps propel the blood, blockage of which leads to disease. It is believed that insertion of needles at various parts of the body determined by astrological calculations can restore balance to the blocked flows, and thereby cure disease.

Experts of this medicine believe that the human body has more than 2,000 acupuncture points connected by 12 pathways or meridians that interact with various organs such as heart, liver and kidneys. Along these meridians, the energy flow rebalances by inserting the needles into specific points.

It is done to help body's natural healing process. It can be effective in treating a number of conditions, like neck and back pain, nausea, anxiety, depression, insomnia, etc.

Acupuncture has numerous positive effects against metabolic diseases, inflammation, digestive issues, respiratory and nervous system problems. In addition, releasing neurotransmitters and hormones also regulates neurochemistry, thus influencing the sensing and cognitive functions.

Some believe that Acupuncture is a pseudoscience; the theories and practices of Traditional Chinese Medicine (TCM) are not based on scientific knowledge, and it has been characterized as quackery.

Note: Now-a-days a number of needleless techniques such as Transcutaneous Electro-Acupuncture, Laser Acupuncture, Sono-puncture, Acutron and Colour puncture are available for patients who are apprehensive of needles

Diseases that May be Treated by Acupuncture: (Courtesy: Ganga Ram Hospital, New Delhi)

1. Diseases of Head and Neck: like migraine headaches, cervical spondylitis.
2. Diseases of limbs and musculature: like muscular pains, rheumatoid and osteoarthritis, low backache, slipped disc with sciatica.
3. Diseases related to digestion: like irritable bowel syndrome, gastritis and constipation.
4. Diseases related to respiratory system: like chronic bronchitis, and bronchial asthma.
5. Diseases related to cardiovascular system: like angina pain and high blood pressure.
6. Diseases related to genitourinary system: like bed wetting in children, frequent urination, enlarged prostate.
7. Diseases related to gynaecological system: like irregular menses, leucorrhoea etc.
8. Diseases related to sexual disorders: like Impotence, Azoospermia.
9. Diseases related to eyes: like optic atrophy & blurred vision.
10. Diseases related to ear, nose & throat: like sinusitis, earache, tonsillitis, laryngitis & nerve Deafness.
11. Diseases related to skin: like Acne, chronic eczema, psoriasis, skin rashes & falling hair.
12. Diseases related to nervous system: including paralysis, polio, epilepsy and coma.
13. Diseases related to psychiatric disorders (including stress related disorders): like insomnia, anxiety, mania, depression, anxiety, schizophrenia and behaviour disorders.
14. Acupuncture also cures addictions: like smoking, alcohol and other addictions.
15. Acupuncture is also helpful in Diabetes and overweight.

16. Laser Acupuncture is extremely useful for cosmetic problems like black circles under the eye, Wrinkles and for tightening the facial muscles.
17. Preventive Acupuncture is also given for patients with family history of Diabetes, Hypertension, and Asthma etc.

ACUPRESSURE

Acupressure is an alternative medicine technique similar in principle to acupuncture. It is based on the concept of life energy which flows through "meridians" in the body. In treatment, physical pressure is applied to acupuncture points with the aim of clearing blockages in these meridians. Pressure may be applied by hand, by elbow, or with various devices.

Acupressure therapy stimulates the body's circulatory, lymphatic and hormonal systems. It helps relieve stress and anxiety, improves sleep, relaxes your muscles and joints, regulates digestive issues, minimises headaches and migraines, and is also beneficial for back pains and menstrual cramps.

CHIROPRACTIC MEDICINE

Chiropractic or Naprapathy is generally categorized as complementary and alternative medicine (CAM), which focuses on manipulation of the musculoskeletal system, especially the spine. Its founder, D.D. Palmer, called it "a science of healing without drugs".

In this type of modality, a qualified and trained person tries to manipulate/adjust the spine of the body or other parts as per requirement to align in a proper form. It is helpful in many forms of pain arising out of joint problems.

The goal of chiropractic medicine is to ease pain, improve body function, and help your body to heal itself naturally.

It may be helpful in following conditions:

1. Low back pain
2. Headaches
3. Neck pain
4. Joint problems in upper and lower body
5. And disorders caused by whiplash

Contraindications:

Spinal manipulation is not recommended for people who have any of the following:

1. Osteoporosis
2. Symptoms of nerve damage or malfunction (neuropathy), such as loss of sensation or strength in one or more limbs
3. Previous spinal surgery
4. Stroke
5. Blood vessel disorders

MAGNETO-THERAPY

It is also known as "Energy Therapy"

The word magnetic therapy comes from the magnet. In this process, the different positive forces of a magnet are taken into account to cure any kind of diseases.

This uses magnetic or electrical fields to treat a number of musculoskeletal problems. It may work for osteoarthritis and other pain conditions. Some studies have even shown that it may help fractures heal faster. There are some contraindications of this therapy such as; Pregnancy, Implanted Pacemakers etc.

Healing magnets of about 200 gausses are considered to be of lower powers and are meant to be used on sensitive and delicate organs and diseases appearing therein like tonsils, eye, nose, etc.

It may be helpful in following conditions:

1. Osteoarthritis and other pain conditions
2. May help fractures heal faster

Contraindication:

1. It is not safe in pregnant women.
2. Contraindicated if a person has implanted cardiac device, use an insulin pump, or take a drug given by patch.

Diseases Curable with Magneto Therapy: (As per Claim of Various Therapists)

A. Chronic ailments with unsatisfactory treatment under other systems:
   Arthritis, Obesity, Hyper acidity, Spondylitis, Baldness, Bronchitis, Sciatica, Greying Hair, Flatulence, Parkinson's Disease, Leukoderma, Ear Discharge, Migraine

B. Ailments where surgery can be avoided:
   Piles, some types of Cancers, Hydrocoele, Fistulas, Cataract, Enlarged Prostate, Corns

C. Aches and Pains:
   Head-ache, Shoulder Pain, Tooth-ache, Sprains, Cuts, Ear-ache, Strains, Wounds, Bach-ache, Abdominal Colic, Insect Bites, Tonsillitis

D. Diseases that have NO permanent cure under other systems:
   Eczema, High Blood Pressure, Asthma, Diabetes, Insomnia

REIKI

Reiki is a form of alternative medicine called energy healing. The experts use a technique called palm healing or hands-on healing through which a "universal energy" is said to be transferred through the palms of the expert to the patient in order to encourage emotional or physical healing.

Reiki is an energy healing technique that promotes relaxation, reduces stress and anxiety through gentle touch.

Here the expert uses body's own natural energy to speed healing. The expert places his hands over your body very lightly to deliver energy to the patient's body. It may improve the flow and balance of the patient's energy to support healing.

THERAPEUTIC ("HEALING") TOUCH

"Non-contact therapeutic touch"

Here the expert uses his own energy to correct the imbalance in patient's energy field. Here the expert does not touch the body. He keeps his hand a little away from the body. It can increase the sense of wellbeing. Till now it has not been authenticated by any research or trials.

It may be helpful in following conditions:

1. In conditions of Anxiety

FEW INDICATIONS FOR ALTERNATIVE MEDICINE:

1. Low Backache
2. Arthritis
3. Bronchial Asthma
4. Skin Ailments
5. Constipation
6. Gastritis
7. Diabetes Mellitus (DM)
8. Conditions of inflammation
9. Cancer
10. Blood Pressure and CVD
11. Anxiety or sleep disorders
12. Menopause

ADVANTAGES OF ALTERNATIVE MEDICINE SYSTEM:

1. Holistic Medicine & Natural, Alternative therapies do not aggravate an already sick, weak & suffering patient, (except as a transient phase when the therapy may release and expel old toxins from the body and detoxify it).
2. They not only act on a physical and local level, but also act on a patient's consciousness, energy fields and psychic bodies to treat & cure him as a whole.
3. They do not cause any drug-induced, drug-related, toxic or drug-resistant conditions
4. It does not lower the immunity.
5. Reducing side effects as they depend upon various Natural way methods over chemical/lab made medicine.
6. More control over health condition.
7. Encourages feelings of well-being, pleasure, positivity.
8. Cost effective compared to conventional medicine.
9. Reliable as they have minimal side effects.
10. Helps in time of post-surgery or post conventional treatment for rehabilitation.
11. Helps in reducing excessive load on hospitals and support in achieving more efficiency in public health care system.
12. Creates more opportunities to students in medical science arena, if more importance and awareness generated.
13. Country's medical tourism has more scope to grow more. (India is ranked 10th out of the top 46 countries in the world in the Medical Tourism Index 2020-21 by Medical Tourism Association.) Resulting in growth of foreign tourist arrival (FTA).
14. All these can lead to exponential growth of alternative medicine in Indian and has scope in reducing the cost of conventional treatment charges enabling more efficient public-health care eco system in India.

DISADVANTAGES OF USING ALTERNATIVE MEDICINE SYSTEM:

1. Has minimal scientific research, resulting less foot fall in such hospitals.
2. As their treatment procedures not suitable for emergency cases, they won't be best options in time of emergency.

3. Takes more time to get benefits of treatment, Resulting loss of interest in patients and family members.
4. Less regulation compared to conventional medicine.
5. Diagnosis can be the main issue in determining patient's health condition.
6. Limited coverage/acceptance by health insurance companies.
7. Even use of herbs and natural methods of treatment, some reactions may worsen the situation.
8. Herbal supplements may be harmful when taken by themselves, with other substances, or in large doses.
9. Concern with fake practitioners.

LIMITATIONS OF ALTERNATIVE MEDICINE:

1. Not advised in life threatening conditions.
2. Cases where surgical intervention is must.
3. Cases who are severely mal nourished.
4. Terminally ill patients.

ACCESSIBILITY: Alternative Medicine may be:

1. more affordable
2. more familiar, or easier to understand
3. more consistent with a person's views or culture
4. closer to where a person lives
5. easier to practice independently

PUBLIC OPINION:

1. *"The Judicious use of Alternative Systems of Medicine is found cost effective and having lesser or no side effects. India stays in rural setup, where medicines from alternative systems can play very big role in curing the primary healthcare problems"*- Shri Narendra Modi ji, Hon'ble Prime Minister, India
2. *"I am also happy to learn that the Council is providing research, education, health services through holistic approach with complementary alternative & traditional medicines for the benefit of the society."*- Late Shri Arun Jaitley, former Minister of Finance, Government of India

BIBLIOGRAPHY, REFERENCES & ACKNOWLEDGMENTS:

1. All India Council of Alternative Medical Science & Research
2. Topical Analysis: Role of Alternative Medicine Systems in Public Health, Published- 8th Apr, 2022 by GS SCORE, New Delhi
3. The Institute of Alternative Medical Science (I.A.M.S.)
4. Bright, P. S. 2000. India's alternative therapies: the cure of modern times. *Junior Science Refresher*, November: 20-27.
5. Stock Jon. 2002. Ayurveda goes global. The Week, July 28: 16-27.
6. Lalit Tiwari, Lok Vigyan Kendra, Almora, India
7. Alternative Medicine: A Recent Overview, by Salima Akter, Mohammad Nazmul Hasan, Begum Rokeya, Hajara Akhter, Mohammad Shamim Gazi, Farah Sabrin and Sung Soo Kim

8. Planet Ayurveda
9. Mansarovar Ayurvedic Medical College, Bhopal, MP, India
10. Ganga Ram Hospital, New Delhi
11. Talking about Complementary and Alternative Medicine with Health Care Providers: A Workbook and Tips, Office of Cancer Complementary and Alternative Medicine, National Institutes of Health, U.S. Department of Health and Human Services
12. Dr. (Mrs.) Sunita Gupta, New Delhi
13. Alternate Medicine Council of India, Mumbai, India
14. Alternative Systems of Medicine in India: An overview by Chandrakant Lahariya
15. "Standard Operating Procedures SOP For Hospitals 2nd Edition" by Dr. Arun K. Agarwal

Chapter - 2

DEPARTMENT OF TRANSPORT – AMBULANCE SERVICES

INDEX

INTRODUCTION:

An ambulance is a vehicle for transportation of sick or injured people to, from or between places of treatment for an illness or injury, and in some instances will also provide out of hospital medical care to the patient. *[From Wikipedia, the free encyclopaedia]*

Ambulance services are the backbone of any hospital. It develops a healthy relationship between hospital and community. The people understand that medical aid is available to them whenever required.

Ambulance services help many people with life-threatening conditions to reach at a hospital or medical aid centre quickly without wasting precious time. Ambulance services should also ensure that some lifesaving treatment is given to the patient even during transport. Paramedics accompanying the ambulance are trained in first-aid to patients and also to emergency care.

Clinical Establishment Act, Standards for Hospital (LEVEL 2), Standard No. CEA/Hospital- 002 reads that;

1. "The establishment shall have provision of transporting patients for transfer/referral/investigations etc in safe manner." and
2. "Ambulance Services may be in-house or outsourced. The Ambulance services shall comply with the applicable local laws, even if they are outsourced."

Well-equipped ambulance(s) with requisite facilities shall be made available round the clock for meeting emergency requirements. The ambulance(s) will also be used on chargeable/free basis for shifting the patient to this hospital and/or to other hospitals as and when need arises.

PURPOSE:

1. To ensure proper and timely transportation of patient to the hospital for appropriate medical attention.
2. To ensure proper transfer of patient from the hospital.
3. Hospital ambulances are mainly for transporting sick patients only.

INFRASTRUCTURE:

1. The hospital has got ---------- (two) well-equipped ambulances at present.
2. More ambulances may be added in near future?
3. The telephone number of emergency reception (it should be a unique number) should be prominently displayed on road side and hospital boards so that if a patient requires ambulance, he can contact that number.

POLICY:

1. The ambulance service provides the first point of access to health care for a wide variety of patient conditions, ranging from life-threatening emergencies to chronic illness and social care.
2. Smoking is prohibited in the ambulance.
3. The MS/In-charge of the hospital will ensure that they are used economically and for the purpose for which they are intended. All requests for ambulance will therefore be sent to the MS/In-charge of the ambulances. In-charge of the ambulances will make one member of his staff responsible to keep track of movements of these vehicles and to check the serviceability of seats, stretchers, fittings, fan etc.

4. The in-charge of the ambulance will ensure that medical equipment and stores normally carried on the ambulance are available according to authorised quantities. He will also detail attendants, if necessary, to accompany patients to and from the hospital.
5. The ambulance will be always kept in running condition.
6. All Ambulance drivers will be BLS trained.
7. Drivers must be in uniform and ID tag when driving the ambulance.
8. All ambulance drivers must have the mobile phone in possession while on duty.
9. Following kinds of ambulances are kept/made available to commensurate the scope of services provided by the hospital.
10. ACLS ambulance with advanced Cardiac life support facility – 1
11. Ambulance shall be parked in area demarcated for ambulances and manned by Basic Life Support trained driver. The access way of ambulance to emergency shall be kept clear all the time. All ambulance drivers shall have (24x7) dedicated official mobile phone for proper communication.
12. Ambulance shall not be used as dead body carriage van.
13. Movement of ambulance is under the control of Hospital Administrator.

TYPES OF AMBULANCES:

As per Health & Family Welfare Department of National Capital Territory of Delhi, Registration of Ambulances, there are following three types of ambulances.

1. **Patient Transport Ambulance:**
   An ambulance used for transporting patients of non-emergency nature.
2. **Basic Life Support Ambulance:**
   The vehicle is equipped to provide basic life support to patients during transport.
3. **Advanced Life Support Ambulance:**
   Such ambulances are equipped to dealing with life-threatening emergencies during patients' transportation and are manned by experienced and qualified personnel.

KEY STANDARDS FOR AMBULANCE SERVICES:

1. Responding to life-threatening calls.
2. Responding to non-life-threatening calls.
3. Getting Emergency drugs and blood for hospital emergency.
4. To provide any such service that the hospital may find deem.
5. Ambulance will not be used for carrying dead bodies except in case where the patient expires during transportation.
6. Ambulance services will be available within city limits and will be restricted to carrying patients to the hospital or transferring patient to the referred medical centre.

STANDARD OPERATING PROCEDURES (SOP):

A. General Procedures:

1. All requests for the ambulance should be sent to the main reception for payment.
2. Advance payment has to be made by the patient for availing ambulance services.

3. Any breakdown should be reported immediately to the officers (MS) and should be rectified as soon as possible.
4. The driver of the ambulance will maintain a logbook, which will be checked & signed by the M.S. on daily basis.
5. In normal circumstances only specified driver will drive the ambulance.
6. Any other person will drive the ambulance in case of emergency only on specific orders by the concerned authorities.
7. Whenever there is a call from patient for Ambulance Service staff should be promptly ready. There will be a team which will go with the Ambulance to bring the patient from the incident spot or to transfer the patient.

TEAM MEMBERS

a. A doctor
b. A Staff Nurse
c. A Ward Boy
d. A Driver

a. Staff Nurse on duty will provide the patient with primary treatment under the supervision of Doctor within the Ambulance to stabilize the vital function. After the patient is transferred from the Ambulance, Staff Nurse on duty will shut the Oxygen Cylinder and will make sure all other electrical switches not in use should be switched off.
b. Ward boy will transfer the patient in and out of the Ambulance carefully, will maintain the cleanliness of the Ambulance and will assist the Staff Nurse.
c. Driver will be responsible for safe driving and will also assist in transfer of the patient as per guidance of doctor and staff nurse.

B. Emergency Calls:

1. The Emergency ambulance call is received in the ED, then the time and Number of the caller is noted down by the ED staff responding to the call and transfer the call immediately to the EMO.
2. The EMO collects the exact address location and landmark etc, from the caller and advices for the precautions to be taken to patient.
3. The Ambulance driver reports to the Emergency Medical Officer (EMO).
4. All the movements of the Ambulance are controlled only by the emergency medical officer. Apart from the Emergency room medical officer the Director, Chief Medical Superintendent and Medical Superintendents can control the movement in conjunction with the Emergency Medical Officer.
5. All the patient calls that are entertained by the hospital are considered load and go situation so the patient is picked up and moved to the hospital as soon as possible.
6. The ambulance driver may assist on all the load-and –go situation in scene of emergency.
7. The ambulance will not move out of the hospital without the EMO concern when patients are being transferred.
8. The EMO summons the Ambulance driver and briefs the Ambulance driver of the location and landmarks etc. On being briefed by the EMO the ambulance driver does all the pre-departure check and brings the ambulance to the front patio of the emergency department.
9. Picks up the Waiting nurse (Refer Transfer of patient policy) in patio and drives to the destination to pick up the patient safely and as fast as possible.

10. The Emergency drugs and the Clinical therapeutic, diagnostic equipment will be kept in the Emergency Department and will be moved into the ambulance only during calls as per the advice of the EMO.
11. The ED staff pharmacist will be responsible for the same.
12. The ambulance driver will have to assist in-shifting of the patient as directed by the EMO.
13. All communications are done from the ambulance to the ground station through the CUG phone in possession with the Ambulance driver.
14. The patient when being brought is wheeled in and loaded in the ED trolley and the Ambulance driver sets back all the system in the ambulance and cleans the ambulance with the assistance of the house keeping personnel inside the hospital. This cleaning operation shall not exceed 20 min.
15. In case of any planned shifting and transfer of the patient all the modalities are worked out by the emergency medical officer in conjunction with the respective departments.
16. The ambulance driver will be informed by the Emergency medical officer and an entry is made in outgoing ambulance register the ambulance driver brings the ambulance to the patio and takes the trolley to the pickup point of the patient inside the hospital and moves the patient accompanied by the nurse/doctor to the ambulance and proceeds.
17. In this operation the Ambulance driver will not be liable to satisfy any clinical documents or requirements.
18. In case of any purchase of pharmacy drugs and Blood done by the ambulance team, the medical officer shall handover the requisite prescription and cash and briefs the ambulance drive as to where and when and how to get it.
19. In case of non-emergency planned pick up of the patient the Ambulance driver may be informed in prior and handed over the trip sheet by the medical officer not exceeding 48 hours in advance.
20. In the Transfer and shifting of the patients, depending upon the condition of the patient a nurse/doctor may accompany the patient.
21. For referral – the referral hospital must be informed before sending the patient. Staff accompanying the patient must be seated at the back with patient. Only one person will be allowed to accompany the patient in the ambulance. Relatives' \ accompanying the patients to do so at their own risk.
22. Sirens – Silent – if the road is empty. Only lights on- for cold cases. Siren only on-if carrying ill case and/or to clear traffic.

STAFFING:

Designation	General Shift 9 am to 6 pm	Shift 1 8 am to 2 pm	Shift 2 2 pm to 8 pm	Shift 3 8 pm to 8 am (Next day)	Reliever	Total
Ambulance Driver	1	1	1	1	From Pool	4
Ambulance Attendant		1	1	1	From Pool	3
Total	1	2	2	2		7

ORGANOGRAM (ORGANISATIONAL STRUCTURE):

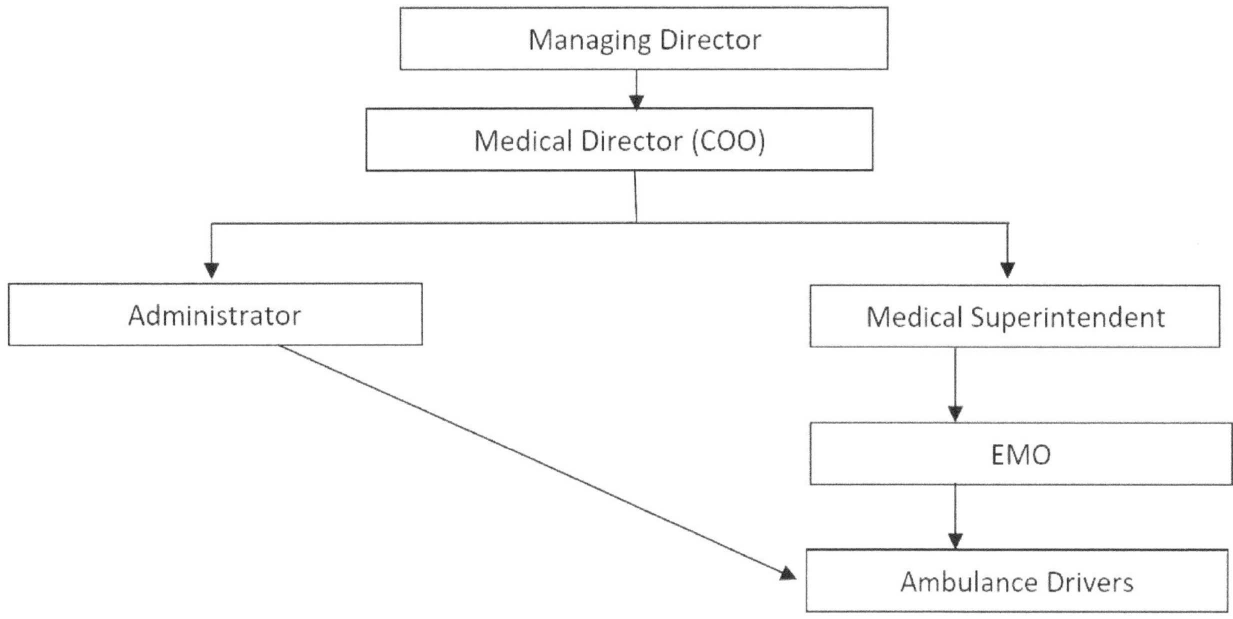

DUTIES & RESPONSIBILITIES:

A. Duties of an Ambulance Driver:

1. He will have a valid driving license for ambulance.
2. He should be an experienced driver who can drive a little faster and can manoeuvre the vehicle even in congested places.
3. He should be able & experienced or will be trained for handling patient, stretcher and other medical equipment.
4. He will keep the ambulance neat & tidy.
5. He will check and/or will ensure that all medical supplies are complete and the ambulance is ready to move in any emergency situation. Checking will be done every day, whether the ambulance has any trip or not.
6. He will maintain a log book properly and up-to-date.
7. He will always be available inside the ambulance or at gate security or at a designated place.
8. It will be duty of EMO to assist the ambulance driver in maintain the medical inventory.
9. He will also help the patient in boarding and de-boarding the ambulance.
10. He will drive the ambulance in a law-full manner.
11. He will try to repair the vehicle, if it breaks down on the way. Otherwise also he will get the ambulance repaired at the specified place/workshop. He will maintain the vehicle as per manufacturer's guidelines.
12. He will be in hospital dress when on duty.
13. He will drive the ambulance to and from the decided place and will not use the ambulance for any other purpose.
14. He will get the ambulance serviced from time to time.
15. He will ensure the safety of all equipment placed inside the ambulance.

16. He will park the ambulance only at the specified location whether inside the hospital or outside the hospital.
17. He will perform all duties as decided by EMO from time-to-time.

B. Duties of an Ambulance Attendant:

1. He will always be available inside the ambulance or at a place identified by the EMO.
2. He will load/unload ambulance equipment.
3. He will assist in boarding and de-boarding of the patient.
4. He will keep a check on the oxygen cylinder and will replace empty cylinder with filled one.
5. He will not discuss patient's medical information with any unauthorised person.
6. He will perform all other duties as directed by the EMO, when not on ambulance duty.
7. He will ensure that the patient is well strapped when ambulance in on move.
8. He will check the ambulance daily in the morning as per "Ambulance Check List."

RESPONSIBILITY FOR MAINTENANCE OF THE AMBULANCES:

1. The ambulance driver shall maintain the ambulance in clean and good condition.
2. The ambulance driver is responsible to maintain 90% of the medical gas (oxygen) to the total storage capacity of Oxygen. If the level of the Oxygen storage goes less than 50% the ambulance driver requests the ED staff to replace a 100% full refilled Oxygen cylinder.
3. The ambulance driver has to ensure the pneumatic pressures of the wheels are within stipulated pressure. If found less it is to be notified and refilled with informing the EMO and a movement entry has to be made in the designated register.
4. The ambulance driver has to upkeep all the non-clinical equipment inside the ambulance if in case of any malfunction it is to be reported to the ED which has to be entered in the designated register.
5. The ambulance driver shall check the brake-oil level, Engine oil level, Wheel pneumatic pressure. Engine coolant, oxygen level, fuel level, siren, lights, UPS charge and the equipment in the ambulance twice every day.
6. The ED Pharmacist will be responsible to maintain the required medicines in the Ambulance. The availability of medicines in the ambulance will be checked by the ED pharmacist at 8:00 am in the morning, the entry of the same would be made in the designated register. Prior to the dispatch of the Ambulance the ED rechecks the medicines in the Ambulance to ensure the availability of all the essential drugs.
7. Once the Ambulance returns, the on-duty ED Pharmacist checks the medicines to replenish any medicine which has been used.
8. The ambulance Driver shall upkeep and maintain all the documentation relating to the ambulance.
9. The ambulance driver shall always maintain the adequate fuel in ambulance and procures diesel as and when it reaches the safe minimum level of stock.
10. The ambulance driver requests for the diesel indents from the designate clerk in the administrative office as and when ambulance diesel stock level goes below the safe stock level. The diesel is got filled from the authorized vendor decided by the Administration.
11. The movement of ambulance for the refill of the fuel is to be notified to the EMO and an entry of the same is made in the designated register.

CHECK LISTS:

A. Checklist Ambulance:

SN	Check	Yes	No
1	Are the services available round the clock 24 x 7?		
2	Is it not used as a normal transport?		
3	Is one driver always available in the ambulance?		
4	Are ambulances fully loaded with drugs and medicines at all times?		
5	Are medical equipment working satisfactorily?		
6	Do ambulances have power backup?		
7	Is logbook properly maintained?		
8	Is the siren of ambulance in working condition?		
9	Are all legal documents [Valid Insurance, Registration Certificate, and PUC (Pollution Under Control) Certificate] up-to-date?		
10	Is ambulance staff vaccinated against Hepatitis B?		

B. Daily Ambulance Inspection Checklist:

SN	Check	Yes	No
Ambulance Equipment			
1	Mobile phone is in place?		
2	Emergency light and siren is in working condition?		
3	Suction apparatus is available and working?		
4	Oxygen cylinder is available and is full (minimum 60%)?		
5	Air conditioner/heater are working?		
6	Log Book is in place?		
7	Removable ambulance stretcher is available?		
8	Ambulance Inverter is working and batteries are fully charged?		
9	Fire Extinguisher is available?		
Ambulance Medicines			
10	Emergency medicines (see checklist no. 05) are available?		
11	Cardiac Monitor is working?		
12	Defibrillator is charged and working?		
13	Spine board is available?		
14	Airways and suction catheters are available?		
15	Stethoscope, BP apparatus are available?		
16	Urinal & Bed pans are available in its compartment?		
17	Intubation Kit is available along with spare blades of Laryngoscope?		
18	Ambu Bag and tourniquet are available?		

C. Checklist Ambulance Working:

SN	Check	Yes	No
1	Is patient consent obtained before putting a patient inside the ambulance?		
2	Are in & out register of the ambulance maintained preferably at security or with Casualty Medical Officer?		
3	Does the driver have valid driving license (Heavy Vehicle) in his possession while on duty?		
4	Is cardiac monitor in working condition?		
5	Is portable ventilator in working condition?		
6	Is defibrillator in working condition?		
7	Is suction apparatus being in working condition?		
8	Are all necessary medicines available as per list?		
9	Are medical/surgical consumables available as per list?		
10	Is glucometer with sugar strips available?		
11	Is water tank checked for water? It should be ¾ full.		
12	Are clean laundry available (*kurta, pyjama*) sheets, blanket?		
13	Did you check the oxygen cylinder for presence of gas? Filled more than 60%)?		
14	Check that a nurse, ward boy/Aya always accompany a sick patient during shifting.		
15	Make sure that siren is not used when the ambulance is without a patient? Pass on standing orders to that affect.		

D. Checklist Ambulance Medicines & Drugs:

SN	Check/Item	Qty	Yes	No
1	Cotton & Gauze pieces			
2	Blood Transfusion Sets			
3	Bandages of various sizes			
4	Intravenous Infusion Sets			
5	Antiseptic Ointments			
6	Antiseptic Solutions			
7	Disposable Syringes with Needles, 2 ml, 5 ml			
8	Leucoplast			
9	Intravenous Fluid (RL)			
List of Important Medicines to be kept inside an Ambulance				
1	Inj. Atropine	3		
2	Inj. Aminophylline	3		
3	Inj. Avil	2		
4	Inj. Adrenaline	4		
5	Inj. Calmpose	1		
6	Inj. Calcium Gluconate	4		
7	Inj. Dexamethasone	1		

SN	Check/Item	Qty	Yes	No
8	Inj. Dopamine Plus	2		
9	Inj. Deriphylline	2		
10	Inj. Digoxin	1		
11	Inj. Eptoin	2		
12	Inj. Fulsed 5ml	1		
13	Inj. Fortwin	1		
14	Inj. Kaplin	1		
15	Inj. KCl	2		
16	Inj. Lasix	2		
17	Inj. MgSo4 25%	1		
18	Inj. Mannitol 100ml	1		
19	Inj. Emset	2		
20	Inj. NTG 25mg	1		
21	Inj. Phenergan	1		
22	Inj. Rantac	2		
23	Inj. Sodabicarb 25ml	2		
24	Inj. Xylocard	1		
25	Inj. DNS	1		
26	Inj. Dextrose 5%	1		
27	Inj. Dextrose 25% 25ml	3		
28	Inj. Dextrose 25% 100 ml	2		
29	Inj. Buscopan	2		
30	Inj. Betaloc	2		
31	Inj. Normal Saline 100 ml	1		
32	Inj. Voveran	2		
33	Inj. Normal Saline 500 ml	1		
34	Inj. Ringer Lactate	1		
35	Inj. Isolyte- P	1		
36	Tab. Disprin	5		
37	Tab. Sorbitrate 5 Mg	5		
38	Tab. Sorbitrate 10 Mg	5		
39	Airway No. – 4	1		
40	Airway No. - 0	1		
41	Bandage 4"	2		
42	Crepe Bandage 4"	1		
43	Crepe Bandage 3"	1		
44	Chest Leads	3		
45	Disposable Needles No. 22	10		
46	Disposable Needles No. 23	5		

SN	Check/Item	Qty	Yes	No
47	Disposable Needles No. 24	5		
48	Disposable Needles No. 26	5		
49	Disposable Syringes 10 cc	5		
50	Disposable Syringes 5 cc	5		
51	Disposable Syringes 2 cc	5		
52	Disposable Syringe Insulin	5		
53	Disposable Gloves No. 7.5	1		
54	Disposable Gloves No. 7	1		
55	Disposable Gloves No. 6.5	1		
56	Distil Water 10 ml	5		
57	Examination Gloves, box	1		
59	E.T Tube No 6.5 & 8	1 Each		
59	Foleys Catheter -14	2		
60	Intracath (Venflon) No. 22	2		
61	Intracath (Venflon) No. 20	2		
62	Microset	1		
63	Nasal Prongs-Adult	1		
64	Face Mask -Adult	1		
65	Scalp Vein -21	1		
66	Scalp-Vein -22	1		
67	Scalp Vein -23	1		
68	Scalp Vein -24	1		
69	Suction Catheter -8,10,12,16	1 Each		
70	Tegaderm	2		
71	Urosac	1		
72	Ryle's Tube No 12	1		
73	Micropore 3"	1		
74	ECG Machine/Cardiac Monitor	1		
75	Defibrillator	1		
76	Ventilator	1		
77	Electric/Foot Suction Machine	1		
78	Linen as per list			

E. Checklist – Equipment for Ambulance – Summary:

SN	Check/Item	Yes	No
A. Ventilation & Airway Equipment.			
1	Suction Apparatus		
2	Oxygen cylinder with Oxygen inhalation apparatus?		
3	Ambu Bag?		

SN	Check/Item	Yes	No
4	Airways of various kinds – Nasopharyngeal & Oropharyngeal?		
5	Pulse Oximeter?		
B. Intubation Aids			
6	Laryngoscope?		
7	Magill's Forceps & Stylet?		
C. Patient Monitoring Devices.			
8	Vital sign monitor?		
9	Defibrillator?		
D. Patient immobilisation Equipment.			
10	Splints?		
11	Collars?		
12	Spine Board?		
E. Dressing Material.			
13	Bandages?		
14	Sterile gauze?		
15	Tourniquet?		
16	Antiseptic Solutions & Ointments?		
17	Hand Sanitizer?		
F. Miscellaneous Medical Sundries.			
18	Stethoscope & BP Apparatus?		
19	Thermometer, Digital?		
20	Ophthalmoscope?		
21	Bed Pans & Urinal Pots?		
G. Linen.			
22	Blanket?		
23	Pillow & Pillow cover?		
24	Bed Sheet?		
25	McIntosh Sheet?		
H. Emergency Medicine.			
26	As per list.		
I. Miscellaneous Items			
27	Mobile phone?		
28	Folding Stretcher?		
29	Legal Papers – Driving Licence, Vehicle Registration Certificate, Vehicle Insurance Certificate, Pollution Certificate (PUCC)?		

KEY PERFORMANCE INDICATORS:

1. Response time
2. Ambulance breakdown time
3. Equipment breakdown time

4. Patient feedback
5. Staff feedback
6. Calls conversion rate
7. Referring doctor feedback

RECORDS MAINTENANCE:

1. Ambulance Log Book – inside the ambulance
2. Ambulance movement Record Register – at the Reception/Emergency

STATIONARY FORMATS:

A. Ambulance Log Book:

Vehicle Registration No.: ....

Date	Details of Journey		Kilometre Reading		K.M. Done	Fuel Received (Lts)	Oil Received (Lts)	Purpose of Journey	Ordering Officer Signature	Driver Signature
	From	To	From	To						

B. Consent Form:

Hospital Name & Address

Informed Consent

Ambulance Transport of a Patient with Serious Medical Illness

Patient Name: .... Age & Sex: .... Date & Time: ....

1. I ______________________________ (attendant of the patient), hereby give my consent for transport/transfer of my patient as stated above, by ambulance, at my own risk, without any liability to the doctors/staff of Ambulance and this hospital.
2. The doctor accompanying along with the patient have explained to me in the language that I understand, about the seriousness, nature of medical illness, present condition and possible prognosis of the disease of my patient.
3. I am fully aware of the risks of transportation of a critically ill patient, including death during transportation. Other risks include delay and discomfort associated with road conditions, transport problems, weather and patient's condition (that are not under direct control of ambulance); extended travel time; fatigue and dehydration; enforced immobility and access in the confined space of an ambulance; reduced availability of medical personnel and medical equipment as compared to a specialized Hospital.
4. The treatment in an ambulance is only of an emergency measure and does not match the full in-hospital treatment.
5. I also give consent for the use of emergency drugs and sedatives etc and any emergency procedure to be carried out on my patient if needed, as applicable, according to the clinical condition, during transportation.

6. I am taking my patient after discharge/on request/against medical advice from one place to other at my own risk.
7. I have been given an opportunity to ask appropriate questions regarding this consent and release and have received satisfactory response to my queries.
8. I also understand that the ambulance service is chargeable as per the ambulance rules and is exclusive of doctor's charges, that would depend upon the number of doctors required to shift the patient, which in turn would depend upon the pre-transfer medical condition of the patient. I shall also pay for the drugs/disposable items used during transfer. The total approximate payment has to paid beforehand and rest of the payments will be paid immediately after reaching destination. A bill will be issued for the payment.
9. In case of death of the patient during transportation from one hospital to another, who is having a medico-legal case (MLC), I authorize the staff of Ambulance, to inform the local police station for the same and take necessary actions. The body of the patient will be handed over to the local police, where the death occurred.

   Only after written appropriate clearance from the police, the body will be handed over to the relatives.
10. I understand that the ambulance van is machinery and it may get some kind of mechanical problem/break down during transport. Everybody, who is present on board should bear it and find out the solution for the same with mutual understanding. I also understand, that the medical equipment (Ventilator, defibrillator, syringe pumps, suction machine, multi-para monitor, laryngoscope, air conditioner, inverter system, sirens and emergency light), installed in the ambulance may get some kind of technical error or may not work properly, there is an alternative for everything in the ambulance, along with an ALS doctor; we have to bear all pros and consequences with mutual understanding for the same. We all are working for the benefit and wish for the safe transport of the patient.
11. I hold complete responsibility, and hereby release the administration, doctors and staff of Ambulance from any medico-legal responsibility in case of any unforeseen eventually/fatality during medical transfer.
12. Moreover, I hereby authorize the staff/doctor of Ambulance, to disclose and release medical information and records concerning the medical assistance, provided to the patient before and during transportation, to the treating physician including Transfer papers and investigation reports.

NOTE: PLEASE READ CAREFULLY THE ABOVE-MENTIONED RULES/PROTOCOLS AND POLICIES OF AMBULANCE" BEFORE SIGNING".

I hereby state that my patient has been transferred/transported satisfactorily on ______________ at _________ am/pm. I am satisfied with the Ambulance services provided to me.

Name and Signature of the Attendant

(Relationship)

C. Patient Transfer Record:

AMBULANCE TRANSFER/TRANSIT RECORD

Date: .... Time: .... Place: ....

Name of the Patient: .... Age/Sex: ....

Name of the attendant: .... Relationship with the Patient: ....

Address: .... Phone: ....

Clinical Diagnosis: ....

Reason for Transfer: .... (Discharged/Referred/DOR/LAMA/Transfer)

Transporting from: .... Transporting to: ....

Doctor/Nursing Staff/Driver Details: ....

MLC No (if applicable): ....

Patient's Clinical condition: (As per details provided by the hospital/General examination)

Patient: Conscious/unconscious; BP: .../...... mmHg Pulse: ...... min. SpO2: ....%

Temp.: ......^{0}F Resp. Rate: ....../min GCS: .... Monitor Pattern: .... CVP: ....

Patient is on: Room Air/O2 Support @ .... Lts./min/BiPAP support/Ventilator support.

Ventilator Settings: Adult/Paediatric/Neonate Mode of Ventilation: ......

Tidal Volume... ml/breath FiO2: ...... % Resp. Rate: ....../min.

PEEP: .... Trigger: ....

IV Access (√/X): Central Line/IV Cannula Arterial Line: Present/Absent

Current Investigation Reports (if present): ABG (date and time)

Ph: ...... PO2: ...... PCO2: ...... HCO3: ...... BE: ...... SpO2: ... Na+: ... K+: ...

Other reports: ....

Current medications/IV fluids on flow

1. IV Fluids ________@ ______ ml/hr.
2. Infusion ___________@ ______ ml/hr/mcg/hr/mg/hr.
3. Infusion __________@ ______ ml/hr/mcg/hr/mg/hr
4. Infusion _________@ ______ ml/hr/mcg/hr/mg/hr.
5. Others ___________________@ ______ ml/hr.
6. Any Sedatives ________________________

(To be filled by the doctor/Medical personal in the ambulance during transport.)

Drugs Given to the patient:

1. .... Time and Reason ....
2. .... Time and Reason ....
3. .... Time and Reason ....

Remarks/any complications/change in patient's general condition/specific observations during transportation:

....

Current Vitals:

Neurological Status: Patient Conscious/Unconscious GCS: _____/15

B.P.: _____/_____mmHg Pulse Rate: ______/min. SpO2: _______% Temp.: ______ °F

Resp. Rate: _______breaths/min CVP: _______cm of H2O

Total Volume In: ______ ml.; Total Volume Out: _______ ml. (Urine/Drains/RT aspiration)

Comments and Remarks:

....

Name and Signature of the Doctor Name and Signature of the Attendant

(Relationship):

Handover taken from .... (Name& Sign)

Handover given to .... (Name & Sign)

BIBLIOGRAPHY, REFERENCES & ACKNOWLEDGMENTS:

1. Dr. Ram Manohar Lohia Combined Hospital, Lucknow 15/1/2008
2. "Standard Operating Procedures SOP For Hospitals 2nd Edition" by Dr. Arun K. Agarwal
3. "Duties & Responsibilities of Hospital Staff" by Dr. Arun Kumar
4. "Checklists for Hospitals" by Dr. Arun K. Agarwal
5. NABH 5th Edition.
6. How To Set Up A Hospital Along with SOPs by Dr. Arun K. Agarwal, Published by Atlantic Publishers & Distributers Pvt. Ltd., New Delhi

Chapter – 3

DEPARTMENT OF ANAESTHESIOLOGY

INDEX:

1. Introduction
2. Description
3. Aim, Vision, Mission
4. Values
5. Super Specialities of this Department:
6. Goals of The Department
7. Types of Anaesthesia
8. Infrastructure
9. List Of Major Equipment
10. List Of Equipment as Per Indian Public Health Standards (IPHS), Government of India
11. Best Practices
12. Services Provided/Offered/Scope of Services
13. Manpower/Staffing
14. Various Checklists of Anaesthesia Services
    a. Checklist Patient Intubation
    b. Checklist Anaesthesia Machine
    c. Checklist Depth of Anaesthesia
    d. Anaesthesia & Surgery Safety Checklist
    e. Anaesthesia Infection Prevention Checklist
    f. Anaesthesia Audit Checklist
15. Duties & Responsibilities
    a. Duties & Responsibilities of an Anaesthetist
    b. Duties & Responsibilities of Anaesthesia Technician/Nurse
16. Key Performance Indicators
17. Stationary formats for this Department
    a. Preoperative Check List (PAC) – By Ward Nurse
    b. Preoperative Check List (PAC) – By Anaesthesiologist
    c. Consent Form:
    d. Anaesthesia & Operation Notes (Short)
    e. General PAC Form:
    f. Anaesthesia & Operation Record (Booklet form)
    g. KPI Data Collection Register: Formats for different QIs

18. SOP – Procedures
    a. Procedure for PAC
    b. Procedure For Obtaining Consent:
    c. SOP for Paediatric Anaesthesia
    d. Administration of General Anaesthesia:
    e. Administration of moderate sedation or monitored anaesthesia care (MAC)
    f. Day Care Anaesthesia:
    g. SOP for Spinal/Regional Anaesthesia
    h. Discharge of From POP/Recovery
19. Post Operative Care with Essential Monitoring
20. Infection Control Practices:
21. Records & Documents Generated/Maintained
22. Subjects For CME/Workshops
23. Teaching Activities
24. Bibliography, References & Acknowledgments

INTRODUCTION:

The term Anaesthesia is derived from the Greek words 'an' meaning "without" and 'aesthesis' meaning "sensation". Thus, anaesthesia literally means **"without sensation".**

Anaesthesiology is a branch of medicine that induces a reversible state of total or partial loss of sensations.

All surgical procedures require partial or complete loss of pain sensation during the procedure. It is achieved by injecting certain drugs or by inhaling certain gases.

Anaesthesiologists contribute significantly to the medical activity from basic sciences to clinical & fundamental research.

To handle this type of science every hospital has a "Department of Anaesthesia".

An advanced "Department of Anaesthesia" is centre to the success of complex and specialized surgeries being performed in this department.

Anaesthesiology department is totally sufficient to meet all type of operative and intensive care requirements of any patient, in the form of comprehensive, compassionate, dedicated, efficient patient care with latest health care techniques.

About 10 to 14 (write number of procedures done in your hospital) procedures are performed on daily basis in this department.

Regular CMEs and workshops are conducted to keep abreast of any developments in this field.

DESCRIPTION:

The Anaesthesia Department in this hospital uses the most advanced equipment and facilities to deliver safe patient-oriented services.

The team consists of educated and trained personnel to deliver services in OTs, ICUs and elsewhere as per need.

The motto is to help surgeons to conduct all procedures safely & successfully. It also takes care of patients during early post operative period.

This department includes:

1. Operation Theatres
2. Pre-Anaesthesia Clinics
3. Hyperbaric Oxygen Therapy Units
4. Pain Relief Clinics
5. ECT Unit of Psychiatric Department
6. Peripheral Units like, MRI, CT, Cath Lab
7. Post Operative Ward
8. ICU (it may also be a part of this department)

AIM:

1. To become a department of excellence in anaesthesia and critical care.
2. To provide high quality, patient centred anaesthesia care.
3. To maintain a professional environment in the department.
4. To provide care on evidence-based knowledge ensuring safe and effective services.
5. To run pain clinic.
6. To provide its expertise to any other department such as ICU, MRI, CT.

VISION:

1. Vision of this department is to serve patients with a human approach.
2. To provide highest quality, evidence-based anaesthesia, pain management and peri-operative medical care by the concerned staff.
3. To combine the services with training of junior staff.
4. To strive to provide efficient, safe services.

MISSION:

1. To respect and value the diversity of the people and communities being served with commitment to responsible stewardship.
2. To prepare the patient for a safe, event less surgery.
3. To deliver services through up-to-date evidence based clinical care, ensuring safe and effective anaesthesia.
4. To take care of post operative pain.
5. To run pain management clinics on OPD basis.
6. To maintain a healthy and meaningful relationship with colleagues and other paramedical staff.
7. To remain a strong, efficient department of this hospital and to remain well versed with latest developments in this science.
8. To provide these services round the clock.
9. Continuing medical education.

VALUES:

- Innovation: To embrace curiosity and evidence and seek new knowledge from diverse perspectives.

- Quality: To strive to set the highest standard of quality in everything we do and constantly challenge ourselves to improve.
- Integrity: To strive to be fair, ethical and transparent in all that we do and in the decisions that we make; we strive to act in the best interests of patients.
- Respect: To demonstrate to our patients, learners and colleagues that we respect value and appreciate them through our words, actions and relationships.
- Accountability: To responsibly use the Department's resources to provide the best quality service possible and strive to exceed expectations as we meet our obligations. We advocate for better health outcomes and understand the importance of giving back to our communities, both locally and globally.
- Equity, Diversity, and Inclusion: In all work and in the way to interact with each other, to strive to remove barriers to equity and create an environment that fosters diversity and inclusion.

SUPER SPECIALITIES OF THIS DEPARTMENT:

1. Cardiac Anaesthesia,
2. Cardiac Surgical Intensive Care,
3. Neuro Anaesthesia,
4. Critical Care Medicine,
5. Onco Anaesthesia

GOALS OF THE DEPARTMENT:

1. Deliver state-of-the-art anaesthesia services in peri-operative care, pain management and critical care; Educate students, residents and fellows;
2. Be recognized for its contributions to the specialty of anaesthesiology through education, research and scholarly activities;
3. Contribute to the success of the Medical School and Medical System;
4. Provide compassionate, ethical patient care;
5. Promote the advancement of the medical discipline of Anaesthesiology and its subspecialties;

TYPES OF ANAESTHESIA:

1. General Anaesthesia (GA): The GA is used for major surgeries. It can cause the patient to lose consciousness.
2. Monitored Sedation: This form of Anaesthesia is usually used for minimally invasive procedures like colonoscopies, and the sedation levels can range from being slightly drowsy to complete unconsciousness.
3. Regional Anaesthesia (RA): It has various nomenclatures given as per site of anaesthesia. This is usually used during childbirth and localized surgeries that are limited to a certain body part like the leg, arm, or abdomen. The affected body part will be numbed, and the patient will be unaware of the pain.
   a. Spinal Anaesthesia: It is used for lower abdominal, pelvic, rectal, or lower extremity surgery. This type of anaesthesia involves injecting a single dose of the anaesthetic medicine into the area that surrounds the spinal cord. This type of anaesthesia is most often used in orthopaedic procedures of the lower extremities.
   b. Epidural Anaesthesia: Though similar to a spinal anaesthesia it involves continually infusing an anaesthetic drug through a thin catheter. The catheter is placed into the space that surrounds the spinal cord in the lower back, causing numbness in the lower body.

4. Local Anaesthesia (LA): Local anaesthesia is given for minor procedures like putting stitches, extracting a corn. The procedure includes injecting the drug in a small area while the patient is awake and alert.

INFRASTRUCTURE:

There are 'x' number of operation theatres including Major, Minor and Emergency operation rooms. Out of this 'x' number of theatres is "Modular OTs".

Each OT is equipped with central oxygen, Nitrous & vacuum. The post operative care area has multichannel monitor, piped oxygen and central vacuum as well as common crash carts in OT and recovery area.

The OT complex is centrally air-conditioned.

The OT complex is situated at the .... floor of the hospital.

A centralized medical gases pipeline supplies medical gases.

Pre and Post operative rooms.

All theatres are well equipped with modern state-of-the-art equipment required to run the services in an ethical manner.

LIST OF MAJOR EQUIPMENT:

1. Anaesthesia Workstation with spare Oxygen & Nitrous cylinders.
2. Anaesthesia Ventilator.
3. Heart Lung Machine.
4. Laryngoscopes, Magill Forceps, Ambu Bags.
5. Set of ET Tubes.
6. Airways, Mouth Prop, Tongue depressors,
7. Central Medical Gases (Oxygen, Nitrous, Carbon di-oxide & Compressed Air) supply or Bulk cylinders of these gases.
8. PFT Machine.
9. Cautery Machines.
10. Monitors, Infusion Pumps, Defibrillator, And Mobile Image Intensifier.
11. Gases Scavenging System.
12. Laminar Flow (it's a part of modular OTs).
13. Fibre optic Laryngoscope.
14. ABG Analyser.
15. ECG Machine.

List of Equipment as per Indian Public Health Standards (IPHS), Government of India:

SN	Name of Equipment	101-200 Beds	201-300 Beds	301-500 Beds
1	Anaesthetic - laryngoscope Magill's with four blades	3	5	8
2	Endo tracheal tubes sets	2	3	3
3	Magill's forceps (two sizes)	6	8	10

SN	Name of Equipment	101-200 Beds	201-300 Beds	301-500 Beds
4	Connector set of six for ETT	6	8	10
5	Tubes connecting for ETT	6	10	10
6	Air way Male/Female	20/10	20/10	20/10
7	Mouth prop*	8	10	10
8	Tongue depressors*	10	12	15
9	O_2 cylinders for Boyles (if no central supply)	10	12	16
10	N_2O Cylinder for Boyles (if no central supply)	10	12	16
11	CO_2 cylinder for laparoscope	2	5	10
12	Anaesthesia machine with ventilator	2	3	4
13	Multi-parameter monitor	2	3	4
14	Pipe line supply of Oxygen, Nitrous Oxide, Compressed Air and suction (desirable)			
15	Defibrillators	1	2	3
16	Infusion pumps			

* To be provided as per need.

BEST PRACTICES:

1. Difficult intubation and advanced airway management.
2. Managing patients with one lung ventilation.
3. Managing required services in the department of emergency.
4. Managing critical patients in ICU.
5. Pain management for the needy patient.
6. To conduct PAC (Pre-Anaesthesia Check-up)

SERVICES PROVIDED/OFFERED/SCOPE OF SERVICES:

The department offers its services to a wide spectrum of medical and surgical indications.

1. Anaesthesia to Elective cases on round the clock basis to patients of all age group.
2. Anaesthesia for Emergency Cases.
3. CPR.
4. PAC.
5. Anaesthesia in other departments; such as for MRI, CT, DSA and ECT of need basis.
6. Resuscitation facility.
7. Day Care anaesthesia services.
8. Training and Fellowship programs.
9. Services are provided to a variety of specialties, such as;
   a. General Surgery
   b. Robotic Surgery
   c. Laparoscopic Surgery
   d. Neurosurgery

e. GI Surgery
f. Urology
g. Joint Replacements
h. Paediatric & Neonatal Surgery
i. Thoracic and Vascular Surgery
j. Obs and Gynae surgeries
k. ENT and Ophthalmology
l. Orthopaedic Surgery.
m. Plastic & Cosmetic Surgery

MANPOWER/STAFFING:

1. A team of 'x' number of anaesthesiologists
2. Senior Residents
3. Junior Residents (MOs)
4. Trained and qualified technicians and Nurses

VARIOUS CHECKLISTS OF ANAESTHESIA SERVICES:

1. Checklist Patient Intubation:

Intubation Checklist

SN	Check	Yes	No
1	There are sufficient indications for an Intubation?		
2	Patient has confirmed his/her identity?		
3	Check for artificial denture.		
4	Are you prepared for a difficult or failed intubation?		
5	Are you ready with the post intubation steps?		
6	Check patient position.		
7	Intubation aids are ready? a. Proper blade length of Laryngoscope. b. Magill's Forceps. c. Stylet/Tube Introducer. d. ET Tubes of proper size. e. Xylocain jelly. f. Guedal airways. g. Tongue depressor.		
8	Suction Machine is working?		
9	Patient's vitals are normal. His/her IV line is running. Look at his monitor?		
10	Anaesthesia machine's working checked?		
11	Vaporisers in anaesthesia machine are full?		
12	If you expect difficult intubation, keep extra staff ready.		
13	Ventilator is ready and checked for its working?		

2. Checklist Anaesthesia Machine:

Check List for Anaesthesia Machines

SN	Check	Yes	No
1	"Log Card" of the machine is maintained? Read the card every day in the morning.		
2	Dry run the machine every day in the morning before taking up a surgery.		
3	There are 2 sources of oxygen available. [Main source of oxygen (piped medical gases) is available. Another alternate source (pin index oxygen cylinder) is also available].		
4	Battery backup is available with the machine (mainly for ventilator)		
5	Hypoxic guard is functional.		
6	Calibrate the oxygen analyser.		
7	See that AGSS (Anaesthetic gas Scavenging System) is functioning.		
8	Check Bain's circuit for its functioning.		
9	Flowmeter bobbins are moving freely?		
10	Vaporisers are adequately filled and filling port is tightly closed?		
11	Ancillary equipment such as Laryngoscopes, Suction machine are in working order?		
12	Monitoring equipment are hooked and working?		
13	Soda Lime colour has been checked and is, OK?		
14	Re-breathing bag is of correct size?		
15	Breathing system (Breathing circuit) has been checked?		

3. Checklist Depth of Anaesthesia:

A. Checklist LIGHT Anaesthesia

Following checks are present if the patient is under light anaesthesia

SN	Check	Yes	No
1	Nystagmus?		
2	Eye position is not central?		
3	Patient can speak/talk?		
4	Patient's body movement are present?		
5	Eye shows signs of lacrimation?		
6	Frequent and spontaneous blinks?		
7	Palpebral reflex is strongly positive?		
8	Muscles are not fully relaxed?		

B. Checklist DEEP Anaesthesia

Following checks are present if the patient is under light anaesthesia

SN	Check	Yes	No	Remark
1	Nystagmus?			No
2	Eye position is not central.			Central
3	Patient can speak/talk.			No
4	Patient's body movement are present.			No
5	Eye shows signs of lacrimation.			Though eyes are moist but less/no lacrimation
6	Frequent and spontaneous blinks.			None
7	Palpebral reflex is strongly positive.			Weekly positive
8	Muscles are not fully relaxed			Fully relaxed

4. Anaesthesia & Surgery Safety Checklist:

Anaesthesia/Surgery Safety Checklist

SN	Check	Yes	No
SIGN IN (Pre-Induction)			
1	Patient has confirmed his/her name, procedure and site of procedure?		
2	Patient is NIL orally?		
3	Intravenous (IV) line is patent?		
4	Intubation checklist completed? ***(Important)***		
5	Head-down position of the operation table is functioning smoothly?		
6	Anaesthesia machine check completed?		
7	Expected complications are identified and communicated to the team?		
8	Resuscitation equipment (Defibrillator, Emergency drugs, Oxygen cylinder and difficult intubation kit, Ambu bag etc) are ready?		
TIME OUT (Pre-Procedure/Pre-Incision)			
1	Patient name and operation again confirmed?		
2	Depth of anaesthesia checked and is, OK?		
SIGN OUT (Recovery)			
1	Post anaesthesia expected complications/problems discussed with recovery nurse?		
2	Post anaesthesia patient management discussed with recovery nurse?		
3	Patient shifted to recovery once he/she is out of anaesthesia?		

5. Anaesthesia Infection Prevention Checklist:

SN	Check	Yes	No
1	Has everybody washed hands before entering a theatre?		
2	Has everybody changed their street clothes and slipper?		
3	Gloves are worn for laryngoscopy and/or IV-line insertion.		

SN	Check	Yes	No
4	Alcohol swab is used on skin at the site of IV insertion.		
5	Used gloves are always removed after the procedure?		
6	Patient's head & jewellery if any is properly covered.		
7	Used medication vials & ampoules are only discarded after the end of procedure.		
8	No wires or IV tubing hang below the level of knee.		
9	Single use items are not reused.		
10	Reusable ointments and other medicines are used taking care of contamination.		
11	Patient drapes are never reused.		
12	Items are never picked up from the floor for use.		
13	Computer peripherals are also disinfected between patients.		
14	Similarly handles of trolleys/carts are also disinfected.		

6. Anaesthesia Audit Checklist: (Courtesy: Geetanjali Sharma (NABH Consultant)

SN	Audit Point	Remarks
1	Are the patients and/or family members explained about the proposed care?	
2	Are the patient and/or family members explained about the expected results?	
3	Are the patient and/or family members explained about the possible complications?	
4	Are the patients and/or family members explained about the expected costs?	
5	Are all patients reassessed at appropriate intervals?	
6	Is staff involved in direct clinical care document re-assessments?	
7	Are Patients reassessed to determine their response to treatment and to plan further treatment or discharge?	
8	Is care delivery uniform when similar care is provided in more than one setting?	
9	Is Uniform care guided by policies and procedures which reflect applicable laws and regulations?	
10	Are care and treatment orders signed, named, timed and dated by the concerned doctor?	
11	Is care plan countersigned by the clinician in-charge of the patient within 24 hours?	
12	Are evidence-based medicine and clinical practice Guiding lines adapted to Guiding patient care whenever possible?	
13	Do documented policies and procedures Guiding the uniform use of resuscitation throughout the Hospital?	
14	Is staff providing direct patient care trained and periodically updated in cardio-pulmonary resuscitation?	
15	Do we capture and record events during a cardio-pulmonary resuscitation?	
16	Is a post-event analysis done by a multidisciplinary committee for of all cardiac arrests?	
17	Are Corrective and preventive measures taken based on the post-event analysis?	
18	Are documented policies and procedures used to Guiding rational use of blood and blood products?	
19	Are the transfusion services governed by the applicable laws and regulations?	
20	Is informed consent obtained for donation and transfusion of blood and blood products?	
21	Does Informed consent include patient and family education about donation?	

SN	Audit Point	Remarks
22	Is Staff trained to implement the policies?	
23	Are transfusion reactions analysed for preventive and corrective actions?	
24	Do competent and trained persons perform sedation?	
25	Is the person administering and monitoring sedation different from the person performing the procedure	
26	Do Intra-procedure monitoring include at a minimum the heart rate, cardiac rhythm, respiratory rate, blood pressure, oxygen saturation and level of sedation?	
27	Are patients monitored after sedation?	
28	Are criteria used to determine appropriateness of discharge from the recovery area?	
29	Are Equipment and manpower available to rescue patients from a deeper level of sedation than that intended?	
30	Is there documented policy and procedure for the administration of anaesthesia?	
31	Do all patients for anaesthesia have a pre-anaesthesia assessment by a qualified individual?	
32	Does the pre-anaesthesia assessment results in formulation of an anaesthesia plan which is documented?	
33	Is an immediate preoperative revaluation documented?	
34	Is separate informed consent for administration of anaesthesia obtained by the anaesthetist?	
35	Does the anaesthesia monitoring include regular and periodic recording of heart rate, cardiac rhythm, respiratory rate, blood pressure, oxygen saturation, airway security and potency and level of anaesthesia?	
36	Is each patient's post-anaesthesia status monitored and documented?	
37	Does a qualified individual apply defined criteria to transfer the patient from the recovery area?	
38	Are All adverse anaesthesia events recorded and monitored?	
39	Do we have Documented policies and procedures guiding the care of patients under restraints?	
40	Do these include both physical and chemical restraint measures?	
41	Do these include documentation of reasons for restraints?	
42	Are these patients monitored more frequently?	
43	Does the Staff receive training and periodic updating in control and restraint techniques?	
44	Do we have Documented policies and procedures guiding the management of pain?	
45	Does the Hospital respects and supports the appropriate assessment and management of pain for all patients?	
46	Are Patient and family educated on various pain management techniques?	
47	Do we have documented policies and procedures for storage of medication?	
48	Are Medications stored in a clean, well-lit and ventilated environment?	
49	Do the Sound inventory control practices guide storage of the medications?	
50	Are Medications protected from loss or theft?	
51	Is Sound alike and look alike medications stored separately?	
52	Is there a method to obtain medication when the pharmacy is closed?	
53	Are emergency medications available all the time?	

SN	Audit Point	Remarks
54	Are Emergency medications replenished in a timely manner when used?	
55	Do we have documented policies and procedures exist for prescription of medications?	
56	Does the Hospital determine who can write orders?	
57	Are orders written in a uniform location in the medical records?	
58	Are medication orders clear, legible, dated, timed, named and signed?	
59	Is Policy on verbal orders documented and implemented?	
60	Does the Hospital define a list of high-risk medication	
61	Are High risk medication orders verified prior to dispensing?	
62	Is Medication verified from the order prior to administration?	
63	Is Dosage verified from the order prior to administration?	
64	Is Route verified from the order prior to administration?	
65	Is Timing verified from the order prior to administration?	
66	Is Medication administration documented?	
67	Do Policies and procedures govern patient's self-administration of medications?	
68	Do Policies and procedures govern patient's medications brought from outside the Hospital?	
69	Are Patients monitored after medication administration and this is documented?	
70	Are Adverse drug events defined?	
71	Are Adverse drug events reported within a specified time frame?	
72	Are Adverse drug events collected and analysed?	
73	Are policies modified to reduce adverse drug events when unacceptable trends occur?	
74	Do we have documented policies and procedures guiding the use of narcotic drugs and psychotropic substances?	
75	Are these policies in consonance with local and national regulations?	
76	Is proper record kept of the usage, administration and disposal of these drugs?	
77	Are these drugs handled by appropriate personnel in accordance with policies?	
78	Do documented policies and procedures govern procurement, handling, storage, distribution, usage and replenishment of medical gases?	
79	Do these policies and procedures address the safety issues at all level?	
80	Are appropriate records maintained in accordance with the policies, procedures and legal requirements?	
81	Are Patient and family rights and responsibilities documented?	
82	Are Patients and families informed of their rights and responsibilities in a format and language that they can understand?	
83	Do the Hospital's leaders protect patients and family rights?	
84	Is Staff aware of their responsibility in protecting patients and family rights?	
85	Is Violation of patient and family rights recorded, reviewed and corrective/preventive measures taken?	
86	Does the Patient and family rights address any special preferences, spiritual and cultural needs?	
87	Does the Patient and family rights respect for personal dignity and privacy during examination, procedures and treatment?	

SN	Audit Point	Remarks
88	Does the Patient and family rights include protection from physical abuse or neglect?	
89	Does the Patient and family rights include treating patient information as confidential?	
90	Does the Patient and family rights include refusal of treatment?	
91	Does the Patient and family rights include informed consent before anaesthesia, blood and blood product transfusions and any invasive/high risk procedures/treatment?	
92	Does the Patient and family rights include information and consent before any research protocol is initiated?	
93	Do the Patient rights include information on how to voice a complaint?	
94	Do Patient and family rights include information on the expected cost of the treatment?	
95	Do the Patient and family have a right to have an access to his/her clinical records?	
96	Is general consent for treatment obtained when the patient enters the Hospital?	
97	Are Patient and/or his family members informed of the scope of such general consent?	
98	Has the Hospital listed those situations where informed consent is required?	
99	Does Informed consent includes information on risks, benefits, alternatives and as to who will perform the requisite procedure in a language that they can understand?	
100	Is the hospital infection control programme documented which aims at preventing and reducing risk of nosocomial infections?	
101	Is there a multidisciplinary infection control committee?	
102	Does the hospital have an infection control team?	
103	Does the hospital have designated and qualified infection control nurse (s) for this activity?	
104	Does the manual identify the various high-risk areas and procedures?	
105	Does the manual outline methods of surveillance in the identified high-risk areas?	
106	Does the manual focus on adherence to standard precautions at all times?	
107	Are equipment cleaning and sterilization practices included in the manual?	
108	Is an appropriate antibiotic policy established and implemented?	
109	Are Laundry and linen management processes also included in the manual?	
110	Are Kitchen sanitation and food handling issues included in the manual?	
111	Are Engineering controls to prevent infections included in the manual?	
112	Are Mortuary practices and procedures included in the manual?	
113	Does the Hospital define the periodicity of updating the infection control manual?	
114	Is verification of data done on regular basis by the infection control team?	
115	In cases of notifiable diseases, is information (in relevant format) sent to appropriate authorities?	
116	Does the Scope of surveillance activities incorporate tracking and analysing of infection risks, rates and trends?	
117	Does the Surveillance activity include monitoring effectiveness of housekeeping service?	
118	Does the hospital monitor urinary tract, respiratory tract, intra-vascular device, surgical site infections?	
119	Is Appropriate feedback regarding HAI rates provided on a regular basis to medical and nursing staff?	
120	Hand washing facilities in all patient care areas are accessible to health care providers?	

SN	Audit Point	Remarks
121	Compliance with proper hand washing is monitored regularly?	
122	Isolation/barrier nursing facilities are available?	
123	Adequate gloves, masks, soaps, and disinfectants are available and used correctly?	
124	Does the Hospital have a documented procedure for handling outbreaks?	
125	Is this procedure implemented during outbreaks?	
126	After the outbreak is over, are appropriate corrective actions taken to prevent recurrence?	
127	Is there adequate space available for sterilization activities?	
128	Are Regular validation tests for sterilization carried out and documented?	
129	Is There an established recall procedure when breakdown in the sterilization system is identified?	
130	Is the hospital authorized by prescribed authority for the management and handling of bio-medical waste?	
131	Is Proper segregation and collection of bio-medical waste from all patient care areas of the hospital implemented and monitored?	
132	Is The Hospital ensuring that bio-medical waste stored and transported to the site of treatment and disposal in proper covered vehicles within stipulated time limits in a secure manner?	
133	Is Bio-medical waste treatment facility managed as per statutory provisions (if in-house) or outsourced to authorized contractor(s)?	
134	Are Requisite fees, documents and reports submitted to competent authorities on stipulated dates?	
135	Are Appropriate personal protective measures used by all categories of staff handling bio-medical waste?	
136	Does the Hospital management make available resources required for the infection control programme?	
137	Has the hospital earmarked adequate funds from its annual budget in this regard?	
138	Does the hospital conduct regular pre-induction training for appropriate categories of staff before joining concerned department(s)?	
139	Does the hospital conduct regular "in-service" training sessions for all concerned categories of staff at least once in a year?	
140	Is Appropriate pre and post exposure prophylaxis provided to all concerned staff members?	
141	Are formats for data collection standardized?	
142	Are necessary resources available for analysing data?	
143	Are documented procedures laid down for timely and accurate dissemination of data?	
144	Do we have documented procedures for storing and retrieving data?	
145	Do appropriate clinical and managerial staff participates in selecting, integrating and using data?	
146	Does every medical record have a unique identifier?	
147	Does the hospital policy identify those authorized to make entries in medical record?	
148	Is every medical record entry dated and timed?	
149	Can the author of the entry be identified?	
150	Are The contents of medical record identified and documented?	
151	Does the record provide an up-to-date and chronological account of patient care?	

SN	Audit Point	Remarks
152	Does The medical record contain information regarding reasons for admission, diagnosis and plan of care?	
153	Are Operative and other procedures performed incorporated in the medical record?	
154	When patient is transferred to another hospital, Does the medical record contain the date of transfer, the reason for the transfer and the name of the receiving hospital?	
155	Does the medical record contain a copy of the discharge note duly signed by appropriate and qualified personnel?	
156	In case of death, Do the medical record contains a copy of the death certificate indicating the cause, date and time of death?	
157	Whenever a clinical autopsy is carried out, Does the medical record contain a copy of the report of the same?	
158	Do the care providers have access to current and past medical record?	
159	Are the medical records reviewed periodically?	
160	Does the review use a representative sample based on statistical principles?	
161	Is the review conducted by identified care providers?	
162	Does the review focus on the timeliness, legibility and completeness of the medical records?	
163	Does the review process include records of both active and discharged patients?	
164	Does the review point out and documents any deficiencies in records?	
165	Are Appropriate corrective and preventive measures undertaken documented?	

DUTIES & RESPONSIBILITIES:

A. Duties & Responsibilities of an Anaesthetist:

1. To provide pre-anaesthetic evaluation and assessment of all cases posted for a surgery.
2. To carry out required anaesthesia procedure.
3. To adjust lists to accommodate surgery cancellation or accommodating new unlisted cases and even emergencies.
4. To ensure that high risk patients have been adequately reviewed and are properly managed.
5. To provide services as an intensivist, in management of critical cases.
6. To ensue clinical management of acute pain services and participation in pain medicine units where applicable.
7. To provide acute resuscitation services for all emergencies.
8. To manage patients in ICU.
9. To follow "Safe Surgery Checklist".
10. Will ensure that 'informed consent' has been obtained in all cases.
11. To supervise the technicians during their working hours.
12. To maintain absolute coordination with the surgical team and the nursing team in the OT.
13. To supervise supply and shortages in drugs, equipment and consumables required in anaesthesia practice in the OT.
14. To actively carry out all difficult protocol with regards to difficult airway, imaging in anaesthesia, regional blocks and newer techniques.
15. To carry out newer and innovative research program with prior planning and approvals.

16. To help maintain statistic and internal audit.
17. To supervise the operation theatre infection control standards and strict asepsis protocols.
18. To document if any sepsis barrier is breeched.
19. To actively participate in all teaching, training and CME programs as prepared and planned by the hospital.
20. To cover and physically involve oneself in the anaesthesia and pain management in odd hours, on calls and duties.
21. To comply with all the SOPs of the department.
22. To supervise/and or fill up all the Anaesthesia records and documents.

Guidelines for Anaesthetist:

1. All patients will undergo Pre-Anaesthetic Check-up (PAC) as per surgeon's reference.
2. PAC should be properly documented in HIS or as a hard copy.
3. Patient's consent (informed consent) will be taken by nurse but anaesthetist must be aware of it.
4. He will check the anaesthesia machine and anaesthesia trolley before starting the procedure.
5. He will himself administer the pre-medication or will make sure that pre-medication has been given by the nurse.

B. Duties & Responsibilities of Anaesthesia Technician/Nurse:

Operate as a member of the anaesthesia team by maintaining equipment and supplies and assisting with sterile procedures.

1. The anaesthesia technician cleans all required machines such as anaesthesia work station, maintains proper inventory on drugs and consumables such as that of medical gases.
2. To check with the OT schedule of procedures planned for that day and to prepare the OT accordingly.
3. To maintain, calibrate all required equipment of anaesthesia department as per hospital policies & protocols.
4. To assist with procedures such as blood transfusion, IV administration and as asked by the anaesthetist.
5. Assists with sterile procedures/surgeries.
6. To keep ready all appliances required to maintain airway.
7. To attach required anaesthesia monitoring devices.
8. To assist in patient positioning.
9. After anaesthesia: to remove airways, transferring patient to post operative area.
10. To properly maintain all records of anaesthesia and get it signed by the concerned anaesthetist.
11. To maintain sterility of the environment.
12. To ensure that the work is completed systematically with attention to detail without damage to equipment or harm to patient/personnel.

Summary:

1. Supervise all drug preparation in the morning.
2. All drugs syringe labelled with coloured code tags.
3. Maintain records of opioids & other reserved drugs.
4. Checking of crash cart/monitor/workstation every day.

5. Maintain all volatile anaesthetic agents.
6. Maintain all other instruments of ANAESTHESIA DEPARTMENT (non-technical work)
7. Helps in wheeling in & out the patient from theatre.

KEY PERFORMANCE INDICATORS: (KPI)

1. Percentage of Modifications of anaesthesia plan
   Formula for calculations:
   No of patients in whom anaesthesia plan was modified (divide by) No of patients who underwent anaesthesia (multiply by) 100
2. Percentage of Unplanned ventilation
   Formula for calculations:
   No of patients requiring unplanned ventilation (divide by) No of patients who underwent anaesthesia (multiply by) 100
3. Percentage of Adverse anaesthesia events
   Formula for calculations:
   No of patients who developed adverse anaesthesia event (divide by) No of patients who underwent anaesthesia (multiply by) 100
4. Percentage of Anaesthesia related mortality rate
   Formula for calculations:
   No of patients who died due to anaesthesia (divide by) No of patients who underwent anaesthesia (multiply by) 100

STATIONARY REQUIRED IN THIS DEPARTMENT:

1. Preoperative Check List (PAC) – By Ward Nurse:

Hospital Name & Address

Anaesthesia & Operation Notes

Patient Name .... Age/Sex................................

Date of Admission.. Date of Discharge...................

Surgeon in Charge...

Preoperative Check List – By Ward Nurse

SN	Check	Notes
1.	Site Preparation is done	
2.	All Jewellery, rings etc are removed	
3.	Artificial denture, any loose tooth, if yes, is removed	
4.	Patient is in OT Suite	
5.	Patient is fasting since	
6.	Urine passed at (time)	
7.	Mensis due date (for female patients)	
8.	Consent below is signed	

Details of Premedication given

SN	Name of Medicines	Dose	Given at	Nurse Signature
1				
2				

Following documents are to be sent along with the patient:

1. Complete Case Sheet
2. All investigations report in original
3. X-Ray/Ultrasound etc plates in original

2. Preoperative Check List (PAC) – By Anaesthesiologist:

Hospital Name & Address

PAC – FORM

page-1

Patient Name: Age/Sex: Ward:

Surgery Advised:

History:

Asthma Bronchitis COPD Jaundice Kidney Diseases

Oedema Feet H.T. Diabetes Mellitus Chest Pain Ex. Tolerance

Previous Operation: If Yes – Why?

Operation: Anaesthesia: Outcome:

Treatment History:

Present Medications:

Any known Allergies:

Pregnancy if Females:

If using?

Contact Lenses Dentures Implants IOL

Page-2 (backside of page-1)

Examination:

G.C. Pulse B.P. CVS Chest

Airway Assessment:

M.P. Scoring Mouth Opening Neck Extension Lose Teeth

Any other Factor/Remark

Investigations:

Hb. TLC DLC KFT RBS LFT

Urine

ECG:

X-Ray Chest

Others:

Advice:

3. Consent Form:

CONSENT FORM

To

.... Hospital Name & Address

I .... S/O, D/O, W/0 ....

hereby consent for myself/relative's .... (Specify relation) operation/procedure under anaesthesia (General/Regional/Local) as deemed fit by the doctors. All the risks and results associated with this operation/procedure have been fully explained to me. I have understood all pros and cons.

I also consent to any alternative measure as may be deemed necessary during the operation.

I am told that in this case the risks are higher because of..

Signature: ....

Name & Address: ....

WITNESS:

4. Anaesthesia & Operation Notes (Short):

Anaesthesia & Operation Notes

Patient Name: .... Age/Sex: ....

Hospital Registration No: .... IPD No: ....

Consultant In-charge: ....

Surgeon In-charge: ....

Anaesthetist In charge: ....

Assistant Surgeon: ....

OT Nurse: .... OT Technician: ....

Pre-operative Assessment & ASA Classification: ....

Anaesthesia: -

Pre-medication (Drug & Dose): ....

Type: .... Route: ....

Respiration (Assisted/Spontaneous): ....

Operation: -

Site Preparation with: ....

Incision: ....

Operative Procedure: ....

Findings: ....

Blood Required: .... Units: ....

Closure Technique: ....

Biopsy taken (Material & Time of sending): ....

Post-operative Diagnosis: ....

Pre-operative Diagnosis: ....

Patient In Time: .... Patient Out Time: ....

Remarks, if any: ....

Signature Chief Surgeon Signature Chief Anaesthetist

5. General PAC Form:

Checklist PAC form (Pre-anaesthesia Check-up)

SN	Check	Yes	No	Remark
1	Consent for anaesthesia taken?			
2	Medical history elicited? for; • Cough • Dyspnoea • Smoking • Alcohol taking • Drug allergy • Hypertension • Diabetes • Vomiting • Diarrhoea • Chest pain • Neck or spine (back) problem • Convulsions/fainting • Bleeding disorders			
3	Vitals have been checked and are within normal limits?			
4	Systemic examination done?			
5	ECG is within normal limits?			
6	Haemoglobin estimation and blood grouping done?			
7	Chest has been x-rayed?			
8	Details of previous surgery and anaesthesia documented?			

SN	Check	Yes	No	Remark
9	Airway assessment done?			
10	Anaesthetist has signed the PAC form?			

Anaesthetist, name, signature and date:

6. Anaesthesia & Operation Record (Booklet form):

Page-1

Hospital Name & Address

Patient Name ____________________

Age/Sex ____________ Ward No./Bed No. ____________ D.O.A. ____________

Address ____________________

Dr. In-charge ____________________

PRIOR TO TRANSFER TO O.T. PLEASE ENSURE PATIENT HAS FOLLOWING:

Case Notes ________ X-Ray ________ Investigations ________

Medicines ________

SN	Check	Yes	No	N.A.
1	Consent form signed?			
2	Site Marking?			
3	Operation site prepared?			
4	Jewellery, wrist watch removed?			
5	Change to theatre gown?			
6	Dentures/Lenses/Loose Teeth removed?			
7	Date of L.M.P. Noted?			
8	Time of last meal/drink?			
9	Time last passed urine?			
10	Pre-medication given?			

Drug				Dose		Doctor Sign	
Route		Time		Given at		Nurse Sign	

CONSENT FORM FOR OPERATIVE/SPECIAL PROCEDURE

To,

The Medical Staff & Management

ABC Hospital

Address

I, ... S/O, D/O, W/O .... hereby consent for myself/son's/ daughter's/wife's/husband's/relative's .... operation under any kind of anaesthesia General/Regional/Local as deemed suitable by doctors. The reason for operation and the likely risks of operation and anaesthesia have been explained to me in language I understand & I accept the risks.

I also consent to such further or alternative operative measures as may be found to be necessary during the course of operation.

I understand that risk of operation in my/my parent's case is high because of

1. .... 2. .... 3. ....

I am ready to take added risk involved in operation.

I understand that facilities better than here may be available at other places. I willingly accept to be treated here. I have been given the opportunity to ask any questions regarding above which I wanted to ask & have received answers to my satisfaction.

I will be responsible for payment of all hospital charges.

Witness: -

Signature .... Signature ....

Name & Address .... Name & Address ....

Page-2

OPERATION SHEET

Name	Age	Sex	Ward/Bed No.	LP No.
Pre-Operative Diagnosis			Post Operative Diagnosis	
Operation				Date
Surgeon	Asstt Surgeon	Anaesthetist	Type of Anaesthesia	

Findings & Operative Procedure:

Post-Operative Orders:

Contd. 3

ANAESTHETIC RECORD

Major Anaesthetic Problems:

Surgical Diagnosis:

Pre-Operative assessment by Anaesthetist:	Weight	Kg
ASA Classification 1……… 2…………… 3………… 4…………… 5…………… E…………	Hb	g/dl
	B.P.	
	Rhythm	
Relevant Medical Conditions/Drug history:	Blood Units	
Pre-medication:	Time Given:	
Anaesthetic techniques:		
Venepuncture/Cannulation Sites:		
Ventilation:	Spontaneous/Controlled	
Breathing Circuit		
Endo-tracheal tube"	Size	Type
Technical Assistant: Name & Signature:		
Nurse:		

Page-4

Time:																					
Drugs & Fluids																					

<table>
<tr><td rowspan="7">B.P. Recording:
200
150
100
50</td><td></td><td></td><td></td><td></td><td></td><td></td><td></td><td></td><td></td><td></td><td></td><td></td><td></td><td></td><td></td><td></td><td></td><td></td><td></td><td></td><td></td></tr>
<tr><td></td><td></td><td></td><td></td><td></td><td></td><td></td><td></td><td></td><td></td><td></td><td></td><td></td><td></td><td></td><td></td><td></td><td></td><td></td><td></td><td></td></tr>
<tr><td></td><td></td><td></td><td></td><td></td><td></td><td></td><td></td><td></td><td></td><td></td><td></td><td></td><td></td><td></td><td></td><td></td><td></td><td></td><td></td><td></td></tr>
<tr><td></td><td></td><td></td><td></td><td></td><td></td><td></td><td></td><td></td><td></td><td></td><td></td><td></td><td></td><td></td><td></td><td></td><td></td><td></td><td></td><td></td></tr>
<tr><td></td><td></td><td></td><td></td><td></td><td></td><td></td><td></td><td></td><td></td><td></td><td></td><td></td><td></td><td></td><td></td><td></td><td></td><td></td><td></td><td></td></tr>
<tr><td></td><td></td><td></td><td></td><td></td><td></td><td></td><td></td><td></td><td></td><td></td><td></td><td></td><td></td><td></td><td></td><td></td><td></td><td></td><td></td><td></td></tr>
<tr><td></td><td></td><td></td><td></td><td></td><td></td><td></td><td></td><td></td><td></td><td></td><td></td><td></td><td></td><td></td><td></td><td></td><td></td><td></td><td></td><td></td></tr>
<tr><td>Drugs:</td><td colspan="3"></td><td colspan="3"></td><td colspan="3"></td><td colspan="3"></td><td colspan="3"></td><td colspan="3"></td><td colspan="3"></td></tr>
<tr><td>Fluids:</td><td colspan="3"></td><td colspan="3"></td><td colspan="3"></td><td colspan="3"></td><td colspan="3"></td><td colspan="3"></td><td colspan="3"></td></tr>
<tr><td>Events:</td><td colspan="3"></td><td colspan="3"></td><td colspan="3"></td><td colspan="3"></td><td colspan="3"></td><td colspan="3"></td><td colspan="3"></td></tr>
<tr><td>Blood Loss:</td><td colspan="21"></td></tr>
<tr><td>Urine Output:</td><td colspan="21"></td></tr>
<tr><td>Posture:</td><td colspan="21"></td></tr>
<tr><td>Recovery:</td><td colspan="21"></td></tr>
<tr><td></td><td colspan="21"></td></tr>
<tr><td></td><td colspan="21"></td></tr>
<tr><td></td><td colspan="21"></td></tr>
<tr><td></td><td colspan="21"></td></tr>
<tr><td></td><td colspan="21"></td></tr>
</table>

Signatures:

Anaesthetic (s) ....

Medical Officer/SR:

OT Nurse:

OT Technician:

Discharge from Recovery at ....

7. KPI Data Collection Register:

Hospital Name & Address

For The Month: __________ Year: ___________

SN	Date	Name of the Patient	Age/Sex	I.D. No.	Plan of Anaesthesia	Anaesthesia Plan changed to (Reason)	Any unplanned ventilation	Any Adverse Reaction of Anaesthesia	Mortality	Sign
Note: It is in Landscape format										

xxxxxxxxxxxxxxxxxx

Indicator: Re-intubation rate

Data Collection Register

Quality Indicator No.: 34							
Indicator: Re-intubation rate							
SN	**Date of intubation**	**UHID No.**	**Patient Name**	**Date & Time of ex-tubation**	**Date & Time of re-intubation (within 48 hours of extubation)**	**Reason for re-intubation**	**Sign**
Note: It is in Landscape format							

xxxxxxxxxxxxxxxxxxxxx

Indicator: Percentage of adverse anaesthesia events

Sr. No.	**Date**	**Patient Name**	**UHID No.**	**Diagnosis**	**Type of anaesthesia planned on PAC**	**Type of anaesthesia administered during surgery**				**Nature of adverse anaesthesia event**	**Reason for adverse anaesthesia event**	**Anaesthetist sign**
						General	**Spinal**	**Local**	**Any other**			
Note: It is in Landscape format												

xxxxxxxxxxxxxxxxxx

Indicator: Percentage of re-scheduling of surgeries

SN	**Date**	**Patient Name**	**UHID No.**	**Name of Surgery**	**Name of Surgeon**	**Scheduled date and time of procedure**	**Date and time when procedure is rescheduled**	**Reason for rescheduling**	**Sign - OT technician/ Anaesthetist/ Surgeon**
Note: It is in Landscape format									

PROCEDURES (SOP):

A. Procedure For PAC:

1. The PAC should be completed on OPD basis itself. But for admitted patients it is done on bedside.
2. Basic vitals such as; weight, height and baseline vitals including BP, HR and SpO2 must be recorded in the PAC form by a trained nurse staff.

3. The ASA classification must be recorded on PAC form.
4. Necessary investigation results should be filled.
5. Female patients are examined as per standard protocol.
6. High risk patients and patients with co-morbid conditions should be referred to respective specialist and their opinion should be documented.
7. The anaesthetist should clearly mention the fasting orders and pre-medications.
8. The attending anaesthetist should sign in the end.

B. Procedure For Obtaining Consent:

1. For consent to be valid it must be voluntary and informed and the person consenting must have the capacity to make the decision.
2. Informed consent should be taken after explaining him all the pros and cons of the procedure by the attending consultant.
3. Adults can give consent by themselves. It should have signature of at-least two witnesses.
4. In case of minors and other cases (mentally ill, unconscious) who cannot consent by themselves, it should be obtained by the legal guardian.
5. If it is an MLC or unknown patient, the left thumb impression of the patient is taken under signature of two witnesses.
6. The nurse in-charge checks for availability of the consent before transferring the patient to OT.

Procedures when informed consent is necessary:

1. All invasive procedures including intra-articular injections.
2. Some procedures such as; Vasectomy, Tubectomy, IUI, IVF, Ultrasound of a pregnant lady require informed consent in advance. Here consent is required from the spouse also.
3. All cases which require sedation in any form.
4. All cases where during the procedure patient can have pain or discomfort.
5. Whenever there is a risk involved or the patient is having any other morbidity.
6. For Dialysis, Blood Transfusion, HIV and Genetic testing and before chemotherapy.
7. In all admissions.
8. Patient has right to refuse a procedure or admission.

C. SOP for Paediatric Anaesthesia:

Purpose:

To ensure safe preparation, safe conduct of anaesthesia and good recovery of paediatric patients.

Scope:

Proper PAC, Transfer of the patient in and out of OT, Informed Consent, Safe administration of anaesthesia, and safe reversal of anaesthesia.

Responsibility:

Anaesthesiologists

OT Technicians

Attending Consultant

Procedure:

A. Procedure for PAC:
   1. In children with co-morbid conditions, paediatrician opinion must be sought.
   2. Neonates should be cleared by a neonatologist.
   3. Treating consultant opinion is also sought.
   4. Children with Upper Respiratory Tract Infection should be rejected or taken with caution.
   5. Fasting Guidelines:

Guidelines	Fasting Time in Hours
Clear Liquids (Fluids without pulp), Tea/Coffee without milk	2 hours
Breast Milk	4 hours
Infant Formula	6 hours
Solid	8 hours

B. Patent should be shifted from ward to the OT in a stretcher with side rails and accompanied with a nurse.
C. PAC should be carried out again. Pre operative Checklist is to be followed.
D. Parents/attendants should be properly counselled.
E. Premedication should be carried out to a minimum and with caution.
F. WHO Surgical Safe Checklist must be followed.
G. Consider of having two well trained anaesthesiologists during the procedure.
H. Anaesthetists have the Neonatal and Paediatric Advanced Life Support Certification.
I. Ensure that laboratory and radiological services are available at that time.
J. Required drugs & equipment for paediatric anaesthesia are available and easily accessible.
K. Defibrillator with paediatric paddles, Paediatric airways, difficult intubation appliances, Resuscitation equipment and drugs.
L. Child should be continuously monitored during the surgery especially for SpO2, Etco2, ECH, HR and temperature.
M. Post operatively all such patients should be continuously monitored for all vital parameters.
N. IV cannula should not be removed before discharge.
O. Proper pain assessment should be carried out.
P. Post op fluid management should be optimum.

D. Administration of General Anaesthesia:

1. Shift in OT on trolley.
2. Confirmation of operating site, procedure, name of patient (matching with identification of tag, file).
3. Application of all required monitoring.
   - Non-invasive mandatory.
   - Invasive at consultant discretion.
4. Induction – Intubation – Maintenance of Anaesthesia
5. Monitoring anaesthesia intra operatively.
6. Recovery assured & confirmed by consultant then shift to recovery room.
7. If shifting of patient on ventilator for elective ventilation. Shift on Bains circuit & oxygen cylinder.

8. Central line, arterial line, PA catheter insertion both in local anaesthesia.
9. Before induction or after induction with peripheral cannula depending upon requirement of individual case is in the discretion of consultant anaesthesia.
10. Urinary catheterization is to be done after induction only and always by surgical team.
11. One female staff is mandatory with female patient in O.T. throughout the time.
12. Drugs selection and dosage of all anaesthetic drugs are as per the discretion of consultant in-charge of Anaesthesia.
13. Changeover of consultant in one case not allowed but in special situation one consultant can take over the case with proper mutual understanding and full over of the case.
14. All adverse reactions related to anaesthesia must be documented.

Procedure:

1. Anaesthesia is to be provided by qualified and trained persons with suitable credentials after taking Informed Consent.
2. Such persons (doctors) are also qualified to monitor and maintain proper hemodynamic state of the patient.
3. Patient is assessed (PAC) before giving any type of anaesthesia.
4. Anaesthetic agent is administered in measured dose enough to achieve desired results.
5. Patients are continuously monitored to keep them at desired level of sedation.
6. These clinicians are also qualified to carry out lifesaving procedures in case of a need.
7. They are also responsible for bringing patients out of anaesthesia after the procedure is over.
8. Anaesthesia has to be given only in properly equipped operation rooms.
9. Patients are monitored in recovery rooms also prior to discharge or shifting.
10. ASA classification is must for every patient.
11. Documentation of whole process in the patient's file is mandatory.
12. Specialised formats are available to document anaesthesia and complete surgical procedure in an established manner.
13. Blood is kept ready or blood bank is asked to be ready, if blood need is anticipated during surgery.
14. As such all procedures are done in OT when the desired blood is available in the blood Bank.
15. At the end of surgery, the patient is shifted to recovery or ICU at the advice of the anaesthetist and surgeon both.
16. Adverse events, if any are documented and reviewed in monthly clinical meetings.
17. Medical Audit is also carried out at random.

Summary

1. Pre-Anaesthetic Evaluation of the Patient: Nil Orally, Informed Consent
2. Prescribing of Anaesthetic Plan
3. Management of Anaesthesia
4. Intra Procedural Monitoring
5. Post Anaesthetic Care

E. Administration of moderate sedation or monitored anaesthesia care (MAC):

1. Informed consent as usual should be taken.
2. Only trained anaesthetist should administer sedation.
3. PAC must be carried out.

4. Intra-procedure monitoring should be same as that for General Anaesthesia.
5. All other parameters that are required should be monitored and recorded.
6. The patient will be shifted either to POP or to the ward after the patient is conscious and responding to verbal command.
7. OT must be ready/prepared to handle any emergency.

Moderate sedation: ASA guidelines

The ASA has produced guidelines that define levels of sedation.

1. Minimal Sedation (Anxiolysis) is a drug-induced state during which patients respond normally to verbal commands. Example: Small amount of fentanyl or midazolam.
2. Moderate Sedation/Analgesia ("Conscious Sedation") is a drug-induced depression of consciousness during which patients respond purposefully to verbal commands, either alone or accompanied by light tactile stimulation. Example: More midazolam or fentanyl.
3. Deep Sedation/Analgesia is a drug-induced depression of consciousness during which patients cannot be easily aroused but respond purposefully following repeated or painful stimulation. The ability to independently maintain ventilatory function may be impaired.

   (Reference: https://www.openanesthesia.org/moderate_sedation_asa_guidelines/)

Moderate Sedation: Procedure

Assessment & Monitoring of the Patient:

1. Pre- procedure:
   - Informed consent is taken.
   - Every patient is assessed clinical and by investigations by anaesthetist or person giving sedation which is similar to PAC.
   - A plan of care is discussed and documented and communicate among all members of team of care givers.
   - It is established that the patient is in physical and psychological condition to undergo that sedation after taking all the potential complications and alternative methods available at hand.
2. Intra-Procedure:
   - One staff member who is not the member of procedure team will continuously monitor the patient.
   - The monitoring includes, monitoring of various vital parameters including but not limited to;
   - Cardiac rhythm & rate, Respiratory rate, BP, SpO2, level of sedation etc.
   - All monitored parameters are documented at every five minutes till the procedure is over.
3. Post Procedure:
   - Monitoring is continued till sedation is over. Here monitoring is to be done every 15 minutes till the patient recovers fully.
   - The patient is only discharged when all vitals are within normal limits.
   - All events are documented in the patient's medical case papers.
4. Following are the responsibilities of persons involved in the care:

SN	Procedure Steps	Responsibility
1	The patient is NIL ORALLY, if advised.	Staff Nurse
2	Only qualified doctor is allowed to order sedation	Consultant
3	All monitoring equipment are readied before start of the procedure.	Staff Nurse

SN	Procedure Steps	Responsibility
4	Informed Consent taken after explaining about the sedation and procedure to the patient/attendants.	Staff Nurse
5	All required drugs are kept at hand. Emergency Resuscitation trolley (crash cart) is at hand.	Staff Nurse
6	Monitoring is done as per SOP explained above.	Team Members
7	Patient is only discharged or transferred after all criteria are met.	Team Members
8	Any adverse event or side effect shall be documented and treating consultant is informed, if he is not the member of the team.	Staff Nurse

F. Day Care Anaesthesia:

1. No sedation/analgesia is practiced by paramedical technicians.
2. All anaesthetic medication administered by consultant.
3. Monitored ANAESTHESIA care is also same.
4. Monitoring non-invasive only.
5. Nausea/vomiting prophylaxis in al patient.
6. Post procedural analgesia is based on NSAIDS in extreme cases and Tramadol given.
7. Discharge from post ANAESTHESIA unit to day care ward (Based Aldrete upon score).
8. Discharge from day care ward in evening after consultant round.
9. Orders always explained to one responsible adult who is going to be with the patient at home.

G. SOP for Spinal/Regional Anaesthesia:

1. Inform the patient regarding the process and take consent.
2. Place the patient in the required position.
3. Wear sterile gloves and prepare the site of injection.
4. Use aseptic techniques during injection.
5. Monitor the patient for vitals as in other type of anaesthesia.

H. Discharge of From POP/Recovery:

Following criteria are used;

a. Activity:
   2 = Moves all extremities voluntarily on command
   1 = Moves two extremities
   0 = Unable to move extremities
b. Respiration:
   2 = Breaths deeply and coughs freely
   1 = Dyspnoeic, Shallow or limited breathing
   0 = Apnoeic
c. Circulation:
   2 = BP + 20 mm of pre anaesthetic level
   1 = BP+ 20-50 mm of pre anaesthetic level
   0 = BP+ 50 mm of pre anaesthetic Level

d. Consciousness:
   2 = Fully awake
   1 = Arousable on calling
   0 = Not responding
e. Oxygen Saturation
   2 = SpO2 > 92%
   1 = Supplemental O_2 requirement to maintain SpO2 >90%
   0 = SpO2 < 92% even with O_2 supplementation
   Once the score is 9 or above, the patient is fit for discharge.
   10 = Total score
f. All patients are kept under observation till the desired score is attained.
g. Patients are transferred/discharge only after written instructions of the anaesthetist.

POST OPERATIVE CARE WITH ESSENTIAL MONITORING:

A. Recovery from General Anaesthesia in Operation Theatre

On the discretion of clinical assessment of consultant anaesthesiologist.

1. Level of consciousness.
2. Return of airway protective reflexes.
3. Free from anaesthetic side effects.
4. Hemodynamic stability.
5. Patient awareness (direct question by consultant).
6. Notes in Anaesthesia sheet.
7. Recovery room instructions are also mentioned i.e., O_2 flow, need of ventilator and shift to ICU.

B. Post Anaesthesia Care

1. Receive patient from the OT
2. Access vitals, level of consciousness, type of operation done. Monitor the patient's SpO2
3. Check airway and adequacy of ventilation
4. Provide oxygen to patient
5. Monitor the BP
6. Monitor ECG if needed
7. Monitor urine output
8. Assess consciousness before sending patient to ward
9. Observe for bleeding from the surgical site
10. Access pain and inform anaesthetist for pain relief
11. Ensure that intravenous fluids/blood are given as per instruction
12. Record BP/Pulse/HR/SpO2 on the chart before sending patient to ward

C. Discharge from Recovery Room:

1. Decision is by consultant anaesthetist
2. Follow modified Aldrete score (>8) for discharge from recovery room

3. Fast tracking is permitted only in special circumstances. (Discretion of consultant anaesthesiologist)
4. For regional ANAESTHESIA motor recovery is not criteria for shifting from recovery room.

INFECTION CONTROL PRACTICES:

1. All the anaesthetists of the hospital should be in contact with ICN and quality cell of the hospital for implementing various infection control practices.
2. Due care must be taken to avoid transmission of infection from the patient to the anaesthetist and vice versa.
3. Hand hygiene practices should be followed as a routine.
4. All anaesthetists will comply by the hospital policies on infection control and waste disposal including sharps.
5. Ensure that all equipment being used by this department are clean and are periodically decontaminated.
6. Use of disposable should be encouraged. All reusable items must be properly sterilized.
7. All invasive procedures must be carried out with due precautions.

RECORDS & DOCUMENTS GENERATED/MAINTAINED:

1. Anaesthesia technique and intra operative monitoring is recorded in ANAESTHESIA record sheet for individual patient.
2. Any deviation from the normal condition is presented as case discussion in morbidity and mortality meet along with surgical department.
3. Pre aesthetic check-up and plan for ANAESTHESIA including consent in written format is there with individual case sheet, which is attached in file.
4. Post operative orders are mentioned in ANAESTHESIA record sheet including post operative analgesia plan.
5. Daily assessment for multi model analgesia (if used) technique and their effects (including adverse effects) are mentioned in patient record file by consultant anaesthetic/in-charge of that individual patient.
6. Anaesthesia audit of individual ANAESTHESIA consultant in-charge is presented in monthly in surgical morbidity and mortality meet.

SUBJECTS FOR CME/WORKSHOPS:

1. Thoracic Anaesthesia.
2. Difficult Airway Management and Airway Management in infants.
3. Mechanical Ventilation.
4. BLS and ALS techniques.
5. Paediatric Anaesthesia
6. ISSP Meet, ISA meet on periodical intervals.

TEACHING ACTIVITIES:

1. The department is involved in teaching undergraduate and postgraduate students of medicine and allied sciences.

2. Teaching nursing and technical staff under its care about best practices in IV Cannulation, Basic Life Support (BLS) and Endotracheal intubation techniques to its junior doctors to enable them to handle emergency situations.

BIBLIOGRAPHY, REFERENCES & ACKNOWLEDGMENTS:

1. Indian Public Health Standards (IPHS)

   Guidelines for District Hospitals (101 to 500 Bedded) Revised 2012 Directorate General of Health Services Ministry of Health & Family Welfare, Government of India
2. "Standard Operating Procedures SOP For Hospitals 2nd Edition" by Dr. Arun K. Agarwal
3. "Duties & Responsibilities of Hospital Staff" by Dr. Arun Kumar
4. "Checklists for Hospitals" by Dr. Arun K. Agarwal
5. NABH 5th Edition.
6. All India Institute of Medical Sciences, New Delhi,
7. SOP for Surgery Department, Ist Edition: August; 2016, Quality Assurance Cell, Delhi State Health Mission, Department of Health and Family Welfare, Government of NCT of Delhi
8. Standard Operating Procedures (SOPs) for (JDW/NRH), Quality Assurance and Standardization Division (QASD) Ministry of Health, Thimphu: Bhutan

Chapter – 4

DEPARTMENT OF BIO MEDICAL ENGINEERING

INDEX

1. Introduction
2. Description
3. Purpose
4. Objectives
5. Staffing
6. Department Organogram
7. Duties & Responsibilities
   a. Bio Medical Engineer
8. Equipment Planning
9. Equipment Maintenance
   a. Routine Maintenance
   b. Breakdown Maintenance
   c. Preventive Maintenance
10. Calibration of Devices
11. Policies & Procedures (SOP)
    a. General Procedures
    b. Equipment Installation
    c. Demonstration & Training
    d. Coding of Equipment
    e. Preventive Maintenance
    f. Breakdown Maintenance
    g. Condemnation Procedure
    h. Equipment Log Card
    i. Calibration of Equipment
    j. Safety Policies
    k. Monitoring of adverse events related to Medical Devices and compliance hazard notices on recalls.
12. Work Flow
    a. Complaint Management
    b. Preventive Maintenance
13. Quality Indicators

14. Check Lists
    a. BME Checklist
    b. Checklist Equipment Management
    c. Checklist Breakdown Maintenance
15. Audit
16. Records Maintained
17. Stationary Formats
    a. Register of Calibration Schedule for Medical Equipment
    b. Complaint Register & Log Book
    c. Equipment Gate Pass
    d. Equipment Log Card/Register: (Format-1)
    e. Log Card/History Card: (Format-2)
    f. Training Record (Training by BME to User Staff)
    g. Calibration Stickers
    h. Format for Collecting Data for KPI
    i. Master Register of Medical Equipment
18. Bibliography, References & Acknowledgments

INTRODUCTION:

Biomedical engineering (BME) is the application of engineering principles and design concepts to medicine and biology for healthcare purposes (e.g., diagnostic or therapeutic). This field seeks to close the gap between engineering and medicine, combining the design and problem solving skills of engineering with medical and biological sciences to advance health care treatment, including diagnosis, monitoring, and therapy. Biomedical engineering has only recently emerged as its own study, compared to many other engineering fields. Such an evolution is common as a new field transition from being an interdisciplinary specialization among already-established fields, to being considered a field in itself. Much of the work in biomedical engineering consists of research and development, spanning a broad array of subfields (see below). Prominent biomedical engineering applications include the development of biocompatible prostheses, various diagnostic and therapeutic medical devices ranging from clinical equipment to micro-implants, common imaging equipment such as MRIs and EEGs, regenerative tissue growth, pharmaceutical drugs and therapeutic biologicals. [Biomedical engineering: From Wikipedia, the free encyclopaedia, *https://en.wikipedia.org/wiki/Biomedical_engineering*]

Health delivery system is very much dependant on modern technology. To maintain a large inventory of technically advanced medical equipment, hospital needs help of biomedical engineers. In a hospital set up, these engineers are responsible for giving their advice on selection of equipment its performance and of course its maintenance.

The Biomedical Engineering Services are responsible for testing, repairing, and maintaining in proper and safe operating condition, the hospital's diagnostic and therapeutic equipment.

The hospital has a separate department to cater to maintenance services of medical equipment. In some hospitals, it may be clubbed with 'Maintenance Department' of the hospital.

This department is fully equipped with men and material to deal with preventive and breakdown maintenance of various medical equipment of the hospital.

DESCRIPTION:

a. The hospital has planned and installed all required medical equipment within its scope of services.
b. Experienced and trained staff is positioned in the respective departments to operate such equipment.
c. BME & Maintenance department to take care of all medical equipment.
d. Training in operation of these equipment is imparted by the engineers of the respective vendors.

PURPOSE:

a. The purpose of this manual is to ensure safe and trouble-free operations of all medical equipment.
b. It provides standard procedures for maintenance, repair and calibration of such equipment.
c. It guides about various activities from selection, purchasing, inspection and maintenance.
d. To advise on planning, scheduling and service contacts of these equipment.
e. It shall also help in investigating any adverse event happening during operation of such equipment.
f. To train user staff in safe and correct operation of equipment.

OBJECTIVES:

a. To ensure functioning of equipment round the clock.
b. To reduce the cost of maintenance.
c. To reduce the downtime.
d. To ensure compliance with regulatory authorities.

STAFFING:

a. Bio Medical Engineers
b. Bio Medical Technicians
c. Assistant/Helper

DEPARTMENTAL ORGANOGRAM:

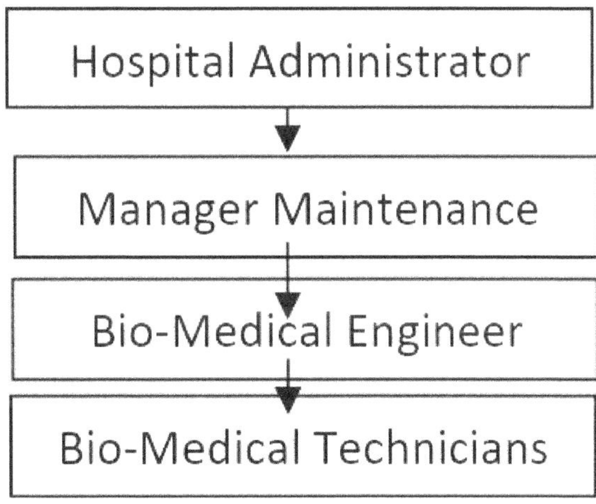

DUTIES & RESPONSIBILITIES:

A. Bio Medical Engineer:

1. To be punctual on duty in a prescribed office dress.
2. To take daily morning round of all departments with a complaint register to ensure proper functioning of all medical equipment.
3. To ensure availability of complaints register in concerned areas (date and time of receipt of complaint, allotment of job, and completion of job.
4. Will advise and assist user staff about application of medical appliances.
5. To carry out all equipment inventory and its Assets coding (in-house floor wise equipment list).
6. To carry out all equipment inventory and its Assets coding (in-house floor wise equipment list).
7. To update Policy and Manual regarding his department.
8. Will check for safety and efficiency of medical equipment while being purchased and also when in use.
9. Will help in installation, calibration and commissioning of such equipment.
10. Will try to repair medical equipment himself if the equipment is not under warranty.
11. To take daily rounds of all departments with medical equipment for routine inspection and noting down maintenance problems.
12. To supervise and carry out planned and breakdown maintenance of all medical equipment in the hospital.
13. To ensure adequate inventory of essential spares.
14. To inform hospital administration of all major and/or minor breakdowns.
15. To coordinate with manufacturers, vendors while doing maintenance of equipment.
16. To update and enter in new service contracts with vendors.
17. To monitor and ensure execution of these service contracts.
18. Log register/card for each costly (definition of costly should be as per the hospital policy) equipment. It should mention the nature of complaint and action taken.
19. Break down time (up time) record register for equipment under AMC & CMC.
20. They will have detailed records of all AMC(s) and CMC(s) of medical equipment.
21. To train nursing and other concerned staff in proper use of the equipment.
22. Will hold training sessions for staff of user department.
23. To advice on medical equipment purchases and to attend such purchase committee meetings.
24. They may be asked to draft specifications of new purchases to float a tender/inquiry.
25. They may be asked to prepare a techno-commercial comparison of bids received.
26. Will carry out reference checks of shortlisted vendors.
27. They will check all new incoming equipment to ensure that they meet set specifications and standards. They will sign the invoices as a token of acceptance of the said equipment.
28. Will be instrumental in its installation and test run while it is still in the custody of the vendor.
29. Ensure periodical calibration of all equipment.
30. Will maintain all quality indicator registers as per NABH standards.
31. Will be responsible for safe custody of various maintenance tools in his/her possession.
32. Will develop/update Standard Operating procedures and checklists of this department.
33. Will advise for Insurance cover (against breakdown & repair) for equipment, if required?
34. To carry out any other duty assigned by seniors.

35. To ensure all equipment quality conformance certificates along with manufacturer test certificates.
36. To prepare and stick to weekly, monthly, annual schedules of inspection and calibration.
37. To carry out preventive and breakdown maintenance for every medical equipment (periodic checks, timely preventive maintenance and response to any breakdown issues including at night and weekend.)
38. To safely keep original equipment manual for all the machines.
39. To ensure checking of compressed air purity from OT and ICU once in a year.
40. To ensure periodical inspection and calibration of utility equipment such as pressure gauze of steam steriliser, temperature gauzes of medication refrigerators.
41. To ensure that all radiological equipment using staff is having TLD badges.
42. To keep TLD Batches record and lead apron screening Record.

Summary:

1. To float inquiry, receive offers, prepare techno-commercial comparison, check vendors' reference and order the equipment as per instructions of the purchase committee.
2. Inspect the received item.
3. Enter in the hospital inventory in the software and/or master register.
4. Install and maintain the equipment. Maintain log registers for all equipment.
5. Try to repair faulty equipment, if not under warranty, AMC, CMC.
6. Is responsible for safe and proper operation of all medical equipment.
7. Ensure AMC/CMC renewal on time.
8. Recommend condemnation of an old equipment.

EQUIPMENT PLANNING:

1. The hospital has a proper equipment planning system that takes in to account the future requirements of the organization in accordance with its scope of services and strategic plans.
2. The plans shall be reviewed periodically or as and when required.
3. All equipment is selected, updated and upgraded by collaborative process.
4. There is involvement of the end-users, management, finance, engineering and biomedical departments in the selection of equipment.

EQUIPMENT MAINTENANCE:

1. Routine Maintenance:

a. The Biomedical Engineer is responsible for the overall management and upkeep of the Bio - medical equipment.
b. Designated staff is responsible for daily maintenance of equipment based on daily monitoring checklist/Weekly monitoring/monthly monitoring.
c. Deficiency details are documented in equipment break down book and the same is communicated to the biomedical engineer.

2. Breakdown Maintenance:

a. All breakdown entries are recorded in the registers.
b. The complaint is registered and complaint number is generated.

c. Bio medical engineer is assigned or directed to the site for rectification as per first line service guidelines.
d. If it is minor break down, corrective actions are taken by the biomedical engineer with the available spare parts in-house within 2-3 hours and the same is documented in the breakdown register with the time of rectification details and it is counter signed by the biomedical engineers who have performed the tests.
e. If the problem is not solved, the complaint is put forward to the service engineer depending upon the warranty/AMC and further plan of action is decided.
f. Average down time depends on the type of breakdown.
g. The details are updated in to the daily breakdown report and follow up is done.

3. Preventive Maintenance:

a. The Biomedical Engineer prepares and maintains a maintenance plan as per the list of available equipment.
b. The Preventive Maintenance of instrument having an AMC contract is done by communicating with Bio-Medical engineer and company engineer.
c. A schedule is prepared by the biomedical department for preventive maintenance as per the manufacturer recommendation.
d. All medical equipment undergoes preventive maintenance at prescheduled period.
e. The concerned department is informed about the schedule of the equipment for preventive maintenance well in advance, so that they can keep the equipment free for required time period.
f. The availability of necessary spares, consumables, tools and necessary materials are ensured through standardisation and/or advance planning, through Stores and guidance by Head of Bio Medical Department.
g. After completion of maintenance (whether preventive or breakdown) the OK report is taken from the user department and also an acknowledgment Is taken from user department.

CALIBRATION OF DEVICES:

1. A list of all instrument/equipment/devices' requiring calibration is prepared and maintained by BME.
2. The list identifies the measurement instruments by name, type, serial number, location, applicable calibration requirements, date of calibration done and calibration due date.
3. The calibration status is updated continuously.
4. Calibration certificate to be obtained from calibration agency with verification marked as O.K./ Not O.K.
5. The same is kept with the biomedical department and copy is provided to the user department. Sticker is displayed on the machine which shows the last calibration date and next due date.

POLICIES & PROCEDURES (SOP):

A. General Procedures:

1. Most of the medical equipment are with AMC to the respective authorized dealers & agencies.
2. The Hospital formulates a Purchase Committee for selection of equipment.
3. BME ensures about service back up, regularity issues and after AMC issues etc.
4. Purchase committee analyses the market value & collects the quotations from the Finance people and negotiates.

5. The Hospital equipment are periodically inspected, calibrated for their proper functioning through authorized service providers.
6. The Hospital deputes qualified & trained personnel for operation and maintenance of the equipment.
7. Preventive and breakdown maintenance of the hospital's equipment shall be done as per the documented procedure. The hospital is having a biomedical engineer to take care of such breakdowns.
8. Individuals who are qualified and available to do preventive maintenance must be identified. A list should be drawn up of personnel who are readily available. Once the personnel have been listed, specific responsibilities should be assigned, perhaps in the form of a work order, giving clear instructions for the task. Each person should have a clear knowledge of his or her responsibilities. Job assignments must correspond to the training, experience and aptitude of the individual.
9. The BME receives call memo from any department which is possessing biomedical equipment for its breakdown and maintenance.
10. Biomedical engineer visits and provides service there itself, if it is under AMC, BME coordinates with service engineer of respective company. If parts repairable or replaceable then he takes permission from Dy MS or MD and get it replaced.
11. In problem solving equipment manual shall be use as a referral tool.
12. If any component is damaged check for availability of the component in the store.
13. Depending upon the availability of the component rectification/information to the purchase department shall be done.
14. The date and time of complain solved shall be documented.
15. If correlated medical equipment problem arises inform to the related service centre and supervise the troubleshooting done by the service engineer.
16. Obtain the signature of the service provider and warrantee if any given to maintain the record.

B. Equipment Installation:

1. All new equipment purchased by the hospital are to be installed by eth supplier or manufacturer.
2. This department makes arrangements for installation and supervises the complete process.
3. It will initiate approval from regulatory authorities, if required.
4. After installation, when equipment is handed over to the hospital, BME takes first charge. He then enters the details in the Master Register.
5. Equipment manuals, accessories and other concerned documents shall be received by the BME, shall be documented and handed over to the departmental head.

C. Demonstration & Training:

1. BME shall arrange with suppliers for proper demonstration and training of installed equipment to existing users.
2. Such first-hand training sessions shall be documented by BME and records shall be maintained.

D. Coding of Equipment:

1. All medical equipment of the hospital shall be listed and coded for easy accessibility and identification.
2. A sticker bearing that code is pasted on the equipment.

3. Coding format is as below;

   Hospital Name in short/Equipment Location (department)/Equipment name in short/Serial number. Example: ABCH/ICU/Defib/001

   Here the hospital name is ABC Hospital.
4. All existing equipment and any new additions shall have these stickers.
5. When any equipment is temporarily shifted to another department, this sticker is not replaced. But if there is any permanent transfer, sticker should be suitably modified.
6. Register shall be maintained by BME documenting such transfers.

E. Preventive Maintenance:

It is a set of activities that are performed on plant equipment, machinery, and systems before the occurrence of a failure in order to protect them and to prevent or eliminate any degradation in their operating conditions.

The maintenance carried out at predetermined intervals or according to prescribed criteria and intended to reduce the probability of failure or the degradation of the functioning of an item.

1. There are two types of equipment in the hospital.
   a. New equipment under warranty/guarantee.
   b. Old equipment under AMC/CMC.
   c. Old equipment under hospital care. (Without any AMC)
2. Preventive Maintenance schedules are prepared by the BME based on manufacturer's recommendations.
3. All equipment under warranty, AMC or CMC are maintained by the concerned vendor. The BME shall contact the respective vendor few days prior to due date.
4. BME shall be responsible for making all arrangements for vendors to carry out necessary maintenance.
5. Departmental head shall be informed in advance and requested to release the equipment for that day. Expected duration of maintenance shall also be communicated to the head of the concerned department.
6. For non-AMC equipment, schedule for PPM is prepared based on manufacturer's recommendations.
7. BME shall ensure availability of necessary spares, consumables and tools.
8. Few days before the scheduled maintenance, departmental head shall be informed and requested to release the equipment. PPM shall be carried out as per convenience of the department.
9. After maintenance whether done in-house or by the vendor, an OK report shall be taken from user department.
10. If required, recalibration has to be carried out.

F. Breakdown Maintenance:

1. In case of breakdown of any equipment, information is given by the user department to BME and the hospital administration.
2. The BME documents the details in the Log card/Breakdown register so that response time and downtime could be monitored.
3. It is verified that whether the equipment is under any warranty or AMC.
4. If it is under maintenance contract by virtue of warranty or AMC, the concerned vendor is contacted and the process is similar to that of a preventive maintenance.

5. If the equipment is not under AMC, then BMC himself carries out the necessary repair, if possible.
6. If the equipment is portable, it is transported to the workshop; otherwise, repair is done at site.
7. If the equipment cannot be repaired by BME in-house, then an authorised service centre is contacted after obtaining permission from the hospital administration.
8. Service engineers of the vendor assess the equipment and submit a financial proposal. The proposal is passed by hospital authorities and then BME gets the job done.
9. Once the repair cannot be carried out or it is uneconomical to rectify the problem, the hospital administration decides about further course of action.
10. Documentation of all process must be done in concerned registers/log cards for analysing indicators.
11. All maintenance activities shall ensure equipment fitness and accuracy.

G. Condemnation Procedure:

Following criteria shall be considered for condemnation of equipment.

- Not reparable
- Not serviceable
- Cost of maintenance is more than the new purchase cost

H. Equipment Log Card:

Log Cards are maintained for every equipment which are costing more than Rs. 10,000/=

I. Calibration of Equipment:

1. Prepare list of equipment needing calibration. Calibration is done for the instruments which require any measuring parameter.
2. Calibration agency has to be finalised. It is either from manufacturer/supplier or a third party.
3. Frequency of calibration is to be documented in individual Log Card.
4. Once calibration is done, certificates are maintained by this department.
5. Calibration sticker shall be pasted on each such equipment.

J. Safety Policies:

1. The In-charge is responsible to observe and making sure that all safety rules are observed in the hospital.
2. All employees will notify any safety hazard which comes in their notice, immediately to Maintenance Department.
3. All concerned staff will ensure that any defective equipment, unsafe working conditions are reported.
4. Ensure that all electrical cables/cords are not lying in passageway.
5. Discourage use of extension cords and multi-plugs.
6. Do not put heavy items on upper shelves.
7. Sharp instruments/items must be stored properly.
8. All electrical equipment should be switched OFF when not in use.
9. SMOKING IS STRICTLY PROHIBITED IN THIS HOSPITAL.
10. Do not store waste items (inflammable or otherwise) in staircases. Discarded cartoons should be stored at specified place to be disposed later on.
11. Exit routes should be clear of all hurdles always.

12. Warning signs should be displayed at all required locations.
13. Working areas should be properly illuminated.
14. Ensure usage of protective garments in specified area and during specified work.
15. All tools should be cleaned and stored at proper place.
16. Take care of earthing in using electrical appliances.
17. Defective or broken tools (ladders etc) should not be used.
18. Metal ladders should not be used while working with electricity.
19. Always wear safety shoes and safety goggles especially while working with Welding machines or while grinding and chipping.
20. Use tag system while repairing a machine.
21. Never overload an electrical circuit.
22. Always use fuse of prescribed specifications.
23. Always qualified staff (depending upon nature of job) will be deployed to carry out the job.
24. The department will respond quickly to any call to repair unsafe conditions.
25. Always keep workshop floor clean and free from objects which can catch fire or are slippery.
26. All electrical appliances must be properly and effectively grounded.

K. Monitoring of Adverse Events Related to Medical Devices and Compliance Hazard Notices on Recalls.

Procedure:

1. The Hospital keeps a record of all recalls initiated by the manufacturer/vendor.
2. If there is any adverse event related to functioning of the equipment, the BME immediately informs hospital administration and contacts the vendor/manufacturer.
3. Further course of action depends on company's engineers' inspection and observation.
4. If the equipment is made ready to use by manufacturer's engineers, a service report is must from the agency.
5. They may also advice for 'Not to use' the equipment till further clarification from the company.

Definitions & Process of Recall:

1. **Correction** means repair, modification, adjustment, relabelling, destruction, or inspection (including patient monitoring) of a product without its physical removal to some other location.
2. **Market withdrawal** means a firm's removal or correction of a distributed product which involves a minor violation that would not be subject to legal action by the FDA or which involves no violation, e.g., normal stock rotation practices, routine equipment adjustments and repairs, etc.
3. Recall means a firm's removal or correction of a marketed product that the FDA considers to be in violation of the laws it administers and against which the agency would initiate legal action, e.g., seizure. Recall does not include a market withdrawal or a stock recovery.
4. Recall strategy means a planned course of action to be taken in conducting a specific recall, which addresses the depth of recall, need for public warnings, and extent of effectiveness checks for the recall.
5. Recalling firm means the firm that initiates a recall or, in the case of a Food and Drug Administration-requested recall, the firm that has primary responsibility for the manufacture and marketing of the product to be recalled.

6. Removal means the physical removal of a device from its point of use to some other location for repair, modification, adjustment, relabelling, destruction, or inspection.
7. **Risk to health** means (1) A reasonable probability that use of, or exposure to, the product will cause serious adverse health consequences or death; or (2) That use of, or exposure to, the product may cause temporary or medically reversible adverse health consequences, or an outcome where the probability of serious adverse health consequences is remote.
8. **Routine servicing** means any regularly scheduled maintenance of a device, including the replacement of parts at the end of their normal life expectancy, e.g., calibration, replacement of batteries, and responses to normal wear and tear. Repairs of an unexpected nature, replacement of parts earlier than their normal life expectancy, or identical repairs or replacements of multiple units of a device are not routine servicing.
9. **Stock recovery** means the correction or removal of a device that has not been marketed or that has not left the direct control of the manufacturer, i.e., the device is located on the premises owned, or under the control of, the manufacturer, and no portion of the lot, model, code, or other relevant unit involved in the corrective or removal action has been released for sale or use.

WORK FLOW:

Work Flow – Complaint Management:

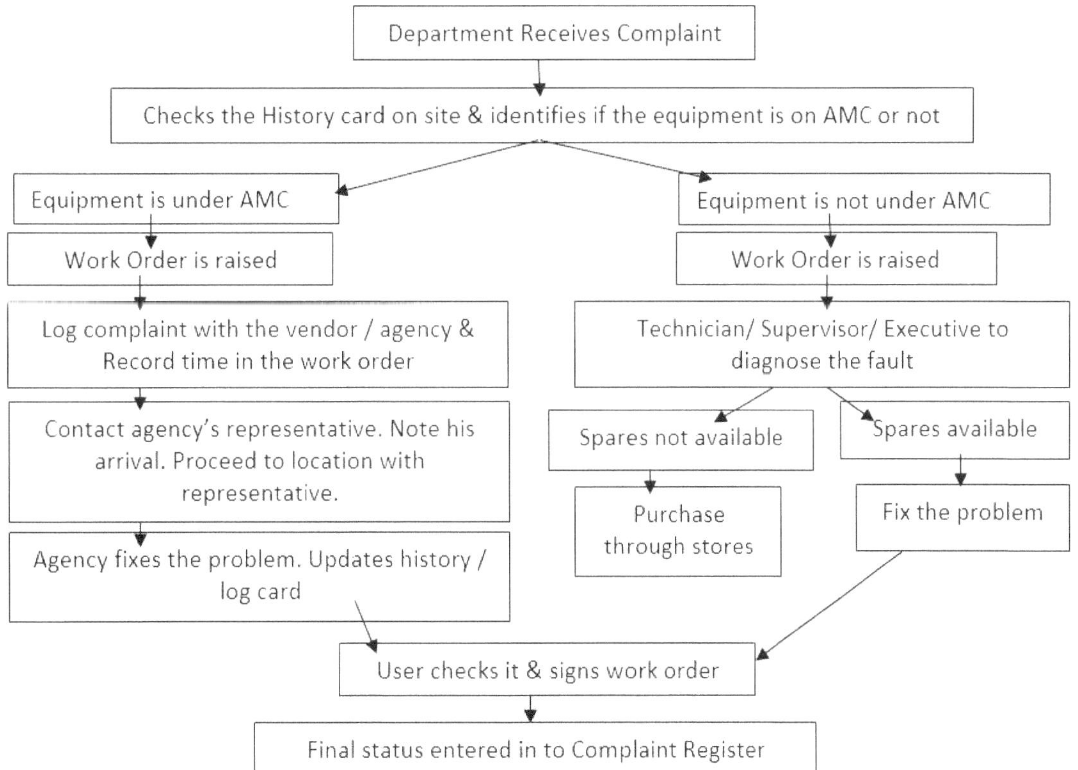

Work Flow – Preventive Maintenance:

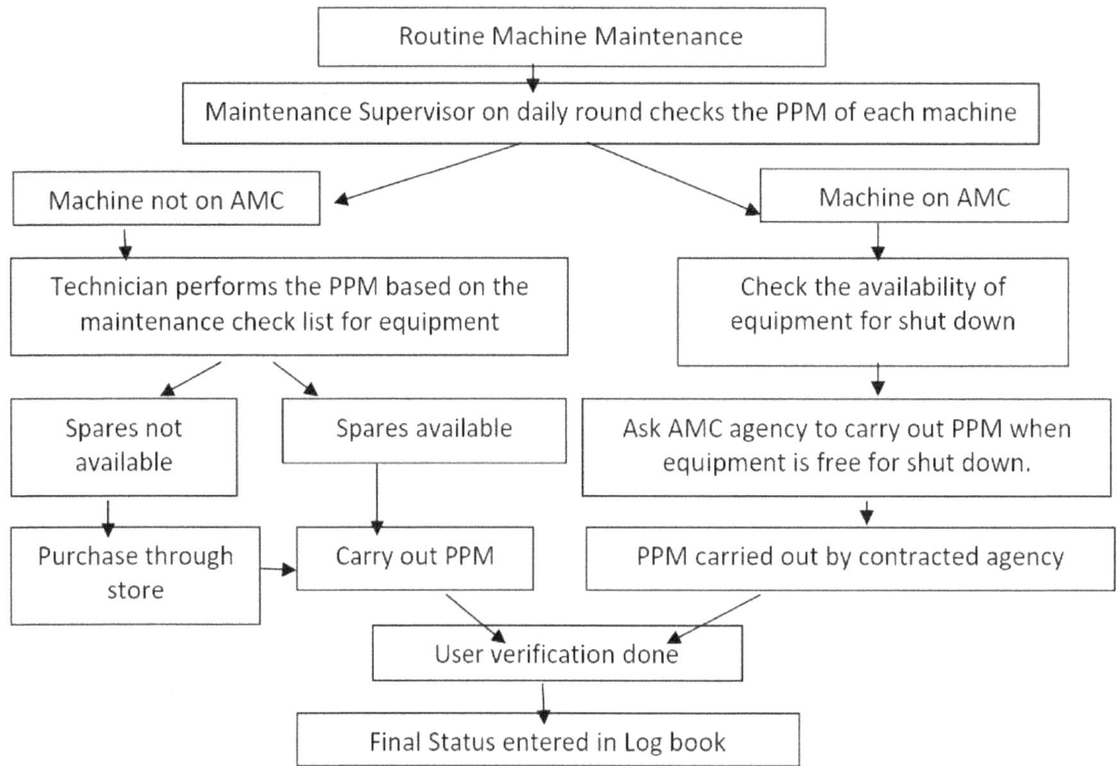

QUALITY INDICATORS:

1. Breakdown Time/Up-time of the Equipment (Down Time Register)
2. Utilisation Rate of Equipment
3. Complaint resolved within 24 hours

   Formula:

   Total number of complaints resolved divided by total number of complaints multiplied by 100 (one hundred)
4. Complaint resolved within 48 hours
5. Complaint resolved beyond 1 week

CHECKLISTS:

A. BME Checklist:

BME CHECKLIST

Date: ....

S.N.	Parameters	Remarks
1	Equipment status in ICU (working/Not working if any)	
2	Equipment status in ECHO room/TMT/EEG (working/Not working if any)	
3	Equipment status in Labour Room (working/Not working if any)	
4	Equipment status in NICU (working/Not working if any)	

S.N.	Parameters	Remarks
5	Equipment status in Second Floor (working/Not working if any)	
6	Equipment status in Dialysis (working/Not working if any)	
7	Equipment status in Emergency (working/Not working if any)	
8	Equipment status in CT & X-Ray (working/Not working if any)	
9	Equipment status in USG (working/Not working if any)	
10	Equipment status in Physiotherapy (working/Not working if any)	
11	Equipment status in Laboratory (working/Not working if any)	
12	Equipment status in the OT (working/Not working if any)	
13	In house PMS Done or Pending (if any)	
14	Any Breakdown/Down time?	
15	Complaint process in case of breakdown	
16	If any Downtime average time for closure of complaint	
17	Percentage of equipment in house Calibration as per schedule	
18	Any machine under repair/insured or not	
19	Any machine sent outside for repair	
20	Names the machine not working, insured/not,	
21	Remarks	

Note: Write details of Equipment not working:

B. Checklist Equipment Management:

SN	Check	Yes	No
1	Do you have a database of all existing medical equipment in your computer or in a register?		
2	Have you classified equipment as (1) Life Support and (2) Routine medical equipment?		
3	Have you made it compulsory in procurement for the vendor to train the hospital employees?		
4	Have you put installation clause in your Purchase Order?		
5	Are you maintaining 'log card' for all costly equipment from the day one?		
6	Are you carrying out preventive maintenance for all medical equipment?		
7	Are you keeping record of all accidents attributed to functioning or malfunctioning of medical equipment?		
8	The hospital has SOP available for action to be taken when medical equipment fails.		
9	Are you still working with obsolete equipment?		

C. Checklist Breakdown Maintenance:

1. Information about a breakdown given to in-charge biomedical engineering department (the Head) by the user department in writing.
2. Complaint details entered in maintenance record register kept with the biomedical department.

3. Find out whether the said equipment is under Guarantee or under AMC/CMC with the supplier.
4. If so, inform the contractor/vendor about the problem, who in turn sends his engineer to repair the equipment.
5. Equipment log card/log sheet is filled at every movement. (The equipment log card is updated). Total interval from the time complaint is made to the time equipment is rectified is recorded.
6. If the equipment is not under service contract, 'the head' looks at the fault. If the engineers can rectify the fault on site, it is done. Records (log card) are maintained.
7. If the equipment is to be shifted to the biomedical department for repair, permission is taken from the hospital superintendent in consultation with user department.
8. Equipment is shifted to the department and repaired. Sent back to user department after repair. All activities are documented.
9. If the equipment is required to be sent outside hospital for repair, written request is made and permission taken from hospital superintendent. Permission letter is kept in records.
10. The item is sent to the workshop on a "Returnable Gate Pass".
11. The head does the follow-up to get it repaired as soon as possible. Once the equipment is received back, it is tested by the biomedical department and then installed in the user department.
12. All activities are recorded in maintenance register and the equipment's log card.

AUDIT:

AUDIT REPORT OF ENGINEERING/MAINTENANCE

AS PER ISO 9001:2008, ISO 14001:2004 & OHSAS 18001

Date of Audit: ....

Auditors: a) ....

b) ....

Auditees: a) ....

Details of Non-Compliances: (No major NCs in the department)

RECORDS MAINTAINED:

1. A Master List of bio-medical equipment.
2. Individual History Card (Log Card/Log Register) of all bio-medical equipment present in the hospital.
3. Calibration Certificate of bio-medical equipment.
4. Calibration Schedule of bio-medical equipment. (Calibration Register).
5. Planned Preventive Maintenance and Annual Maintenance Schedule of the equipment.
6. Maintenance Register (Preventive & Breakdown details).
7. AMC/CMC Register.
8. Training record of all employees.
9. Complaint Register.
10. Breakdown Slips.

STATIONARY FORMATS:

1. Register of Calibration Schedule for Medical Equipment:

Register for Calibration Schedule for Medical Equipment

Equipment	Monitors			Ventilator			X _ Ray Machine			Etc
Month	Schedule	Actual	Sign	Schedule	Actual	Sign	Schedule	Actual	Sign	
January										
February										
March										
April										
May										
June										
July										
August										
September										
October										
November										
December										

2. Complaint Register & Log Book:

Complaint Register & Log Book (Register)

Medical Equipment:

For Bio Medical Engineer:

Equipment Name	Department	Model Sr. No.	Company Name	Nature Of Complaint	Complaint Date	Complaint Time	Response Date	Response Time	Completion Date	Completion Time	Expenses	Engineer Name	Signature BME
Note: It is in Landscape Format													

3. Equipment Gate Pass:

Equipment Gate Pass (Returnable)

Date: ....

OUT GOING SLIP/GATE PASS

Please allow (Name of the equipment :)...

To be taken by Mr.: ....

To (place): ....

For (reason): ....

Time out: ....

HOD/In-charge: .... Authorised signatory: ....

Details at the time of in:

(To be entered at security gate)

Date In: ....

Time in: ....

4. Equipment Log Card/Register: (Format-1)

Log Card

Page-1 (Front side of the card)

EQUIPMENT LOG BOOK/CARD	
Name of the Hospital	
Description of the Machine	
Located at (place)	
Model No.	
Installed on (date)	
Warranty Starts on (date)	
Summarise the main specifications	
Accessories Supplied along with the Machine	
Anything Pending	
Manufacturer's Address & Telephone Numbers (contact details)	
Indian Supplier's Address & Telephone Numbers (contact details)	
Contact Details of Vendor who supplied	
Service Engineer, Name & Cell Nos	
Preventive Maintenance Schedule	
AMC/CMC details	

Page-2 (or back side of the card)

Name of the Equipment – Location

SN	Date	Complaint	Informed to ?	Action taken (Date)	Details of repair	Cost of repair	Sign

5. Log Card/History Card: (Format-2):

Name of the Equipment:					
Location:					
Make & Model:					
Serial Number:					
Purchase Date:					
Installation Date:					
Assets Code:					
Manufacturer/Dealer Address & Contact Numbers:					
SN	**Preventive Maintenance Details**		**Company Engineer Sig.**	**B.M.E. Sig.**	**Breakdown Details with Date, Time & Expenses**
	Done Date	**Due Date**			

6. Training Record (Training by BME to User Staff):

Hospital Name & Address

TRAINING RECORD

Equipment Details: ....

Name: .... Model: ....

Make: .... Sr. No.: ....

Date & Time of training: ....

Department & Floor: ....

Name of the trainer: ....

SN	Staff/Technician Name	Department/Floor	Signature

(Signature of the Bio-Medical Engineer) (Signature of the Trainer)

7. Calibration Stickers:

Calibration Record/Status	
Name of the Equipment	
Model No./Serial No.	
Date of Calibration Done	
Date of Calibration Due	
Name & Contact no. of the Service Engineer	
Signature of BME	

8. Format for Collecting Data for KPI:

Equipment Downtime Record Register

Equipment Down Time										
Sr. No.	Name of Equipment	Name of department	Date when the Equipment was down	Time when the Equipment was down (T1)	Date when the Equipment becomes functional	Time when the equipment becomes functional (T2)	total number of hours when equipment is non functional (T1-T2)	Reason for non-functioning of equipment	Signature
Note: The register is in a Landscape Format									

9. Master Register of Medical Equipment:

SN	Equipment Name	Model	Serial No.	Accessories included	Supplier's Name, Address & Contact No.	Location	Hospital ID Code	Remarks
Note: It is in Landscape format or both pages of the register are used.								

BIBLIOGRAPHY, REFERENCES & ACKNOWLEDGMENTS:

1. Indian Public Health Standards (IPHS)
   Guidelines for District Hospitals (101 to 500 Bedded) Revised 2012 Directorate General of Health Services Ministry of Health & Family Welfare, Government of India
2. "Standard Operating Procedures SOP For Hospitals 2nd Edition" by Dr. Arun K. Agarwal
3. "Duties & Responsibilities of Hospital Staff" by Dr. Arun Kumar
4. "Checklists for Hospitals" by Dr. Arun K. Agarwal
5. Stationary Formats. By Dr. Arun K. Agarwal
6. Hospital Manual. DGHS, Ministry of Health & Family Welfare, GOI

Chapter – 5

DEPARTMENT OF CARDIOLOGY

INDEX

   d. Cardio Vascular Technician
   e. ECG/ECHO Technician
   f. Perfusionist/Cardiac Pump Technician
21. Daily Audit
22. Various Checklists of Cardiology Services
   a. Checklist for OPD Consultation.
23. Stationary Formats Used in This Department
   a. Consent Form for ECHO/(TOE)
   b. Consent Form for T.M.T.
   c. U.S/ECG/ECHO/TMT/PFT Record Register
   d. TMT Consent & Report Format
   e. Cardiac Clinic Record
   f. Consent for Stress ECHO/TEE
   g. Consent for TMT:
   h. Informed Consent Angioplasty/Angiography/Balloon Valvotomy:
   i. ECHO Reporting Format:-1
   j. ECHO Reporting Format:-2
   k. Foetal ECHO Report Format
24. Drugs For Cardiology Department
25. Records/Documents in Cath Lab
26. Bibliography, References & Acknowledgments:

INTRODUCTION:

The Cardiology Department provides complete cardiac care under its roof. It includes both elective and emergency services. The services are backed by state of art equipment.

This department is dedicated to providing a holistic approach to treat the cardiac ailments utilizing the expertise of best doctors at an affordable price and meant to give the best possible service to the people of this region.

The hospital provides highest standards in heart care services. The services are backed by latest equipment and well qualified, trained, experienced faculty. The hospital caters to a wide spectrum of society. Nursing in the CCU is on 1:1 basis.

Health checks up schemes are offered to general public. The purpose of these tests is to examine the apparently normal people so as to pick up any abnormality at its incubation stage and thus take remedial measures.

Emergency services are provided round the clock including transport facility.

All range of complex coronary interventions is managed such as Left main coronary artery interventions, Post CABG graft interventions etc.

The hospital provided outpatient as well as inpatient services.

OUTREACH PROGRAMS:

The hospital regularly carries out free heart check-up camps in nearby areas and also in distant locations. In these camps a cardiologist examines all cases and some tests such as ECG, Blood test, are done free of cost.

AIM, VISION & MISSION:

1. To provide professional ethical patient care.
2. To provide all types cardiology services, under one roof.
3. To organize CME programs and conferences.
4. To achieve excellence in patient care, teaching and research.
5. To promote quality clinical research.

AIM:

1. To provide most modern services in various fields of cardiology to patients at affordable cost.
2. To provide all types of services in cardiology under one roof.

VISION:

1. To provide world-class services to every citizen of India.
2. To continue delivering quality cardiac care through our professional staff, scientific approach to the diverse communities we serve.

OBJECTIVES:

- The Department of Cardiology strives to provide quality cardiac care to all patients irrespective of their economic class.

HIGHLIGHTS OF THE DEPARTMENT

1. Round the clock availability of a Cardiologist.
2. Comprehensive Cardiac Rehabilitation Program.

INFRASTRUCTURE:

A. **OPD:**

It is located on ground floor in the main OPD complex.

B. **Cardiac Lab:**

It is located on First Floor of the hospital.

It has following facilities;

Echo, TMT, Holter, etc

C. **IPD:**

ICCU:

The Intensive Cardiac Care Unit (ICCU) has 6 beds with the cardiologists available round the clock and nurses in one-to-one ratio.

CTVS ICU:

The Cardio Thoracic & Vascular Surgery Intensive Care Unit (CTVS ICU) has 6 beds with cardiologist available round the clock and nurses in two-to-one ratio.

Step Down Ward:

The Step Down ICCU has 12 beds and the settled patients will be taken from CTVS ICU, ICCU and Cath Lab.

PLANNING POINTS:

Non-Invasive Cardiology Diagnostics:

a. The size of the TMT room should be about 280 sq. ft.
b. Change room provision near ECHO.

FACILITIES:

1. Daily OPD
2. ICCU & HDU
3. Fully Equipped Cardiac Ambulances with Doctor (Round the clock)
4. Blood Banks (Round the clock)
5. Pharmacy (Round the clock)
6. Cardiac Rehabilitation centre
7. Department of Radiology
8. Fully equipped Pathology Laboratory

DIAGNOSTIC FACILITIES

1. ECG
2. Coronary Angiography
3. Digital Subtraction Angiography (DSA)
4. Cerebral & Peripheral Angiography
5. Electrophysiological Studies
6. Electrolyte Machines
7. Blood Gas Measurement
8. Echocardiography & Stress ECHO
9. Treadmill Test (TMT) & Holter
10. Muga Test

THERAPEUTIC FACILITIES

1. Neonatal Cardiac Surgery
2. Coronary Artery Bypass Surgery
3. Valvular Surgery
4. Valve Repair & Replacement
5. Vascular Reconstruction
6. Aneurysm Repair
7. Carotid Artery Surgery
8. Coronary Angioplasty/Stenting
9. Radio Frequency Ablation

10. Peripheral Angioplasty/Stenting
11. PTMR
12. Valvuloplasty & ASD Closure
13. Pericardiocentesis
14. Pacemaker Insertion

SPECIALITY CLINICS:

a. Congenital Heart Disease Clinic
b. Preventive Cardiology & Lifestyle Clinic
c. Valvular Disease Clinic
d. Arrhythmia Clinic

AILMENTS TREATED:

1. Ischemic Heart Disease (IHD)
2. Heart Failures
3. Valvular Heart Diseases
4. Hypertension
5. Cardiac Rhythm Abnormalities.
6. Congenital heart problems
7. Vascular problems

COMMON CARDIAC PROBLEMS:

1. Acute chest pain (ischemic heart disease/Acute cardiac syndrome)
2. Acute and chronic hypertension (Giddiness)
3. Acute pulmonary oedema
4. Congestive cardiac failure
5. Acute arrhythmias/Cardiac arrest
6. Brady arrhythmias

CARDIOLOGY PROCEDURES AND DIAGNOSTIC TESTS

1. ECG
2. Echocardiography (Including TEE)
3. Tread Mill Test (TMT)
4. Holter (Ambulatory ECG Monitoring)
5. Ambulatory B.P. Monitoring
6. Angiography
7. Angioplasty
8. Thrombolytic Therapy
9. Temporary Pacemaker (T.P.I.)
10. Blood Tests (Cholesterol, Triglycerides, Urea, Electrolytes, etc)
11. Nuclear Cardiology - Thallium Scanning (Myocardial Perfusion Scintigraphy)

12. Cardiac CT (CT Angiography)
13. MRI Angiography
14. Troponin Blood Tests
15. Chest X-Ray
16. Tilt Test

LIST OF SOME EQUIPMENT:

1. ECG machine computerized
2. TMT Machine
3. Echocardiography Machine
4. Cardiac Monitor
5. Ventilators (Adult & Paediatric)
6. Pulse Oximeter
7. Cath Lab
8. IABP (Intra-Aortic Balloon Pump)
9. Tilt Table
10. ABG Machine
11. Defibrillators
12. Infusion Pump/Syringe Pump
13. Nebuliser
14. Peak Expiratory Flow Rate (PEFR) Meter

SERVICES PROVIDED:

1. Angiography
2. Angioplasty
3. PMI- Pacemaker Implantation
4. ICD- Intracardiac Defibrillators
5. CRT- Cardiac Resynchronize Therapy
6. BMV- Balloon Mitral Valvuloplasty
7. BPV- Balloon pulmonary valvuloplasty
8. ASD- Device closer
9. VSD- Device closer
10. PDA- Device closer
11. Peripheral Angioplasty (Renal, Carotid, Iliac)
12. IVC fitter
13. Cardiac Rehabilitation
14. Preventive Cardiology
15. Follow up care

PAEDIATRIC CARDIOLOGY:

Paediatric cardiologists broadly treat congenital heart disease (present at birth), arrhythmias (variations in heartbeat rhythm) and disturbances of circulatory function.

The initial assessment performed by the paediatric cardiologist might start with a physical examination using a stethoscope, after which more detailed investigations may be suggested.

Patients often present with complex diagnostic and medical problems and after the initial assessment, the paediatric cardiologist then chooses an optimal management plan. They work closely with a wide range of specialists as part of a multidisciplinary team to assess and treat patients.

Paediatric cardiologists play a vital role in the teaching of medical students, doctors, GPs, nurses and paramedical staff. Most are also involved in research.

Role of a Paediatric Cardiologist:

To provide the highest quality cardiology care for the children.

To provide expertise in all areas of paediatric cardiology services available to all ages – from the unborn to the adult with congenital heart disease.

To value compassionate care and service.

Paediatric cardiology includes:

1. Cardiac Catheterisation and Catheter Intervention
2. Cardiac Pacing, Electrophysiology and Ablation
3. Foetal Cardiology
4. Adolescent and Adult Congenital Heart Disease
5. Advanced Echocardiography
6. Transplantation Cardiology
7. Pulmonary Hypertension
8. Advanced Imaging (MRI and CT)

CARDIAC REHABILITATION:

The cardiac rehabilitation is much more than just controlled exercises. It is advice on lifestyle changes and continued medication after discharge.

Regular exercise, particularly those forms of endurance exercise which enhance cardiovascular fitness, may have a role to play in the prevention of **atherosclerotic disease**. It is important to emphasize, however, that exercise is not free from danger both to the musculoskeletal and the cardiovascular system. This is particularly true for middle aged individuals – especially, coronary prone persons – who suddenly take up vigorous exercise after years of minimal physical activity. Physicians and other professionals need aid in guiding a concerned public to avoid these problems

It is insured that each patient with ACD (Acute Coronary Syndrome) attends rehabilitation program being run by the hospital. The program includes exercises and advice on lifestyle changes.

It is advised that one near relative should also attend the program along with the patient. The program helps in reducing recurrence and prevention of disease in other family members.

The program includes;

1. Advise on diet
2. Role of exercise
3. Methods of stopping tobacco and alcohol use
4. Yoga & Meditation

CARDIAC REHABILITATION PROGRAM at Mahatma Gandhi Medical College And Hospital, Sitapur, Jaipur)

https://www.mgmch.org/departments/cardiac-care

Most people who have undergone bypass surgery benefit from participating in a structured, comprehensive cardiac rehabilitation program. People who participate in cardiac rehabilitation usually have appointments several times per week in a hospital or clinic, allowing the person to live and sleep at home. The potential benefits of rehabilitation include an improvement in heart function, a lowering of the heart rate at rest and during exercise, and a reduced risk of dying or developing complications from heart disease.

There are several components to cardiac rehabilitation, including exercise, reducing risk factors, and dealing with stress, anxiety, and depression. The benefits of cardiac rehabilitation are seen only when this multifactorial approach is used. In other words, one component alone is not enough.

Exercise — Exercise has consistently been shown to improve cardiovascular health. Importantly, the first step in starting to exercise is to determine the potential risk of heart and/or blood vessel complications from exercise. This is usually done by undergoing a monitored exercise test on a treadmill. Although nearly everyone can exercise safely after discharge, the intensity and duration of exercise should be adjusted according to the severity of a person's heart disease.

Risk categories for exercise — Risk categories are a way of describing a person's risk of cardiovascular (heart-related) complications related to activity. Each category has a unique requirement for supervision and exercise restrictions. People in risk category A are generally healthy, do not require medical supervision during exercise, and have no limitations on the duration or intensity of exercise. Conversely, people in exercise category 'D' have strict limits on activity and should not exercise, even with close medical supervision. Most people who have had bypass surgery are in category B or C.

- Class A – Individuals who are apparently healthy and in whom there is no evidence of increased heart-related risk with exercise.
- Class B – Individuals with established coronary heart disease that is stable. These individuals are at low risk of heart-related complications with vigorous exercise.
- Class C – Individuals who are at moderate or high risk of heart-related complications during exercise. Examples of people who would be in this category are those who have had several heart attacks and those who have chest pain at a relatively low level of exercise. Patients with certain positive findings on an exercise test may also be in this group.
- Class D – Individuals with unstable disease should not participate in an exercise program.

Exercise - During cardiac rehabilitation, a trained clinician will work with the patient and the patient's main healthcare provider to develop an exercise program that is safe and beneficial. The program will consider the patient's fitness level, heart health, any physical limitations, the amount, intensity and duration of exercise needed to improve heart health, and the need for supervision.

- Type of exercise – The exercise should use large muscle groups and include aerobic exercise. Walking, jogging, cycling, rowing, and stair climbing are some examples.
- Frequency – The recommended frequency of exercise is three to five times a week.
- Content and duration – It is important that each session consist of a 5- to 10-minute warm-up phase, a conditioning phase of at least 20 minutes, and a 5- to 10-minute cool-down phase. Eliminating the cool-down phase can increase the risk of heart-related complications.
- Intensity – One of the most important components of the exercise prescription is the intensity of exercise. This is based upon the patient's heart rate or the level of exertion. A number of formulas exist to calculate the appropriate maximum heart rate for each patient.

- The patient gauges the level of exertion during an activity by rating it on a standardized scale called the rating of perceived exertion (RPE). Moderate-intensity exercise (an RPE of 12 to 13) is needed to achieve cardiovascular health benefits. The benefits of very high intensity exercise are small; intense exercise is not recommended because it leads to muscle fatigue and increases the risk of physical injury and cardiovascular complications.
- Exercise progression – Over time, most people can gradually increase the level of exercise in the workout. Beneficial exercise can also be built in to the daily routine by taking a brisk walk or enjoying active play with children or grandchildren.

Supervision –

- Patients who are in Class C should be in a medically supervised program where the electrocardiogram (ECG) is monitored during exercise. Advanced life support equipment (e.g., a defibrillator, medications, personnel trained to use this equipment) should be on hand. This level of supervision should continue for at least 8 to 12 weeks.
- Lower-risk patients (Class B) benefit from a medically supervised, ECG-monitored program for the first 6 to 12 sessions. Following this, a home-based exercise program is safe and effective.

REDUCE CARDIAC RISK FACTORS

- A number of factors increase the risk of developing or speeding the progression of heart disease. Reducing or eliminating these risk factors can be helpful, even if a person already has heart disease or has had a heart attack. Strategies to reduce risks are discussed below.
- Follow a heart healthy diet — Diet counselling is helpful for people who need to lose weight or reduce cholesterol levels. A registered dietician is the best person to consult about foods that are helpful and harmful, appropriate portion sizes, total calorie recommendations, and realistic ways to change bad eating habits.
- Most cardiac rehabilitation programs have a dietician who is knowledgeable and experienced in advising people who are recovering from a heart attack.
- Stop smoking — Cigarette smoking significantly increases the risk of coronary heart disease and heart attack, and stopping smoking can rapidly reduce these risks. One year after stopping smoking, the risk of dying from coronary heart disease is reduced by about one-half and the risk continues to decline with time. In some studies, the risk of heart attack was reduced to the rate of non-smokers within two years of quitting smoking.
- Cardiac rehabilitation programs can recommend a treatment to help stop smoking, such as group programs; nicotine patches, gum, or nasal spray; or a prescription medication.

(Courtesy: Mahatma Gandhi Medical College and Hospital, Sitapur, Jaipur)

STANDARD OPERATING PROCEDURES (SOP):

A. Patient with Chest Pain of less than 12 hours:

1. The patient presents within 12 hours of onset of pain?
2. History is suggestive of Ischemia?
3. In ECG "ST" is elevated?
4. Get the Cath lab ready.
5. The patient is willing for Angiography/Angioplasty?
    - Explain risks and benefits of the intervention.
    - Take consent.
    - A quick ECHO may be done, if time permits.

- Carry out part preparation.
- Shift the patient to the Cath lab with all papers (Case sheet and investigations).
- Perform the procedure.
- Shift the patient to CCU
- Medication as per cardiologist advice.
- Discharge when stable – as per doctor advice

6. The patient is unwilling for an intervention?
   - Thrombolyse after taking consent.
   - Start treatment as advised.
   - Check: BP (if less than 100 mm of Hg), Heart rate (more than 100/minute), patient is unable to lie flat, pericardial effusion seen on ECHO.
   - Again, counsel the patient for interventional procedure.
   - But stabilise the patient before taking any intervention.

B. Patient with Chest Pain but without ECG Changes:

1. Carry out laboratory test.
2. Tropin T is negative?
3. Keep under observation
4. Repeat ECG and Trop T test every 6 hours.
5. If ECG shows changes or Trop T becomes positive?
6. Advice for angiography/angioplasty.

C. SOP for Conducting ECG

Purpose:

To conduct ECG to rule out any cardiac abnormalities

Scope:

Patients prescribed for ECG

Responsibility:

Cardiologist

Procedure:

1. Patient walks in with invoice/Dr. Prescription & Record details of patient: name, age, sex, registration no in ECG register
2. Explain the procedure to the patient about the test and prepare the patient for the test
3. Apply ECG jelly at the defined locations and attach limb leads
4. Connect four limb leads to right foot, left foot, right hand and left hand namely and six chest-leads to specific location on chest namely V1, V2, V3, V4, V5, V6
5. Record patient details in ECG machine-name, age, sex registration number
6. Record ECG graph
7. Handover the report to the patient and record in the ECG register
8. In case of breakdown of the machine, log command to equipment breakdown call register with details of breakdown and inform

Routine ECG: The Placement of the Precordial Electrodes:

LEAD V1	Placed over the fourth intercostal space immediately to the right of the sternum.
LEAD V2	Placed over the fourth intercostal space immediately to the left of the sternum.
LEAD V3	Placed on the chest exactly midway between the lead V2 & lead V4 electrode position.
LEAD V4	Placed over the fifth intercostal space in the midclavicular line.
LEAD V5	Placed at the same horizontal level as lead V4 but on the anterior axillary line.
LEAD V6	Placed at the same horizontal level as lead V4 & V5 but on the mid axillary line.
LEAD RA	Placed at the wrist of the right arm.
LEAD LA	Placed at the wrist of the left arm.
LEAD RL	Placed at the right foot.
LEAD LL	Placed at the left foot.

Notes:

1. ECG with right sided chest leads done for dextrocardia & suspected right ventricular infarction.
2. The lead placement for chest leads V1 to V6 is done in same location on the opposite side of the chest.

D. SOP for Conducting HOLTER Test

Purpose:

To conduct Holter test for ruling out cardiac abnormality

Scope:

Patient prescribed Holter

Responsibility:

Cardiologist

Procedure:

1. Patient walk in with invoice, prescription & Record details of patient name, age, sex, Registration no, address in HOLTER register
2. Give instructions and explain the procedure to the patient about the test and prepare the patient for the test
3. Paste ECG electrode on specific location on chest and connect chest leads on it.
4. Tie up the HOLTER recorder belt around the patient's waist
5. Patient change the dress and leaves with connected HOLTER recorder for 24 hrs. & do ECG recording
6. Explain to the patient about event entries
7. Patient comes back the next day at the same time for HOLTER recorder removal
8. Disconnect HOLTER record & flash card and INSERT IN FLASH CARD READER
9. Review of report readings by cardiologist and sign off.
10. Hand over the report to patient & update in HOLTER register
11. In case of the breakdown of the machine, log complaint to equipment breakdown register with details of breakdown and inform BME

	AHA colour	Channel	Lead	Location
A	Red	CH1(+)	mv5(+)	Fifth intercostals. Space at the left axillary line.
B	White	CH1(-)	mv5(-)	Right clavicle, just lateral to the Sternum
C	Brown	CH2(+)	mv1(+)	Fourth intercostal space. At the right sternal edge
D	Black	CH2(-)	mv1(-)	Left clavicle, just lateral to the sternum
E	Orange	CH3(+)	mv3(+)	Equidistant between the normal locations for precordial leads V2 and V4.
F	Blue	CH3(-)	Mv3(-)	Mid-sternum at the level of clavicles
G	Green	Ground		Lower right chest wall

E. SOP for Conducting Exercise Stress ECHO:

Purpose:

To conduct Exercise Stress Echo to rule any cardiac abnormalities

Scope:

Patient prescribed for stress Echo

Responsibility:

Cardiologist

Procedure:

1. Patient walk & Record details of patient name, age, sex, and registration no, address in Echo register
2. Explain the procedure to the patient about the test and prepare the patient for the test
3. Take consent from the patient
4. Record Blood pressure. Stress Echo conducted only on normalized BP up to 150/90 of mm hg)
5. Record details of patient data in stress Echo machine/TMT monitor-name age, sex, registration number
6. Conduct test by applying jelly and probe on specific location
7. Save pre stress Echo images of patient
8. Make proper connection of ten leads (4 limb leads and 6 chest leads) on specific location
9. Record Supine ECG
10. Follow Bruce Protocol & Modified Bruce protocol (refer protocols and given) + Conduct test by applying jelly and probe on specific location
11. Save post exercise Echo images of the patient
12. Remove lead, wipe jelly, patient change the dress and leaves
13. Review Echo report with pre and post images by cardiologist and sign off
14. Hand over the report to patient & update in echo register
15. In case of breakdown of the machine, log complaint to equipment break-down and inform BME

Routine ECG: The Placement of the Precordial Electrodes:

LEAD V1	Placed over the fourth intercostal space immediately to the right of the sternum.
LEAD V2	Placed over the fourth intercostal space immediately to the left of the sternum.
LEAD V3	Placed on the chest exactly midway between the lead V2 & lead V4 electrode position.

LEAD V4	Placed over the fifth intercostal space in the midclavicular line.
LEAD V5	Placed at the same horizontal level as lead V4 but on the anterior axillary line.
LEAD V6	Placed at the same horizontal level as lead V4 & V5 but on the mid axillary line.
LEAD LA	Left shoulder
LEAD RA	Right shoulder
LEAD LL	Lower edger of the rib cage in the left side
LEAD RR	Lower edge of the rib cage in the right side

Notes:

1. ECG with right-sided chest leads done for dextrocardia. The lead placement for chest leads V1 to V6 is done in same location on the opposite side of the chest.
2. ECG Three limb leads: Lead LA- Left shoulder
   Lead RA- Right shoulder
   Lead LL- Lower edge of the rib cage in the left side

F. SOP for Conducting PFT (Pulmonary Function Test):

Purpose:

To conduct pulmonary function test (PFT) to rule any pulmonary dysfunctions

Scope:

Patients for prescribed for MT

Responsibility:

Pulmonologist

Procedure:

1. Patient walks in with invoice Dr Prescription & update details of patient: name, age, sex, registration no. in PFT register.
2. Explain the procedure to the patient about the test and prepare the patient for the test
3. Record height and weight of the patient
4. Record details of patient data in PFT machine, name, and Record details of patient data in stress Echo machine/TMT monitor-name age, sex, registration number
5. With the help of disposable mouthpiece, patient breaths deeply and blows forcefully during PFT test
6. Review PFT graph by pulmonologist and sign off with stamp & send back in cardiology department

G. SOP for Conducting Treadmill Test (TMT):

Purpose:

To conduct Treadmill test to rule any cardiac abnormalities

Scope:

Patients prescribed/Opted for TMT

Responsibility:

Cardiologist/Technician

Procedure:

Modified Bruce Protocol:

1. Patient has to walk on treadmill modified Bruce protocol. After every 3 minutes for 3 stages speed will be same 1.7 mile/hereafter 4th stage speed will be 2.5,3.4,4.2,5.0 mile/hr and grade (00, 5.0, 10, 12, 14, 16, 18%) increases in every stage along with B.P and ECG are continuously recorded
2. Terminate test after achieving end point of TMT. End point of TMT significant ECG changes
3. Stop the treadmill record the recovery till the ECG change converted to baseline ECG
4. Remove the leads, patient change the dress and leaves.
5. Review the TMT graph by cardiologist and sign off, handover the report to the patient and update in the TMT register

KEY PERFORMANCE INDICATORS (KPI):

Indicators may be developed for the hospital in consultation with the cardiologist and quality cell of the hospital.

Few Indicators are as follows;

1. **Percentage of mortality within 1 year following IHD:**

   Formula: Number of deaths in any setting that occurred within one year of hospital admission with a primary diagnosis of IHD divides by Number of individuals hospitalised with a primary diagnosis of IHD and then multiply by 100.
2. **Total Cardiovascular Mortality Rate:**
3. **Percentage of patients prescribed Aspirin on discharge after Ischemic Heart Disease (IHD)**

   Formula: Numbers of patients prescribed Aspirin divide by Number of total discharges of IHD patients multiply by 100
4. **Timing of thrombolytic procedure for patients with IHD:**

   Formula: Numbers of minutes from time of arrival at hospital to time of administration of the thrombolytic divide by Number of patients with confirmed IHD receiving thrombolytic later

   Note: Similarly, KPI can be developed for CABG or other cases.
5. Number of reporting errors/1000 investigations
6. Rate of re-dos.
7. Percentage of Reports co-relating with clinical diagnosis
8. Average waiting time for diagnostic services.
9. Percentage of patients whose waiting time is more than … minutes.
10. Rate of re-admission

STAFFING:

There must be at least one female staff in this department during working hours.

1. Cardiologist
2. Cardiac Technicians (ECG Tech, ECHO Tech, etc)
3. Cardiac Nurses
4. GDAs and Helpers

DUTIES & RESPONSIBILITIES:

A. Cardiologist Doctor:

Duties are similar in nature to that of any specialist consultant.

1. Cardiologists must assess their patients holistically that is going through their medical history, and physical examination and investigations to create a treatment plan.
2. To interact with the patient's family and respond to patient questions.
3. To order and carry out procedures related to his speciality such as cardiac catheterization, angiograms, or echocardiograms.
4. To treat cardiac disorders.
5. To guide patients and relatives about prevention measures.
6. To explain the risks of prohibited activities to patients
7. To carry out screening for early detection.
8. To maintain medical documents as per hospital policy.
9. To communicate effectively with patients, physicians, staff, and administration.

B. Cardiac Technical Supervisor:

Are following but not limited to;

1. Is responsible to the cardiologist or head of the Cardiology department.
2. To supervise work of all other technicians and to assign their duties.
3. To recruit, train and retain cardiac technicians in the department.
4. To periodically submit appraisal reports of junior staff.
5. To listen and resolve staff & patient related issues.
6. To ensure complete patient satisfaction.
7. To supervise working of various both invasive & non-invasive procedures like TMT, ECHO, ECG, Cath Lab & Holter etc.
8. To ensure proper maintenance of all equipment of this department.
9. To make necessary arrangements for repairing of faulty equipment.
10. To help in purchase of new cardiac equipment for this department.
11. To carry out all administrative work of the department.
12. To perform other duties as asked by seniors.

C. Cardiac Technician

1. To be punctual on duty in proper uniform.
2. They work under direct supervision of a cardiologist.
3. They may be put on rotational duties. They will be "on call" also.
4. To ensure and organise patients' related appointments.
5. Will be responsible to schedule the tests so as to reduce the waiting time of OPD patients to a minimum.
6. To take written consent before any procedure after checking identity of the patient before taking up the examination.
7. To ensure good history taking of a patient going to be examined by the doctor.
8. To prepare patients (to explain entire procedure to reduce patient's anxiety and to get his/her cooperation) for doctors to examine or conduct tests.

9. To attach the required equipment (TMT, ECHO, ECG) to the patient's body with the electrodes just placed.
10. To monitor and record patient vitals.
11. To complete the test as per cardiologist's instructions.
12. To ensure good record keeping and ensuring g its confidentiality.
13. To interact with patient and his/her family members to answer their queries and contact the cardiologist in case of doubt.
14. To conduct various on-invasive cardiac tests, such as ECG, Echocardiograph, TMT, PFT (Pulmonary Function Test) etc independently using available equipment.
15. To prepare reports of various diagnostic tests for review/interpretation by doctors.
16. To send test reports to RECEPTION for further distribution.
17. To assist doctors in carrying out their duties and in performing various procedure.
18. They may also be trained and asked to assist in Cath Lab, Pulmonary lab operations.
19. To ensure proper billing before taking up a patient for consultation or investigation, procedure.
20. To maintain good interpersonal relationship.
21. To ensure proper maintenance and timely repair of equipment put under his/her care.
22. To indent and receive supplies required in this department.
23. To maintain and update records of all procedures carried out as per policies of the hospital.
24. To ensure full assistance to Sonologists whenever asked for.
25. Will be responsible for proper maintenance of all equipment placed under his control.
26. To perform other duties as asked by seniors.

D. Cardiovascular Technician

1. They work as direct assistant to cardiologists.
2. They conduct/help in conducting both invasive and non-invasive tests.
3. To call patient from waiting area to the examination/procedure room.
4. To make patient comfortable on the procedure table.
5. To identify and counsel the patient.
6. To explain the patient about the impending procedure.
7. To take his/her consent in writing.
8. Duties are same as that of other Cardiac Technicians & Cath Lab Technicians.

E. E.C.G./ECHO TECHNICIAN

An ECG technician is expert in conducting/helping doctors to conduct various cardiovascular tests such as TMT, PFT, Holter, ECHO etc.

1. To be punctual on duty.
2. To be in uniform or proper dress while on duty.
3. Should perform shift duties whenever asked for. He/she may be put 'on call' duties also.
4. To be responsible for ECG recording and Holter monitoring of patients.
5. To assist doctors (Cardiologist) in his work.
6. To do and/or assist doctors and staff in conducting various other non-invasive tests such as TMT, ECHO, PFT etc.
7. To ensure patient's safety and comfort during total process.
8. To check that proper billing has been done.

9. To take written consent after checking and confirming the patient's identity.
10. To explain entire procedure to the patient to reduce patient's anxiety and to get his/her cooperation.
11. To prepare patient for the test and to attach ECG electrodes to patient's body.
12. To start machine, take the print-out and complete the test.
13. To diagnose an emergency and call the doctor immediately.
14. To do all paper work related to his job. To maintain records as per hospital policy and procedure.
15. To maintain good interpersonal relationship.
16. To attend emergency cases immediately.
17. To maintain equipment, such as ECG Machine, Defibrillator, TMT, Holter, ECHO) in working order at all time.
18. To clean machines/equipment and its accessories and keep in good condition.
19. To inform seniors if an equipment needs further attention.
20. To record patient vitals as per instructions of a doctor.
21. To keep inventory of consumables and non-consumable items.
22. They may be asked to assist doctors in other procedures as well such as Angiography, Angioplasty, Pacemaker insertion etc.
23. Any other duty assigned by seniors.

F. Perfusionist/Cardiac Pump Technician:

1. Will ensure that perfusion related services are available in the hospital at all times.
2. Responsible for managing and operating heart-lung machine during surgery.
3. Will make sure that the Heart Lung machine is in working order before start of any surgery.
4. Will always be coordinating with the anaesthetist.
5. Responsible for setting up and testing of heart-lung machine to ensure its proper functioning according to the specifications.
6. Will prepare, administer and monitor all required medications.
7. Should be able to Interpret blood gas results so that machine can be adjusted accordingly.
8. Responsible for its operation and changing settings as per surgeons & anaesthetists' instruction.
9. Responsible for monitoring various physiological & metabolic parameters during surgery.
10. Responsible for assuring patient's safety.
11. Will ensure that air does not enter into the patient's cardiovascular system.
12. Will ensure;
13. Adequate blood flow.
14. Adequate blood pressure.
15. Adequate oxygenation of blood.
16. Adequate blood temperature.
17. Will remove tubing's from the patient after surgery only after the patient's condition has stabilised.
18. Will constantly monitor the patient during surgery.
19. Will ensure sterility of consumables being used.
20. Will observe standard aseptic precautions.
21. Shall maintain good and clear communication with other members of the team.
22. Will ensure completion of all relevant medical records.
23. Will maintain the machine in working order including its cleaning.

24. Will indent and receive consumable stocks.
25. Will supervise and manage all inventories related to his/her services.
26. He/she can be put on duty in ICCU (Intensive Cardiac Care Unit) and in Cath labs.
27. Will provide IABP (Intra-Aortic Balloon Pump) support in the hospital where ever required such as Cath Lab, OT and may be in CT.
28. Will maintain quality assurance in all patient care services.
29. Will be responsible for proper maintenance of the machine in coordination with the biomedical engineer.
30. Will be on call duty round the clock.
31. Will carry out other duties similar in nature and appropriate to his skills as per instructions of seniors.

DAILY AUDIT:

SN	Audit Point	Remark
1	Cleaning of area?	
2	BMW Management?	
3	Equipment Cleaning done?	
4	Hazard identification checklist Completed?	
5	Medicine storage & labelling with open and expiry date?	
6	Random Check on Medicine Expiry?	
7	Personal hygiene of staff?	
8	Autoclave Sets Expiry?	
9	Fridge and room temperature?	

Remarks:

Signature of senior staff/Area In-charge:

Signature of auditor:

VARIOUS CHECKLISTS OF CARDIOLOGY SERVICES:

A. Checklist for OPD Consultation:

SN	Checks	Remark
1	What are your symptoms and how long you have them?	
2	Factors worsening your symptoms (Exercise, alcohol, stress, your position, etc)	
3	Factors reliving your symptoms (Rest, Food, Sleep, etc)	
4	Frequency of these symptoms?	
5	Any associated medical problem?	
6	Present medication?	
7	Any family history of cardiac ailment?	
8	Have you heard about any treatment of your illness?	

STATIONARY FORMATS USED IN THIS DEPARTMENT:

1. Consent Form for ECHO/(TOE):

Hospital Name & Address

Consent for ECHO/TOE/Stress ECHO

I .... S/O, W/O, D/O Sh. .... C.R. No. .... hereby gives consent to have Echocardiogram/ Transesophageal Echocardiography Test, which has been advised by my physician and to be conducted on me.

I understand that this test is necessary to evaluate my heart disease. However, I may request that the test be discontinued at any time for any type of discomfort to me during the test.

However, I understand that just as with other diagnostic tests there are possible potential risks associated with this test such as (I) Burning pain, (ii) Chest discomfort, (iii) Rare cases of rupture at oesophagus (1 in 10,000), (iv) Arrhythmia's (1 in 5000), (v) Death (1 in 10,000) have been reported/or may occur.

Signature of patient	Witness:
Name	Name:
C.R. No.	Signature:
Date	Relation:

2. CONSENT FORM FOR T.M.T.:

Hospital Name & Address

Consent for TMT

Patient Name:

Height: Weight:

I .... consent to have an exercise (stress) test, which has been advised by my physician, administered and conducted on me.

I understand this is designed to evaluate the presence or absence of significant heart disease and/or to evaluate the efficiency of my current therapy, and/or to measure my physical fitness for work and/or sport.

I understand that I will walk on a motor driven treadmill. During the performance of the exercise test, my ECG will be monitored and my blood pressure will be measured and recorded at periodic intervals. The exercise will be progressively increased according to the standard schedule. However, I may request that test be discontinued at any time. Every effort will be made to conduct the test in such a way as to minimize discomfort and risk. However, I understand that, just as with other diagnostic test there are possible potential risks associated with the exercise test. These include weakness, transient light-headedness, fainting, chest discomfort and shortness of breath, leg cramps and palpitations. On rare occasions (approximately 2 to 3 per 10,000 tests) heart attacks (myocardial infarction) or even sudden death (approximately, 1 per 1,00,000 tests) may occur.

Signature of patient	Witness:
Name	Name:
C.R. No.	Signature:
Date	Relation:

(8) US/ECG/Etc/Record Register

ABC Hospital

3. U.S/ECG/ECHO/TMT/PFT Record Register:

SN	Patient Name	Age/ Sex	Consultant	Referred By	Test Details	OPD/ IPD	Receipt No./IPD No.	Amt Rs.	No. Of Films/ PG Paper		Remark/ Test Report Short
									Used	Wasted	

PG = Photographic Paper used in computer printers for printing ECHO Photos

The register has following columns using both right & left side of the register:

1. Serial No.
2. Patient's Name
3. Age/Sex
4. Consultant
5. Referred By
6. Test Details (e.g., TMT/PFT/ECG/US/Echo)
7. OPD No./IPD No.
8. Receipt No/Room No.
9. Amount (Rs.)
10. No. of P.G. paper; Used/Wasted
11. Remark/Test Report Summary

4. TMT Consent & Report Format:

Hospital Name & Address

TMT CONSENT & REPORT FORMAT

Page-1

Name ____

I hereby give my consent for exercise test to be done on me. The details of the test and possible complications have been explained to me:

Witness: ________________ Patient Signature

Dated: __________________

Page-2

EXERCISE ECG

Patient Name:	Age/Sex:
Lab No.:	Reg. No.:
Clinical Diagnosis:	
Resting ECG	
Medications:	Protocol:
Duration of Test:	Stage:
Maximum Predicted Heart Rate:	85% Max.:
Heart Rate Achieved:	% Age of Predicted Heart Rate:
Test Terminated (END Point):	
Pressure Rate Product:	METS:

Description	Time (Min.)	Heart Rate (BPM)	B.P. (mm Hg.)	Symptoms
Control Recumbent				
Control Standing				
Hyperventilation				
Stage 1				
Stage 2				
Stage 3				
Stage 4				
Stage 5				

ECG ABNORMALITIES EXERCISE PHASE

Stage	ST-T Changes	R Wave	Arrhythmia
Stage 1			
Stage 2			
Stage 3			
Stage 4			
Stage 5			

ABNORMALITIES DURING RECOVERY

____

____

Page-3

FINAL IMPRESSION

1. ________________ Exercised for ________ (minute) on Bruce Protocol at a work load of ________________ Mets and achieved ___ % of max. predicted HR.

   Exercise was terminated due to ________________
2. Resting ECG revealed ________________
3. No. significant ST-T changes were observed during exercise test. Developed asymptomatic/ symptomatic ________ mm ST depression/elevation in lead ________ during stage ______ at HR of ________________ BPM, which progressed to ________

   ST-T changes reverted to basal pattern after ________________ of recovery period.
4. No significant arrhythmia was observed during stress test ________________
5. Normal HR and BP response to exercise. No S3/S4 heard.

IMPRESSION:- Normal stress test (negative for reversible myocardial Ischemia)

Dr. ________

Consultant Cardiologist

5. Cardiac Clinic Record:

Hospital Name

Dated ____________________

CARDIAC CLINIC RECORD

Patient Name: .... UHID No.: ....

Presenting Complaints: .... (give proper space)

History: ....

Page-2 (either on back of 1 or separate page)

Family History: ....

Personal History: ....

Diet History: ....

Durg History: ....

Surgical History: ....

Page-3

PHYSICAL EXAMINATION

Wt. (Kg): .... Height (cm): .... Pallor: .... Jaundice: ....

Appearance : .... Build: .... Neck Swelling: ....

Clubbing: .... Oedema: .... Lymph nodes: ....

JVP (cm): .... Pulse Waves: .... Cyanosis: ....

Pulse/Minutes: .... B.P. (mm Hg): Rt. Arm: ...... Lt. Arm: ....

Peripheral Pulses: ....

Precordium: .... Parasternal left: ....

Apex Beat: .... PMI: ....

Other Pulsations: ....

Heart Sounds: ....

Chest: ....

Abdomen: ....

CNS: ....

Other Systems: ....

Page-4

Clinical Diagnosis: ....

Treatment Advised: ....

Signature: ....

Page-5

Detailed Management: ....

Page-6

Test		Date	Date	Date	Date
BLOOD CHEMISTRY					
Sugar: Fasting	mg/dl				
: Post Prandial	mg/dl				
: Random	mg/dl				
Urea	mg/dl				
Creatinine	mg/dl				
Uric Acid	mg/dl				
Cholesterol	mg/dl				
Triglycerides	mg/dl				
HDL	mg/dl				
VLDL	mg/dl				
LDL	mg/dl				
Bilirubin Total	mg/dl				
Conjugated	mg/dl				
Unconjugated	mg/dl				
Proteins: Total	Gm/dl				
Albumin	Gm/dl				
Globulin	Gm/dl				
Sodium	meq/dl				
Potassium	Gm/dl				
Chloride	meq/dl				
SGOT	meq/dl				
SGPT	Units				
CPK	Units				
LDH	Units				
Acid Phosphatase	Units				
Calcium	mg/dl				
Magnesium	mg/dl				
Drug Levels	(specify)				

Haematological Investigations:

		DATE	DATE	DATE	DATE
Haemoglobin (Gm%)					
R.B.C. count/cmm					
P.V.C. (%)					

		DATE	DATE	DATE	DATE
W.B.C. Total count/cmm Polymorphs (%) Eosinophils (%) Lymphocytes (%) Basophils (%) Monocytes (%)					
Abnormal Cells (specify)					
Platelet Count/cmm					
Reticulocytes (%)					
Other Parameters not mentioned above					
ESR (Wintrobe) mm/1 hr					
Prothrombin Time (sec) Control					
Patient					
Bleeding Time (sec)					
Clotting Time (sec)					
Blood Group					
Urine					
Stool					
Sputum					
Others					

Page-7

MICROBIOLOGY AND IMMUNOLOGY

CULTURE/SENSITIVITY (SPECIFY)

Test	Date	Date	Date	Date	Date
ASLO (titre)					
CRP (mg)					
A'Dnase (titre)					
Others (titre)					
Rheumatoid Factor					
LE Cells					
ANF					
Others (Specify)					

Surgical Operation Details: ....

Page-8

E.C.G. Record

Date	Rhythm Rate	Axis	PR	QRS	R/S	Q	S-T	Diagnosis

X-Ray Record:

Date	Observations

Page-9

Laboratory Investigations

Investigation	Date	Brief Report
Graded Exercise Test (TMT)		
Colour Doppler (TEE)		
Vascular Doppler		
Holter (24 Hours)		
Radionuclide Studies		

Page-10

Electrophysiology: ....

Cardiac Catheterisation & Angiography: ....

Page-11

Date	Progress Report

****

6. Consent for Stress ECHO:

Hospital Name & Address

Department of Cardiology

CONSENT FOR THE STRESS-DOBUTAMINE ECHO/TEE INVESTIGATION

I,..S/0, W/o, D/o Sh.. having CR No................., CVC No ...., hereby consent to STRESS-DOBUTAMINE ECHO. INVESTIGATION, which has been advised by my physician and to be conducted on me.

I understand that this test is necessary to evaluate my heart disease. However, I may request that the test be discontinued at any time for any type of discomfort to me during the test.

However, I understand that just as with the other diagnostic tests there are possible potential risk associated with this test such as (i) Chest Pain (1 in 100) (ii) Chest Discomfort (1 in 100) (iii) Tachycardia (1 to 50) (iv) Ventricular Tachycardia (1 in 1000) (v) Death (1 in 10,000) have been reported (or may occur).

Signature: ....   Name: ....

Witness: ....   Name: ....

7. Consent for TMT:

CONSENT FORM FOR T.M.T.

Ht _____Wt _____.

I .... consent to have an exercise (stress) test, which has been advised by my physician, administered and conducted on me.

I understand this is designed to evaluate the presence or absence of significant heart disease and/or to evaluate the efficiency of my current therapy, and/or to measure my physical fitness for work and/or sport.

I understand that I will walk on a motor driven treadmill. During the performance of the exercise test, my ECG will be monitored and my blood pressure will be measured and recorded at periodic intervals. The exercise will be progressively increased according to the standard schedule. However, I may request that test be discontinued at any time. Every effort will be made to conduct the test in such a way as to minimize discomfort and risk. However, I understand that, just as with other diagnostic test there are possible potential risks associated with the exercise test. These include weakness, transient light headedness, fainting, chest discomfort and shortness of breath, leg cramps and palpitations. On rare occasions (approximately 2 to 3 per 10,000 tests) heart attacks (myocardial infarction) or even sudden death (approximately, 1 per 1,00,000 tests) may occur.

Signature: Date:

Witness: Signature:

8. Informed Consent Angioplasty/Angiography/Balloon Valvotomy:

Hospital Name & Address

Department of Cardiology

INFORMED CONSENT FOR ANGIOPLASTY/VALVOTOMY

I, the undersigned understand that Mr./Ms. .... (Name of the patient) my .... (Relationship) named above, is suffering from .... (Diagnosis) and needs angioplasty/coronary stenting/balloon valvotomy.

It has been explained to me by doctors that this procedure carries a .... % risk to life. I also understand that there may be complications like, acute MI, thrombo-embolism, unconsciousness, neurological deficit, stroke, and bleeding & allergic reaction to contrast material. In the case of coronary angioplasty, 20-30% patients are expected to have a recurrence of symptoms over a period of 6 months to one year. Valvular stenosis treated by balloon dilatation may recur over a period of months to years. Rarely, in the case of angioplasty/coronary stenting, acute closure of the target vessel may occur and in the case of balloon valvotomy acute valvular regurgitation or bleeding may occur necessitating emergency surgery.

The risk in the case of my patient is high because..

I have fully understood the above risks and despite these I give unconditional consent for ....of..................................... ....

Signature — Signature of Patient/Guardian

Name of Doctor — Name in Capitals

9. ECHO Reporting Format:-1

ECHO REPORT

Name: .... Age: ... Sex: ... Height: ... Weight: ...

C.R. No.: ... Echo No.: ...

Study Date: ......

Reason for Study: .... (HTN, R/O CAD)

Interpretation Summary

NO RWMA, LVEF = (55%)

Normal Cardiac Chamber Dimensions:

TRIVIAL MR, TRIVIAL AR, TRIVIAL TR.

NO THROMBUS/PERICARDIAL EFFUSION.

Left Ventricle:

(The left ventricle is normal in size. There is no thrombus. The left ventricular ejection fraction is normal.)

Left Atrium:

(The left atrium is normal in size.)

Right Ventricle:

(The right ventricle is normal in size)

Right Atrium:

(The right atrium is normal.)

Aorta:

(The aortic root is normal.)

Pulmonary Artery:

(The pulmonary artery is normal.)

Pericardium:

(There is no pericardial effusion.)

Aortic Valve:

(Mild aortic sclerosis is present with good valvular opening. The aortic valve is tri-leaflet. There is trace aortic regurgitation.)

Mitral Valve:

(The mitral valve leaflets appear normal. There is no evidence of stenosis, fluttering or prolapsed. There is trace mitral regurgitation.)

Tricuspid Valve:

(The tricuspid valve leaflets are thin and pliable and the valve motion is normal. There is trace tricuspid regurgitation.)

Pulmonary Valve:

(The pulmonic valve leaflets are thin and pliable, valve motion is normal.)

M-Mode/2-d Measurement & Calculations:

LVID: …… (4.07) LA Dimension: …… (2.30)

LVIDs: …… (3.220 AO root dimension: …… (2.50)

FS: … (20.8) ACS: ……… (1.60)

Time Measurements:

Doppler Measurements & calculations:

Ao V2 max: …… (131 cm/sec) TV V2 max: …… (40.0 cm/sec) PV V2 max: … (73.0 cm/sec)

MV E point: …… (117 cm/sec)

Echo Photos……… to be pasted here.

Interpreted by: … Dr. ………………… on date ……… At …… (time)

10. ECHO Reporting Format:-2

Hospital Name & Address

ECHOCARDIOGRAPHY REPORT

Page-1

Name……………………………………………………………………………………………Age/ Sex…………………

Registration No……………………………………OPD/IPD……………………… Bed……………………

Cardiac Lab No………………………………………Date…………………………………………………

Referred by…………………………………………………………………………………………… ……………………

Clinical Diagnosis…………………………………………………………………………………………

Procedures:

M-MODE/2D/DOPPLER/COLOUR/CONTRAST

Measurements:	Reported Value	Normal Value
Aortic Root Diameter	________________ cm	2.0 – 3.7 cm < 2.2 cm/M^2
Aortic Valve Opening	________________ cm	1.5 – 2.6 cm
Right Ventricular Dimension	________________	0.7 – 2.6 cm < 1.4 cm/M^2
Right Ventricular Thickness	________________	0.3 – 0.9 cm
Left Atrial Dimension	________________ cm	1.9 – 4.0 cm < 2.2 cm/M^2
Left Ventricular ED Dimension	________________ cm	3.7 – 5.6 cm < 3.2 cm/M^2
Left Ventricular ES Dimension	________________ cm	2.2 – 4.0 cm
Interventricular Septal Thickness	ED _______ ES _______	0.6 – 1.2 cm
Left Vent. PW Thickness	ED _______ ES _______	0.5 – 1.0 cm
IVS/LVPW	________________	
INDICES OF LEFT VENT. FUNCTION :		
Mitra E-Septal Separation	________________	< 0.9 cm
Minor Axis Shortening	________________	24.42 %
LV Ejection Fraction	________________	60 ± 6.2 %

Imaging:

M mode examination revealed normal movement of both mitral leaflets during diastole (DE = ……(1.7 cm), EF = ……(87 mm/sec). No SAM, or mitral valve prolapse is seen. Aortic cusps are not thickened and closure line is central. Tricuspid valve is normal. Aortic root is normal is size. Pulmonary valve is normal. Dimensions of left ventricle, and left atrium are normal.

2D imaging in PLAX, SAX and apical 4 'C' views revealed a normal sized left ventricle. Movement of septum, posterior and lateral walls is normal Global LVEF is ……(60%). Mitral Valve opening is normal. No evidence of mitral valve prolapse is seen. Aortic valve has three cusps and its opening is not restricted. Tricuspid valve leaflets move normally. Pulmonary valve is normal. Interatrial & interventricular septa are intact. No intracardiac mass or thrombus is seen. No pericardial pathology is observed.

PASTE RELEVANT IMAGES HERE

Page-2

Doppler:

MV	______(87)____________	cm/sec	MR	__________(Nil)________
AoV	______(82)____________	cm/sec	AI	__________(Nil)________
TV	______(60)____________	cm/sec	TR	__________(Nil)________
PV	______(95)____________	cm/sec	PI	__________(Nil)________

Colour Flow:

Colour flow mapping revealed presence of normal intracardiac flow characteristics. No valvular regurgitation or intracardiac shunt was observed.

Final Diagnosis:

2D colour Doppler examination of .... (Name of the patient) revealed:

1. No regional wall motion abnormality.
2. LVEF = 60%
3. No pericardial effusion/clot/intracardiac mass.

Dr.................................

Consultant Cardiologist

It is study of images and not a final diagnosis. Please correlate the findings clinically.

For interpretation by Registered Medical Practitioner only. Not for Medico-legal Purposes.

11. Foetal ECHO Report Format:

Hospital Name & Address

FOETAL ECHO REPORT

Name: .... Age/Sex: ....

CR No.: .... OPD/IPD No.: .... Date: ....

Referring Doctor: ....

Date of Test: .... Date of Reporting: ....

Investigation: FOETAL ECHOCARDIOGRAPHY

Results:

2 Atria - - - - - - seen/..............

2 Ventricles - - - - - - seen/..............

2 AV Valves - - - - - - seen/..............

2 Great Vessels - - - - - seen/..............

Both seem normally related with normal flow/...........

PFO present/...........

Flow visualized across the interventricular septum/...........

Foetal Heart Rate - 140/min/...........

All the above parameters are within normal limits for this gestational age/........................

Result: ....

Advise: Repeat foetal ECHO after 32 weeks.

Radiologist

(Dr......................................)

It is study of images and not a final diagnosis. Please correlate the findings clinically.

For interpretation by Registered Medical Practitioner only. Not for Medico-legal Purposes.

DRUGS FOR CARDIOLOGY DEPARTMENT:

Following drugs must be available at hospital pharmacy/in the department for patients of this department.

Clopidogrel Tablet 75 mg	Diltiazem Tablet 60 mg
Glyceryl Trinitrate Sublingual Tablet 0.5 mg	Glyceryl trinitrate Injection 125 mg/5 ml
Isosorbide-5- mononitrate Tablet 10 mg	Diltiazem SR Tablet 90 mg
Isosorbide-5- mononitrate SR Tablet 30 mg	Isosorbide dinitrate Tablet 5 mg
Isosorbide dinitrate Tablet 10 mg	Atenolol Tablet 50 mg, 100 mg
Metoprolol Tablet 25 mg	Metoprolol Tablet 50 mg
Amiodarone Tablet 100 mg	Amiodarone Injection 50 mg/ml
Amlodipine Tablet 2.5 mg	Amlodipine Tablet 5 mg
Amlodipine Tablet 10 mg	Hydrochlorothiazide Tablet 50 mg
Hydrochlorothiazide Tablet 12.5 mg	Hydrochlorothiazide Tablet 25 mg
Labetalol Injection 5 mg/ml	Labetalol Tablet 100 mg
Labetalol Injection 20 mg/2 ml	Methyldopa Tablet 250 mg
Methyldopa Tablet 500 mg	Enalapril Tablet 10 mg
Enalapril Tablet 2.5 mg	Enalapril Tablet 5 mg
Captopril Tablet 25 mg	Lisinopril Tablet 5 mg
Verapamil Tablet 40 mg, 120 mg	Verapamil Injection 5 mg/2 ml
Ramipril Tablet 2.5 mg/5 mg	Telmisartan Tablet 40 mg
Digoxin Tablet 0.25 mg	Digoxin Tablet 250 mg
Dobutamine Injection 50 mg/ml	Dopamine Injection 40/ml
Protamine Injection 50 mg/5 ml	Noradrenaline Injection 2 mg/ml
Enoxaparin LMWH Injection	Clofibrate Tablet 500 mg
Streptokinase Injection 15 lac/vial	Streptokinase Injection 7.5 lac/vial
Fenofibrate Tablet 40 mg, 160 mg	Atorvastatin Tablet 10 mg
Atorvastatin Tablet 40mg	Sodium nitroprusside Injection 10 mg/ml
Alteplase Powder for Injection 20 mg	Alteplase Powder for Injection 50 mg

RECORDS/DOCUMENTS IN CATH LAB:

1. Procedure Register
   - Inventory Register
   - Medicine Consumption Register
   - Consent forms of - TPI, PPI, AICD, IABP, CAG, PTCA & PTRA.
   - Undertaking forms
   - Pre & post procedure check list
   - Radiation protection guide lines.
   - Pharmacy Indent forms.
   - AMC/Maintenance records.

BIBLIOGRAPHY, REFERENCES & ACKNOWLEDGMENTS:

1. Mahatma Gandhi Medical College and Hospital, Sitapur, Jaipur https://www.mgmch.org/departments/cardiac-care
2. Standard Operating Procedure (SOP) for those presenting to the Emergency at the Department of Cardiology King George's medical University Lucknow.
3. "Standard Operating Procedures SOP For Hospitals 2nd Edition" by Dr. Arun K. Agarwal
4. "Duties & Responsibilities of Hospital Staff" by Dr. Arun Kumar
5. "Checklists for Hospitals" by Dr. Arun K. Agarwal
6. Standard Operating Procedures (SOP) For Hospitals In India: Complete with Stationery Formats Used in Various Departments in a Hospital– 19 July 2022 by Arun K. Agarwal
7. "Cardiac Rehabilitation, Adult Fitness and Exercise Testing", By Philip K. Wilson, Paul S. Fardy, Victor F. Froelicher
8. Six Sigma Multispeciality Hospital, Nasik, India
9. Duties and Responsibilities of a Perfusionist. Brian Schwartz, CCP September 2, 2003;
10. Shalby Hospital, Mohali, Punjab, India

Chapter - 6

DEPARTMENT OF CARDIOLOGY – CATH LAB

INDEX

INTRODUCTION:

Cath lab is a specialized laboratory with diagnostic imaging equipment where the cardiologist diagnoses and treats the patient who suffers from obstruction of their blood vessels, in particular the vessels of heart (Coronary Artery Disease). The cardiologist first has to localise the obstruction area of the blood vessel, referred to as stenosis, measure its length & width & finally enlarge the blood vessel.

The localization of stenosis is done by a special tube called catheter. For inserting the catheter, the cardiologist makes a small opening in one of the patient's blood vessels, on the accessible area of the body such as right thigh. Through this opening catheter is inserted & then guided towards heart. The femoral artery is associated with local complication up to 3%, so more interventions are moving towards the radial artery as an alternative site.

Disadvantages of the radial artery include small vessel calibre and different learning curves for cardiologists. The catheter is guided using fluoroscopy which means, inserting low dose of contrast fluid via the catheter known as dye and exposing the patient's region of interest to low intensity X-Ray fluoroscopy to visualize the position of catheter's tip within the patient's body in real time.

When the catheter reaches the heart area, the cardiologist performs an exposure, which means inserting high dose contrast fluid & exposing the relevant region of the patient's body to high intensity X-rays.

The exposure provides accurate images of the blood vessels as it is important to localise the stenosis. Images acquired are displayed on a monitor for further analysis. Next a stent is deployed via the catheter's guide were. The stent is a special thin aluminium (special metal) cylinder that can be enlarged in order to correct the stenosis.

During the intervention, the cardiologist uses different systems situated in adjoining room of the Cath lab.

The intervention room houses the X-Ray system and the patient's monitoring system.

The control room houses the patient data logging system and reviewing work station for studies.

The need for increased efficiency of Cath lab requires the integration of theses system. The goal of integration is to reduce the number of cumbersome systems, tasks & personnel required in Cath lab and are to reduce intervention time. Therefore, we are using integrated Cath lab.

Besides coronary interventions we do Temporary Pacemaker Implantation, Permanent Pacemaker Implantation, AICD Implantation, IABP, Valvuloplasty etc in the Cath lab.

The Cath lab functions round the clock. The hospital has performed more than 50 angiographies and about 25 angioplasties in a month. It is staffed with trained and dedicated nurses and technicians. Procedures are mainly done through trans-radial route but femoral route is also used in some cases. The post procedure stay is reduced in radial procedures.

OBJECTIVES & SCOPE:

Usability of this integrated Cath lab can be simply described in 3 words: -

1. **Effectiveness:** It refers to the accuracy means absence of mistakes or errors and completeness of the intervention.
2. **Efficiency:** It refers to the expenditure of physical & human resource (time, people & materials) for a particular task in relation to effectiveness.
3. **Satisfaction:** It refers to the freedom from discomfort and positive attitude towards the Cath lab systems.

This hospital has state of art Integrated Cath Lab

ORGANISATION STRUCTURE:

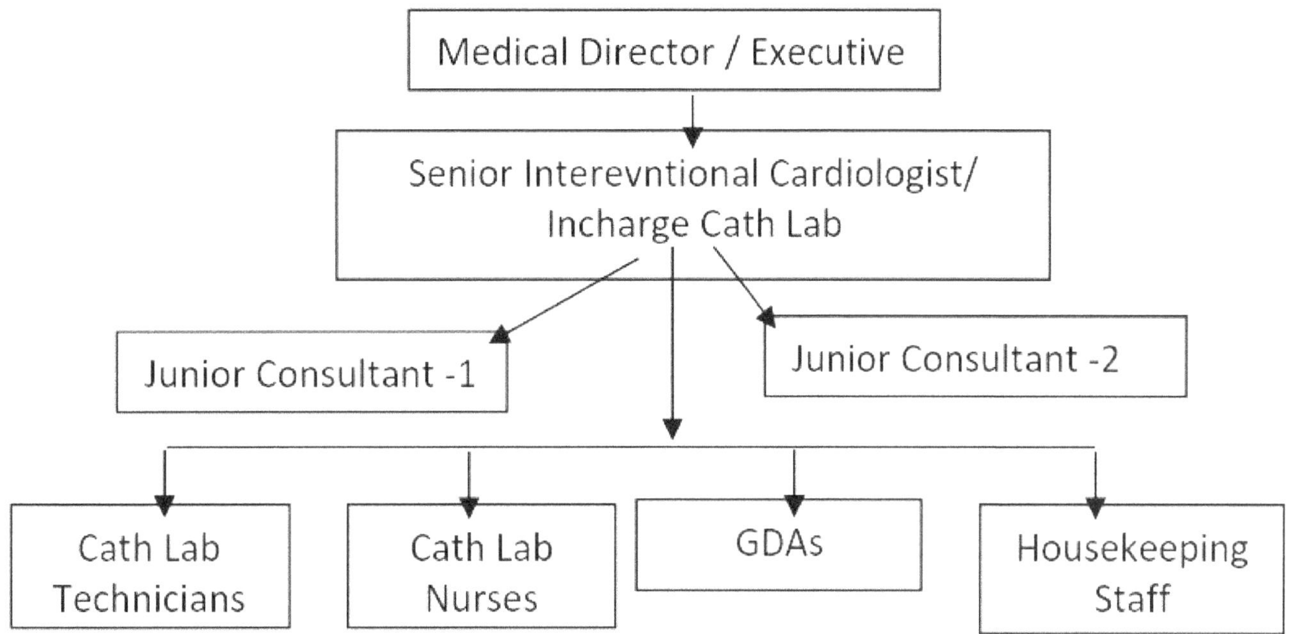

DUTIES & RESPONSIBILITIES:

1. HOD Cath Lab:

HOD is responsible for overall functioning of the Cath Lab which includes maintenance of strict aseptic standards, Cath lab techniques, discipline & handle any emergency arising.

1. He is responsible & guides other people for the safety & comfort of the patient.
2. He intervenes immediately, in any breakdown or trouble & assigns other people to take corrective measures.
   a. Overall functioning of Cath Lab equipment & instruments.
   b. Responsible for maintaining highest standards of asepsis & sterility.
   c. Maintain discipline & atmosphere of comfort amongst staff members.
   d. Corrective measures when any emergency arises.

2. Cath Lab In Charge:

1. He is responsible for assigning duties for nursing & non nursing persons working under him.
2. He is also responsible for strict asepsis & antisepsis, supervision of equipment & prepares staff to deal with any emergency.
3. Safety & comfort of staff & patients is taken care of by him.
   a. Ensure proper functioning of Cath Lab equipment.
   b. Sterility & proper supply of sterile goods.
   c. Assignment of duties for technical & nursing staff.
   d. Assign clinical help & Anaesthetist.

e. Ensure safety & comfort of the patient.
f. Regularly checks indents & inventory records.
g. Supervises autoclaving of hospital supply.
h. Ensure infection control measures & adequate corrective measures are taken.
i. Maintain discipline.
j. Ongoing Formal & Informal training of staff members.
k. Orientation programs for new staff.

3. Technician In-charge/Technicians:

1. They work under direct supervision of invasive cardiologists.
2. To operate cardiac catheterisation equipment (Cath Lab).
3. To enter protocol data in the Cath lab computer.
4. To position the patient on the table.
5. To work with cardiologist in assisting them in various diagnostic and therapeutic procedures.
6. To operate the machine to help cardiologist put the guide wire/catheter.
7. To assist in open heart surgeries, pacemaker implantation, angiographies, angioplasties and other related procedures.
8. To comfort the patient before, during and after the procedure.
9. To work in coordination with other team members.
10. To ensure proper sterile environment.
11. To ensure that all equipment is in working order before start of a procedure.
12. To record vitals of a patient.
13. To follow WHO 'Surgical Checklist' during a surgery.
14. To prepare all instruments required for a procedure.
15. To assist in cardiac emergency and ICCU/post angioplasty, post-operative departments.
16. To keep record of procedures performed in this department.
17. To ensure manufacturers guidelines while operating an equipment.
18. To carry out administrative duties as scheduling appointments and marinating files.
19. To ensure completion of records and registers.
20. To ensure that all radiological safety precautions are taken.
21. To ensure compliance of all BARC/AERB regulations.
22. To ensure proper functioning and upkeep of equipment.
23. Should be able to do preventive maintenance and calibration of the machine.
24. To perform trouble shooting procedures for cardiac equipment.
25. To be responsible for preventive maintenance of equipment of this department.
26. To coordinate with other maintenance agencies and company's engineers.
27. To perform other duties as assigned by seniors.
28. To ensures regular inventory supplies & record keeping of the same.
29. To receive sterile sets from CSSD & sending packed set to CSSD.
30. To handle monthly stocking.
31. To check daily crash cart & emergency drug & its record maintenance.
32. Disposal & waste management of Cath Lab.
33. Proper cleaning/Disinfection of Cath lab & regular functioning as for period

34. Registering all untoward incidences of Cath lab & reporting it to Cath Lab in charge for corrective measures.
35. Co-ordination between cardiologist & surgical teams for various procedures.
36. Once the patient is in Cath Lab, he ensures that the patient is not left alone & tries to gain confidence.
37. Maintenance of all documents & records Cath Lab.
38. Maintenance of lead aprons, thyroid shield & other protective garments.

4. Cath Lab Nurses:

1. Nurses in the Cath Lab are responsible for receiving the patients from CCU or Ward & Then to make them ready for procedure. Preparation of trolley, cleaning and autoclaving are their responsibility.
2. They are accountable to in charge Cath lab.
   a. Taking over of the patient, equipment & documents
   b. Preparing patient for procedure & making them comfortable and alley their anxiety.
   c. Preparation of trolley for procedures.
   d. Assisting cardiologist for procedures.
   e. Immediate pre & post procedure care.
   f. Shifting of the patient from Cath lab to CCU & handing over the patient charge to CCU sister.
   g. Maintaining records of swabs, instruments & other things.
   h. Assisting Cath Lab technicians in managing Cath lab. and officiate his/her presence.

LIST OF PROCEDURES PERFORMED IN THE CATH LAB:

1. Angiography
2. PCI in Acute Coronary Syndrome.
3. Multi Vessel angioplasties including left main stenting & Bifurcation lesions.
4. Selective heart chambers & vessels studies for CHD.
5. Selective contrast Angiography for left ventriculogram.
6. Valvuloplasty's – Mitral & Aortic
7. Device Closures of ASD & VSD.
8. Carotid Artery Angioplasties.
9. Renal Angioplasties.
10. CABG graft Angioplasties.
11. Umbrella device insertion in cases of DVT.
12. Catheter Therapy of Co-arctation of aorta.
13. Endovascular repairs of abdominal & thoracic Aneurysm.
14. Selective vessel & Heart chamber pressure recording.
15. Selective vessel & Heart Chamber blood sampling for Oximetry, Carboxy & Oxyhaemoglobin.
16. Blood gas analysis
17. Cardiac output measurements by thermodilution method.
18. Cath Studies for shunt detection & grading.
19. Right heart Catheterisation with multiple oxygen saturation & QP/QS determination.
20. Temporary & Permanent pacemaker implantation.
21. Pericardiocentesis.

22. Pulmonary Artery Catheter (Swan Ganj) Placement.
23. Balloon Arterial Septostomy.
24. Retrieval of foreign bogy from heart & great vessels.
25. Trans septal puncture procedure.
26. IABP insertion.
27. AICD Implantation.

Note: All of the above angiograms may be performed in conjunction with radiographic film devices, including single cine-fluoroscopy, cut film rapid sequence Angiography & rapid sequence & spot film cameras or digital imaging.

Procedure performed in Cath Lab can be classified under 3 categories:

1. **Emergency cases:**
   a. Like cases which are acute myocardial infarction. As soon as they are diagnosed, they are taken immediately for intervention. (The hospital follows golden hour rule to savage myocardium)
   b. In cardiogenic shock – IABP is inserted on emergency basis along with other requires intervention.
   c. Pericardial tamponade causing hemodynamic compromise are taken immediately for pericardiocentesis.
   d. In case of complete heart block or sinus arrest, immediately temporary pacemaker implantation is done.
   e. Post PCI dissection causing homodynamic instability is taken urgently for intervention.
2. **Elective cases:**
   a. Majority of procedure falls into the category. They are planned procedure for unstable/Stable Angina, PPI, Cath Studies etc. They are thoroughly investigated & prepared before procedure & are planned accordingly.
3. **High risk cases:**
   a. They are cases with hemodynamic instability, review dysfunction, Haematological complication. Patient with multiple metabolic disorders, with pulmonary oedema, arrhythmias, pulmonary embolism.
   b. As this centre is a tertiary level hospital, all above mentioned cases are taken care of in Centre.

ADMISSION CRITERIA:

Symptoms of;

1. Angina
2. Dyspnoea on exertion
3. Heaviness in chest
4. Discomfort in chest
5. ECS-ST/T changes for ischemia
6. Myocardial infarction
7. BIOMEDICAL MARKERS
   1. Trop-T
   2. Trop-I
   3. Raised CPK-MB

PREVENTION & TREATMENT OF PROCEDURAL COMPLICATION:

Here are the most common complications during procedures in Cath Lab & an approach to anticipate & handle them.

1. It is important to know your patient especially for interventional cardiologist who is going to perform the procedure.

   It is done by carefully reviewing the patient's records. Through (Haemostasis', renal Dysfunction, Potential problems with diabetes, patency of vascular access) check & anticipation of history of drug allergy (contrast reaction)
2. Assess the PCI indication to calculate the clinical benefits which is the primary objective of the PCI.
3. Judge the interventional risk: Clinical, hemodynamic & Angiographic. Integrate risk assessment in the predefined strategy.
4. Predefine your strategy:
   a. Interventional Strategies: -
   b. Guiding Catheter- size & curve.
   c. Guide wires?
   d. Direct Stent?
   e. IABP assist device?
   f. Need for surgical back-up?
   g. Which drugs?
   h. Should know you own boundaries.
5. Informed consent:
   a. Complete information about risk complications & benefits
   b. Describe about the therapeutic benefits.
   c. Discussion about the expected day time outcome.
   d. Obtain a written/signed informed consent.
6. Severe Vascular Access:
   a. Try to treat artery from first stick.
   b. Haemostasis between failed attempts by asking for help.
   c. Stop procedure in case of bleeding until it is controlled.
   d. Try radial if femoral is difficult to puncture (PVD)
7. Work according to strategy:
   a. Apply your planned strategy.
   b. Working with 2 operators, anticipating difficulty.
   c. Work from simple – more complex strategy.
   d. Be calm & patient.
   e. You need to be fit.
8. Communicate & Observe:
   a. Continuous communication with patient & observes time regularly.
   b. Avoid unrelated & unnecessary conversation in Cath Lab during intervention.
   c. Anticipate & quickly correct the discomfort.
9. Prepare & know how to treat common complications e.g.:
   a. Vascular access injury
   b. Guiding catheter or wire induced dissection at aorto-coronary or Coronary Artery.
   c. Perforation.

d. Foreign body loss.
e. Critical wire loss across a lesion

10. Look for hidden complication:
    a. Patient is always right – look, observe & think about complication which are hidden e.g.: aorta dissection, contrast reaction, retroperitoneal bleed
12. Step in Peace.
    a. Obtain excellent angiographic images for a final judgment.
    b. Do not leave angiographic uncertainties unsolved.
    c. Ensure a secondary prevention programme.
    d. Stress the crucial role of the dual antiplatelet therapy.

PATIENT SHIFTING PROTOCOL (FROM CATH LAB TO ICU/WARD):

SN	PROCEDURES	RESPONSIBILITY
1	Inform the ICU/Ward before shifting the patient from Cath Lab	Nurse & Ward Boy
2	Checking of monitor and ventilator and keeping them ready if needed by the technician	Technician
3	After checking the vitals and having the orders, monitor leads are disconnected and the patient is shifted from the Cath table to the stretcher. In case of criticality shifted along with the monitor.	
4	Shifting the patient to the stretcher in comfortable position and covered with proper sized bed sheet	Nurse and Technician
5	Staff Nurse/technician is always accompanied with the patient when patient is shifted from the Cath Lab to ICU/Ward, in case of female patient female staff accompanies her.	
6	Handover the patient to the ICU/ward sister, check the vitals and informed to the Cardiologist	Nurse staff Nurse.
7	Patient is attached to the monitor as advised by cardiologist	Ward/ICU Staff Nurse
8	Give details of procedure	
9	Handover all documents to ICU/Ward	Cath Lab

SHEATH REMOVAL PROTOCOL:

Steps:

1. Remove the dressing & apply betadine
2. Start I/V fluid (N.S) (Amount depending on Ejection fraction)
   Note: Keep atropine/Morphine/Mephentin/Hydrocortisone injection ready
3. Give 2% xylocaine around sheath.
4. Remove arterial sheath first by pulling the sheath and keep firm pressure distally to allow spurt of blood and then press femoral artery proximally.
   Note: Keep a close watch on BP/HR
5. Removal femoral vein sheath (if required) after 4-5 min of arterial sheath removal.
6. Keep firm pressure over grain for 15-20 min post angiography & 30-45 min post angioplasty
7. Check the distal pulses e.g., Posterior tibial, dorsalis pedis etc.

8. Apply pressure dressing with dynaplast.
9. Keep sand bag over groin for 1-2 hrs for post angiography & 4-6 hrs for post angioplasty
   Note: Avoid sheath removal if blood pressure: Higher than 180/110 and lower than 100/60

PRECAUTIONS FOR PREVENTING/CONTROLLING INFECTION:

1. Air cleaning of Cath lab.
2. Wash floor with soap followed by Carbolization.
3. Regular fumigation and Carbolization is done specially before PPI, Device closure etc.
4. Hand washing with soap water and disinfectants between touching two patients and before procedure.
5. Barrier nursing by wearing gloves and mask.
6. By keeping minimum trafficking in cath lab.
7. All disposable items are sent for ETO.

RADIATION PROTECTION PROTOCOLS:

1. A radiation protection protocol is followed as per guide lines proposed by National Council on radiation protection and measurement stated in report no-102 (Annexure enclosed)
2. Education on radiation hazard, safety & its prevention are continuously done by training & awareness programmes of Cath lab staff.
3. Strict measures are taken to avoid unnecessary radiation exposure for patient as well as Cath Lab staff.
4. Strict adherence to formulated guidelines & procedure manuals.
5. Only those staff members who are required in the Cath Lab room during procedure are allowed to remain in side.
6. All the members, who are in Cath Lab during procedure are provided with protection devices like lead aprons with minimum thickness of 0.25mm lead equivalent, lead gloves (0.35 mm of lead equivalent, thyroid lead shield and portable lead shields.
7. Operators are standing behind an overhanging lead screen barrier whenever possible.
8. Those staff who are moving around the room during procedure are wearing wrap around protective garments.
9. Whenever possible operating consultant & staff step back from the table & behind protective shield, during cine radiography & serial radiographic procedures. This action decreases the exposure by a factor of 3 or more.
10. Minimum staff is allowed in Cath lab during cine of Angio to minimize exposure.
11. Exposure to radiation is reduced by reducing exposure & minimizing fluoroscopy & cine screening time.
12. Operators are kept at distance from the radiation beam. Doubling the distance between the primary beam and operator reduces the exposure by a factor of four.
13. Oblique views & steep angulation views increase the exposure so they are used only when better visualization is required. 600 angulation gives 3 times more dose of radiation then 300 angulation for minimum time.
14. We are following our set guidelines & radiation safety protocols & staff is complying with those rules.
15. Regular maintenance calibration & replacement of malfunctioning equipment are done.
16. Radiation counter (TLD Counter – Geiger counter) are used by all members in Cath Lab & is interrogated every 3 months & advice given accordingly.
17. If any procedure is required on pregnant patient especial precaution are used like lead shields and minimal exposure times is practiced.

18. Finally for all practical purposes all medical exposures are kept as low as reasonably achievable, consistent with obtaining the required diagnostic information.
19. **No dose greater than 3 rem should be allowed a 3 months period.**

WASTE MANAGEMENT:

All the waste items are disposed of by following the colour coding of the dustbins as follows.

1. Red Bin: Pus and blood-soaked dressing.
2. Yellow Bin: Human tissue, body parts, biotechnology waste, swabs, dressing & bandage which is finally sent for incineration.
3. Black Bin: General waste, paper, kitchen waste, wrapping paper, cans which finally go for municipal dump.
4. White Plastic Bags: Plastics, blood bags, urine bags, drains, IV sets & globes which are finally goes for shredding or dumping.

Quality Assurance Activities in Cath lab:

1. Employee safety: (Radiation and infection safety protocol followed. Kindly refer- infection control manual and Radiation safety manual).
2. Patient safety: (Radiation and infection safety protocol followed, kindly refer- infection control manual and Radiation safety manual).
3. Environmental surveillance done every monthly.
4. Preventive maintenance and calibration of all equipment (Refer Bio medical engineering Manual).
5. Quality indicators: Maintained by Cath Lab are

LIST OF CONSUMABLES IN CATH LAB:

ECG Electrodes	I.V. Set	Pressure Line, 50/200 cm
Syringes with leur lock 50, 20, 10, 5, 3 cc	Manifold	Disposable Needles 26 G/26.5 G
Jelco 18/20/22	Contrast Omnipaque	Disposable Needles 23 G/23.5 G
Femoral Puncture Needle 18 G	Contrast Visipaque	Disposable Needles 18 & 22 G
I.V. Cannula 18/20/22 G	Computer CDs	Three-way stopcock
Three-way extension 10 cm/50 cm	Inflation Device	Surgical Blade No. 11/21/10/15
Surgical Gloves No. 6/6.5/7/7.5/8	Easy Catch	Sheath Radial 4/5/6 fr
Diagnostic Catheters	Guide Wire	Sheath Femoral 5/6/7 fr
Inj. Atropine	P.T.C.A Wire	Inj. Adrenalin
Inj. Avil	P.T.C.A Balloon	Inj. Heparin
Inj. Efcorlin	Inj. Emeset	Inj. Rantac
Inj. Lasix	Inj. Betaloc	Inj. Cordarone
Inj. N.T.G 25mg	Inj. Norad	Inj. Glyco-P
Inj. Isolin	Inj. Dilzem	Inj. Lox 2%
Normal Saline 100 ml/500 ml/1000 ml	Inj. Taxim	Inj. Nikoran 2 mg/48 mg
Guide Wire 0.32-150/35-150 J/S Tip	Inj. Pantodac	Guide Wire 0.35-260/35-260
Guide Wire 0.35-260/35-260 J/S Tip	Inj. RL 500/1000 ml	Inj. DNS 500/1000 ml

ECG Electrodes	I.V. Set	Pressure Line, 50/200 cm
Inj. Dobutrax	Inj. Dopamine	Betadine solution
Tab. Ecosprin	Inj. Augmentin	Coronary Stents
I.A.B.P Balloon		

KEY PERFORMANCE INDICATORS (KPI):

Indicators may be developed for the hospital in consultation with the cardiologist and quality cell of the hospital.

Few Indicators are as follows;

1. **Percentage of PTCA performed in IHD patients:**
   Formula: Total number of PTCA performed in a given period divide by total number of patients with IHD presented in emergency ward/OPD in that period, divide by 100
2. **Timing of PTCA for patients with IHD:**
   Formula: Time in minutes from arrival at the hospital until the beginning of the PTCA divide by Number of patients with confirmed IHD receiving a PTCA within 12 hours after arrival to the hospital
3. **Percentage of repeat PTCA within 30 days of discharge in one year:**
   Formula: Numbers of patients having a second PTCA within 30 days of discharge divide by Number of PTCA performed during that period, multiply by 100
4. **Percentage of mortality following PTCA:**
5. **Percentage of Re-infarction after PTCA:**

Note: Similarly, KPI can be developed for CABG or other cases.

1. Number of reporting errors/1000 investigations
2. Rate of re-dos.
3. Percentage of Reports co-relating with clinical diagnosis
4. Average waiting time for diagnostic services.

DAILY AUDIT:

SN	Audit Point	Remark
1	Cleaning of area?	
2	BMW Management?	
3	Equipment Cleaning done?	
4	Hazard identification checklist Completed?	
5	Medicine storage & labelling with open and expiry date?	
6	Random Check on Medicine Expiry?	
7	Personal hygiene of staff?	
8	Autoclave Sets Expiry?	
9	Fridge and room temperature?	

Remarks:

Signature of senior staff/Area In-charge:

Signature of auditor:

VARIOUS CHECKLISTS OF CATH LAB SERVICES:

A. Check List for ANGIOPLASTY/ANGIOGRAPHY:

Patient Name:	Age/Sex:	
Diagnosis:		
SN	**Check**	**Yes/No**
1	Lab test report attached (TLC/DLC, Hb, Blood Group, RBS, Urea, Creatinine, Electrolytes, SGPT, SGOT, BT/CT, PT, HIV, HBsAg)?	
2	ECG present?	
3	Height & Weight recorded?	
4	Chest X-ray present?	
5	Consent Taken?	
6	Part prepared?	
7	Patient is Nil Orally	
Signature of the Resident Doctor/Technician:		

B. Cath Lab Safety Check List:

To be filled by the Cath Nurse/Cath Technician

Patient Name: ....

Procedure Name: ....

Date & Time: ....

Consultant Name: ....

Nurse/Technician Name: ....

Diagnosis: ....

Note; All answers must be in "YES"

SN	Check Point	Remark
1	Patient/Relative has been explained about the procedure?	
2	Patient identified by two identifiers?	
3	Procedure Confirmed?	
4	Team Members confirmed?	
5	Consent Signed?	
6	Allergies any? If yes describe:	
7	Medications given? Aspirin, Clopidogrel, Atorvastatin,	
8	Any other medication?	
9	Antibiotic given? If yes start time:	
10	Investigation reports done & reviewed?	
11	Implants/Equipment available?	
12	Relevant Images Reviewed?	

Signature of Nursing Staff:

Signature of Technician:

Signature of Cardiologist:

C. Cath Lab Utilisation:

Total Functional Hours	Number of hours utilised	Utilisation Rate

Prepared By: .... Approved By: ....

RECORDS/DOCUMENTS:

1. Procedure Register
2. Inventory Register
3. Medicine Consumption Register
4. Consent forms of - TPI, PPI, AICD, IABP, CAG, PTCA & PTRA.
5. Undertaking forms
6. Pre & post procedure check list
7. Radiation protection guide lines.
8. Pharmacy Indent forms.
9. AMC/Maintenance records.

BIBLIOGRAPHY, REFERENCES & ACKNOWLEDGMENTS:

1. Mahatma Gandhi Medical College and Hospital, Sitapur, Jaipur

   https://www.mgmch.org/departments/cardiac-care
2. Standard Operating Procedure (SOP) for those presenting to the Emergency at the Department of Cardiology King George's medical University Lucknow.
3. "Standard Operating Procedures SOP For Hospitals 2nd Edition" by Dr. Arun K. Agarwal
4. "Duties & Responsibilities of Hospital Staff" by Dr. Arun Kumar
5. "Checklists for Hospitals" by Dr. Arun K. Agarwal
6. Standard Operating Procedures (SOP) For Hospitals In India: Complete with Stationery Formats Used in Various Departments in a Hospital– 19 July 2022 by Arun K. Agarwal
7. Six Sigma Multispeciality Hospital, Nasik, India
8. Shalby Hospital, Mohali, Punjab, India
9. BBC Heart Care Pruthi Hospital, Punjab, India
10. Rockland Hospital, Manesar, India
11. Duties and Responsibilities of a Perfusionist. Brian Schwartz, CCP September 2, 2003

Chapter – 7

DEPARTMENT OF DENTISTRY

INDEX

    c. Procedure for Taking OPG
    d. Procedure for Dental Chair
    e. Procedure for RVS
    f. Risk Management
22. Standards in Dental Practice
23. Principals of Dental Practice
24. Various Checklists
    a. Checklist Dental Department
    b. Checklist Dental Department Planning
    c. Checklist Dental Services
    d. Checklist patient satisfaction Survey
    e. Check List for Purchasing an Equipment
    f. Checklist for Infection Control
25. Key Performance Indicators (KPI)
26. Daily Audit Points
27. Out Reach Programmes
28. Topics for CMEs/Conferences/Workshops
29. Stationary Formats
    a. Agreement For Outsourcing Dental Services: (Format-1)
    b. Agreement For Outsourcing Dental Services: (Format-2)
30. Guidelines For Patients:
    a. How to Prevent Cavities?
    b. How Frequently One Should Brush Teeth?
    c. Dietary Guidelines
31. Bibliography, References & Acknowledgments

INTRODUCTION:

Teeth are a very important part of the body, for good health starts with good oral health. The general well-being is associated with good oral health.

Dentistry is the branch of medicine that is involved in the study, diagnosis, prevention, and treatment of diseases, disorders and conditions of the oral cavity, maxillofacial area and the adjacent and associated structures and their impact on the human body.

Dental services include conservative dentistry and endodontics, oral and maxillo-facial, periodontal treatments and other common dental treatments.

The Department of Dentistry deals with the diagnosis and management of patients with dental diseases and trauma. The department works in collaboration with other clinical specialties like the Departments of ENT and Surgery.

The hospital also has a State of the art fully equipped dental implant centre which regularly conducts continued dental education (CDE).

The department of dental sciences is a multispecialty dental clinic. It is fully equipped with latest technology and facilities. It offers affordable dental treatment with national standards.

The team of dental surgeons include experienced Periodontist, Prosthodontist, Endodontist, Pedodontist and Orthodontist.

AIM, VISION & MISSION:

The motto of this department is to provide efficient and quality dental services to the community. It shall provide services in the field of diagnosis, treatment and prevention of oral diseases. In a hospital set up the department does not function independently but is a part of other clinics being run by the hospital.

AIM:

1. To provide these services to one and all irrespective of religion, caste or creed.
2. The focus of the department of Dentistry is to provide comprehensive dental care to its patients.
3. To extend high class and concurrently affordable Dental services to all strata of society.

Vision:

1. To be nationally recognised as a leader in patient care and service in the field of Dental Sciences.
2. To emerge as department of excellence by providing competent and compassionate dental services that are affordable to rural, poor and common people.
3. To offer patients high-quality dental treatment and to provide excellent oral health care and create an awareness regarding preventive measures.

Mission:

1. 'Oral health care for all'
2. To use innovative techniques in treating dental disorders.
3. To provide Dental treatment in large scale.
4. To create awareness about poor oral hygiene among common people.
5. To conduct social outreach programs and provide specialty services.
6. To achieve professional excellence in Dentistry by updating recent trends and innovations.
7. To conduct free dental camps for the needy to increase dental awareness and also to address dental problems among them
8. To continuously improve on departmental standards in providing best quality of preventive and curative Dental services.

INFRASTRUCTURE:

The department of dentistry of this hospital is having Dental OPD with two dental chairs.

It has all the required instruments and equipment to deal with all routine and complex dental problems.

EQUIPMENT:

A. Dental Equipment:

1. Dental chair Unit complete with foot control with;
   a. Hand Pieces: Air rotor hand pieces (Standard), Micro motor hand piece (Straight & Contra angle), Motorised Suction machine, Oil Free noise free air compressor
   b. Light Cure Unit

   c. Ultrasonic Scalar
   d. Dental X-Ray Unit
   e. Radio-Visio-Graph (RVG)
   f. Glass Bead Steriliser
   g. Doctor Stool
2. OPG Machine

B. Dental Instruments & Appliances:

Dental Mirrors	Dental Tweezers	Explorers (Dental Probes)
Hand Scalars	Extracting Forceps	Dental Elevator
Periosteal Elevators	Saliva Ejector	Mouth Prop
Amalgam plugger	Cement Spatula	Mallet (Hammer) & Chisel
Double ended curettes	Mortar & Pastel	Dental Wire Cutter
Dental Burrs	Excavators	Burnishers
Dental Files	Suction Tips	Dap pen dish- Glass/Ceramic
G.P. Point No. 15 to 80		
Cotton Forceps (Cotton Wool Holder)		
Dental Probes including Periodontal Probe		
Cheek, Lip, Tongue retractor		
Glass Slab 6" x 3" x 8-10 mm in thickness		

C. Prosthodontic Instruments:

Articulators	Blow torch	Bunsen burner
Callipers	Face bow	Fox plane
Glass mixing slab	Lecrons carver	Mixing bowls
Wax knife	Wax spatula	Wax carver
Willis's gauge		
Spatulas for mixing dental plaster		
Spatulas for mixing impression materials		

D. Dental Laboratory:

1. Crowns and Bridges
2. Metal Free Ceramics
3. Implant Prosthesis
4. Partial Dentures & Complete Dentures

E. General Equipment:

1. Dual/Multi frequency Apex locater
2. CBCT (Cone Beam Computer Tomography)

3. OPG
4. Amalgamator Motorised

SUB SPECIALITIES:

1. Endodontic
2. Oral and maxillofacial surgeons
3. Orthodontists
4. Periodontists
5. Pedodontist or Paediatric Dentist
6. Prosthodontist

SERVICES OFFERED & PROCEDURES CARRIED OUT:

The Department not only offers quality basic dental care to the rural and urban population but also provides specialized care.

Services provided can be classified under following heads.

1. Preventive Dentistry: Complete dental check-up. Comprehensive treatment plan to take care of disease already present and advice on how to prevent further dental problems.
2. Conservative Dentistry: Teeth with Cavities (Carious) are treated filled using tooth coloured filling materials.
3. Paediatric Dentistry:
4. Prosthodontics: Dental Implants, Fixed Bridges, Removable Dentures.
5. Periodontics: Routine Scaling, deep subgingival Scaling, Gingivectomy & Bone augmentation.
6. Oral & Maxillofacial surgery: Extraction of impacted tooth, Wisdom Tooth, Cysts and Tumours of the Jaws, Maxillofacial Trauma & TM joint disorders.
7. Orthodontics: to correct teeth deformity, cleft lip and palate correction.
8. Dental Implants: to replace extracted or missing tooth.
9. Cosmetic Dentistry: Bleaching and Whitening.
10. **Laser Dentistry:** LASER dentistry is a minimally invasive treatment option that is now available for a wide variety of procedures in dental practice. LASER dentistry is used in the treatment of oral mucosal lesions, root canal procedures, periodontal procedures, prosthodontic procedures, bleaching and other conservative dental treatments.

Some of the services are listed here.

1. Dental extractions & Dental Implants,
2. Root canal treatment (RCT) including Painless single sitting Root Canal Treatment,
3. Fillings (Restorations),
4. Crowns & Bridges,
5. Scaling & Polishing
6. Dentures (complete or partial),
7. Intra Oral X-rays
8. Light Cure Treatment & Crowning
9. Prosthetic treatment,
10. Tooth Impaction, Flap, Malocclusion,

11. Cosmetic Dentistry (Tooth Whitening)
12. Braces,
13. Minor Surgical Procedures:
    a. Dental Abscess,
    b. Apicectomy, Gingivectomy and, Removal of cyst etc.
    c. Fracture Wiring
4. Periodontal surgeries,
5. Prosthodontia (Trauma including vehicular accident),
6. Maxillo-facial and periodontal surgeries,
7. Sub mucus fibrosis (SMF),
8. Subluxation and arthritis of Temporo-mandibular Joints,
9. Pre-cancerous lesions and Leucoplakias,

OPD SERVICES

1. Extractions:

Introduction:

Dental extraction is dreaded by the patients almost more than any surgical procedures due to pain phobia

The extraction of teeth is a minor surgical procedure involving the bony & soft tissues of the oral cavity. A great majority of dental extractions can be carried out as routine procedure in the dental office however Hospitalization is required for some patients who are poor surgical risk for their systemic problems.

Indication for extraction of Tooth:

1. Periodontal disease accounts for the most-common cause for tooth extractions when the support of the tooth is destroyed & success of periodontal therapy is not there the tooth has to be extracted even if the patient desires to save the tooth.
2. Dental caries and its squeal.
3. Non-vital tooth with acute or chronic pulpitis where root canal treatment is not possible for various reasons are indicated for extraction.
4. Teeth with infected pulp that has led to peri-apical disease where teeth are not treatable by endodontic procedures with or without apicoectomy.
5. Teeth mechanically interfering with placement of partial dentures & bridges.
6. Over retained deciduous teeth that may deflect or prevent the normal eruption of permanent teeth.
7. Some teeth require extraction during the course of orthodontic treatment e.g., therapeutic extraction of the teeth line promotes is carried out for gaining space during realignment of the malposed teeth.
8. Malposed teeth whose realignment is not possible by orthodontic technique are indicated for extraction.
9. Serial Extractions – Few deciduous teeth are extracted in chronological order to provide enough space for permanent success to achieve stability of the dental arch.
10. Retention of impacted & un-erupted teeth is sometimes responsible for facial pain, TMJ problems and bony pathology. Impacted teeth are considered responsible for malocclusion and are indicated for removal.
11. Supernumery teeth are also indicated for extraction for the same reason as mentioned above.
12. Teeth in the line of fracture- this has been a controversial subject for many years. A tooth in the line of fracture should be extracted if it is fractured a source of infection or interfering with fracture solution or healing of the fracture.

13. Teeth with fractured roots especially if root is fractured in the coronal half.
14. In patient of oral malignancy where radiation therapy is to be given, the teeth which cannot be maintained in sound condition are indicated for extraction.
15. Teeth that are causing bony pathology like osteomyelitis or neoplasm etc. should be extracted.

Contraindications for extractions

A. Local Factors:
   1. Acute infection with on uncontrolled cellulites.
   2. Acute pericoronitis especially in selection to mandible third molar because of the fact that it has direct access to spaces in the neck.
   3. Acute infections like gingivitis and stomatitis.
   4. extractions of maxillary premolars and molars is contraindicated in acute maxillary sinusitis
   5. Tooth embedded in malignant growth is not extracted since it leaves behind a non-healing wound.
   6. Extraction of tooth from irradiated jaw may develop osteoradio necrosis because of low vascular supply & hence is not-generally carried out.

B. System Factors
   1. Uncontrolled Diabetes Mellitus.
   2. Cardiac problems.
   3. Pregnancy.
   4. Bleeding Disorders.
   5. Medically compromised patient.
   6. Patient on steroid therapy.
   7. Renal failure.
   8. Psychosis and neurosis.
   9. Patient on anticoagulant therapy.
   10. Patient with liver disorders.
   11. Patients with toxic goitre.

Anaesthesia:

Local Anaesthesia is the best and safest method for most of the ambulatory patients reporting for extraction. General Anaesthesia is used in cases where multiple extractions are to be carried out and the local Anaesthesia is not indicated for systemic and local reason. There patient should be intubated and oropharynx is packed off completely before carrying out the extraction.

Complications Involved in extractions

1. Fracture of tooth
2. Alveolar bone fracture.
3. Maxillary tuberosity fracture.
4. Mucosal tear.
5. Oro- antral opening.
6. Tooth pushed into spaces of neck.
7. Neural Injuries.
8. Injury to soft tissues.
9. Haemorrhage.
10. Injuries to the adjoining teeth.

Post-Extraction complications

1. Post-operative Haemorrhages.
2. Pain and swelling.
3. Dry socket.
4. Osteomyelitis.
5. Bacteraemia.
6. Precipitation of systemic problem.

2. Impactions:

A tooth should be termed as impacted only if the root formation is completed and yet it has not erupted fully up to the final position.

A tooth may remain un-erupted or partially erupted in the mouth. A partially erupted tooth may be mal-positioned in the dental arch, erupting buccally or lingually to the arch.

Frequency of impaction:

1. Maxillary third molars.
2. Mandibular third molars.
3. Maxillary canines
4. Mandibular premolars
5. Mandibular canines
6. Maxillary premolar
7. Supernumerary teeth
8. Maxillary central incisors
9. Maxillary lateral incisors.

Complication Associated with Impaction:

1. Infection.
2. Pain.
3. Fracture of jaw.
4. Trismus.
5. Chronic cheek biting.
6. Mal-alignment of other teeth.
7. Other complications.

3. Fractures of Maxillo-facial Region:

A fracture is a break in the continuity of a bone when stretched or bent beyond its elastic limit.

Signs and Symptoms of fracture:

1. Patient will have oedema of the face.
2. Presence of ecchymosed on the face i.e., subcutaneous haemorrhage leading to discoloration of the face.
3. Deformity of face leading to facial asymmetry.
4. Disturbance in occlusion.
5. There is abnormal mobility of the fragment when the arch is broken.
6. There is difficulty in opening the mouth leading to loss of function.

7. Loss of sensation over the face e.g., Numbness of the side of the lower lip is due to inferior alveolar nerve involvement whereas the involvement of the infra orbital nerve will be responsible for the numbness of the upper lip.
8. Patient may be having bleeding from the mouth, nose, and eye.
9. Subconjunctival Haemorrhage is suggestive of fracture involving the bony orbit.
10. There may be CSF rhinorrhoea i.e., CSF leak through the nose and CSF otorrhoea i.e., leak from the ear.

Radiological examination

The following radiographs are generally advised.

Extra oral radiographs.

1. Posteroanterior (PA) view of mandible.
2. Right and left lateral oblique view of mandible. There are advised for left body & ramus of the mandible.
3. X-ray for the temporo-mandible joint area both in open and closed mouth position.
4. Orthopantomography reveals complete mandible from condyle to condyle.
5. Posteroanterior (PA) view maxilla in water's position is advised for fracture of the maxilla.

Intraoral Radiographs:

1. Intra oral periapical radiographs help to diagnosis the alveolar fractures.
2. Occlusal view of the mandible to see split fractures in body of the mandible.
3. Occlusal view of the maxilla to see any midline split & fractures of the palates.

Treatment of fractures of the Mandible

1. Reduction:
   It is 2 types.
   a. Closed reduction:
      i. Reduction by manipulation.
      ii. Reduction by traction.
   b. Open reduction.
2. Fixation:
3. Immobilization:
4. Mobilization of Jaws: after the fractured bone has healed

Techniques of wiring

1. Gilmer's direct method of wiring.
2. Ivy eyelet wiring or interdentally eyelet wiring. Multiple loop wiring.
3. Arch –Bar wiring.
4. Risdon's method of horizontal wiring.

Splints

Cast metal splints acrylic cap splints and gunning splints are used for fixation and immobilization of the fractured mandible especially in the body region.

1. Cast-Metal Splints
2. Acrylic cap splints
3. Circumferential wiring
4. Gunning splints.

External Pin Fixation:

Tran Osseous Wiring:

Intra Osseous Wiring:

Use of lag screws and bone plates:

Indication for bone plating:

1. Where there are absolute contraindications to intermaxillary fixation/wiring e.g., Epileptics mentally retarded patients.
2. When patients want to return back to work early.
3. Edentulous jaws where there is loss of bone segment & need of maintaining the gap or grafting is indicated.
4. In sub condylar and angle fractures of the mandible, when the joint is required to be functionally active.

Contraindications for bone plating:

1. In heavily contaminated fractured where there is active infection and discharge.
2. In badly commented fractures where open reduction may pose risk of compromising the vascularity.
3. In children having mixed dentition when there is a danger of injury to the developing tooth germs.
4. Presence of gross pathological abnormalities in the bone.

4. Osteomyelitis of the Jaw:

Osteomyelitis is the inflammation of the soft tissue of the bone namely marrow spaces of the spongiosa and the haversian system of the cortex.

Osteomyelitis more frequently occurs in mandible than in maxilla in an adult. Whereas in infants more bone is available in the maxilla then in the mandible hence maxilla is more commonly involved.

Classification of Osteomyelitis

a. Acute Osteomyelitis:
    1. Pyogenic osteomyelitis in infants and nurslings.
    2. Acute infective Osteomyelitis in young children.
    3. Acute infective Osteomyelitis in adults.
b. Chronic Osteomyelitis:
    1. Chronic suppurative Osteomyelitis.
    2. Chronic Sclerosing Osteomyelitis.
    3. Garre's Osteomyelitis.
c. Chronic Osteomyelitis associated with systemic diseases.
    1. Tuberculosis of the jaw.
    2. Syphilis of the jaw.
    3. Actinomycosis of the jaw.
d. Necrosis of the jaw due to
    1. Chemicals
    2. Electro-coagulation.
    3. Radiation.
e. Dry socket.

Management:

The management lies in good antibiotic cover. Culture and sensitivity tests should be done as early as possible when the pus is available abscess formed may be incised and drained Inta-orally to lessen the toxaemia. If sequestration this occurred it should be removed. In addition to the surgical management, the patient should be put on good nutritious diet. Dehydration should always be taken care of in this age group.

5. Apicoectomy:

In case of root canal filling has been done pre-operatively an intra oral periapical X-ray should be taken to determine the accuracy of filling and level at which the root should be cut. The design of muco-periosteal flap to be raised should be such that it must have an adequate exposure of the periapical pathology good vascularity of the margin of the flap should be supported by healthy bone when replaced back. However, the design of the flap is purely the choice of the surgeon. The muco-periosteal flap should not be reflected beyond the muscle attachment or beyond the defect to avoid a massive post-operative haematoma. After the flap has been raised, a window in to the periapical defect is made in the absence of any perforation in the bone. If the perforation is present opening is enlarged with rongeur forceps chisel or burs to provide an adequate exposure. The root-apex is identified. A double ended curative or a large excavator is used for curettage of the periapical granuloma. If a cyst is present, it should be enucleated using a periosteal elevator or curettes. The root apex is resected using a flat fissure bur at a level in order to remove all pathological tissue attached to the root-apex. The procedure should not be carried out with a chisel as it causes invaluably the luxation of the tooth. The bevelling of the cut surface of the root towards the labial plate of bone helps in making a retrograde filling and sealing of the apex. In case the filling has not been done pre-operatively the root canal should be cleaned and filling is done at this stage. If a retrograde filling in silver amalgam is required. An inverted cone bur is used to undercut the cavity for retention of the amalgam. The area is made dry and silver amalgam filling is done. If a Gutta Percha filling had been done through conventional coronal approach, the apical seal is obtained by cutting the excess filling and burnishing the canal.

6. Enucleation of Cyst:

Cyst:

A cyst is a sac like pathological structure occurring either in hard or soft tissues of the body, containing liquid or semi-solid which is surrounded by a wall of connective tissue and is usually lined by epithelium.

Classification:

A. Congenital cyst (Brachial cleft-type).
   1. Thyroglossal cyst and epidermoid cyst.
   2. Dermoid cyst and epidermoid cyst.
   3. Brachiogenic cyst.
B. Development Cyst:
   1. Non – Odontogenic cysts:
      a. Fissural type:
         i. Incisive canal cyst.
         ii. Nasoalveolar cyst.
         iii. Globulo maxillary.
         iv. Median Cyst.

b. Retention Type:
   i. Mucocele
   ii. Ranula.

Other Cysts:

1. Odontogenic Cyst:
2. Periodontal Cyst:
3. Gingival cyst
4. Lateral cyst.
5. Periapical Cyst
6. Residual Cyst.
7. Primordial or follicular cyst:
8. Dentigerous or eruption Cyst.
9. Central type.
10. Lateral type.
11. Circumferential type.
12. Multiple type.
13. Kerato cyst
14. Haemorrhagic or traumatic bone cyst
15. Neoplastic variety [ameloblastom]

Diagnosis of cyst:

- Radiological Examination
- Aspiration
- Histopathological Examination

Management of cyst:

The various operative used for treatment of various types of cysts are based on the following principles.

1. Elimination of cystic lining along with its contents.
2. Decompression of the intra cystic pressure.
3. Elimination of cystic lining.
4. Preservation of the teeth.
5. Preservation of important anatomical structures.
6. Preservation of recurrence of cyst.

Operative procedure:

1. Enucleation of the cyst and primally closure.
2. Enucleation and open packing.
   - With removal of the tooth.
   - With tooth conservation.
   - Combined with Caldwell-luck operation.
   - Combined with fixation of the pathological fracture.
3. Marsupialization
4. Combination Procedure: - Marsupialization followed by enucleation after the cavity shrinks.

7. Marsupialization of Cyst:

Also called "partsch operation" It is indicated in excessively large cysts where there are chances of doubtful enucleation. It involves deroofing of the cyst along with adjoining bone and muco-periosteum so that the cystic lining becomes continuous with the lining of the oral cavity.

Indications for Marsupialization

1. If the cyst is very large and placed in an inaccessible area from where complete enucleation is not possible.
2. Large cysts that have weakened the bone and there is a fear of pathological fracture if enucleation is tried.
3. Dentigerous cysts in younger patients where a chance for eruption of an un-erupted tooth is there.
4. In large cysts when there are chances of entering into adjacent paranasal sinuses or nasal cavity.
5. A large cyst where there are chances of damage to the neurovascular bundle if enucleation is tried.

Post-operative Complications:

1. Oedema or post-operative swelling.
2. Infection
3. Haematoma formation.
4. Neural Injuries.
5. Oro-antral Fistula.
6. Oro nasal opening.
7. Fracture of the bone.

8. Abscesses:

Tooth abscess Definition: -

A tooth abscess is an infection of the tooth or root of the tooth.

Causes:

The cause of a tooth abscess is an infection. So, the question in looking at the cause of tooth abscess, is how did the infection get there?

Common Causes of tooth abscess:

The infection was there when the tooth had dental work performed on it; such as a crown, or root canal, or filling. Normally the tooth had been compromised by infection through a cavity in the tooth. The germ, that would later go on to form the tooth abscess, was NOT completely killed off when the tooth was repaired. Secondly, the cause of a tooth abscess may be time delayed. If it has been a while since the tooth had work on it - then, for some reason the tooth abscess germ, which was there, is now out of control and has now formed a tooth abscess.

Symptoms:

There are several tooth abscess symptoms:

The tooth abscess symptoms in a dead tooth - A tooth where the nerves have been removed or died - tend to follow stages, based on the extent of the swelling of the tooth abscess. An early tooth abscess symptom is the feeling that the tooth may be becoming loose, even though the tooth shows very little movement at all. This symptom may last about two days.

A slightly later indicating tooth abscess symptom is the feeling that the tooth is sitting a bit higher than usual - caused by the tooth abscess's infection pus build up - its swelling or enlargement

- underneath the tooth, which raises the tooth to slightly rise up. The symptom of pain caused by the tooth abscess may or may not be present at this time. The later stage symptom of a tooth abscess is a combination of the symptoms of pain, discomfort and sometimes the feeling that the tooth is about to explode - I have a crown, so this feeling that the tooth is swelling and trapped by the crown is very real.

In the real late stages, tooth abscess symptoms include, when left untreated, the tooth abscess infection will eat away the jaw near it, cause the teeth to drop out. In the very last stage, the tooth abscess symptoms include not only the disfigurement of the face through the compromise of the soft facial bones, but also often in death, as the tooth abscess infection can spread throughout the body, causing heart attack and so on.

The tooth abscess symptoms in a live tooth are normally sharp pain on contact with fast airflow, such as breathing in and out really, really fast through the teeth. The air enters the cavity and irritates the abscess. Generally, if a tooth reacts painfully to cold fluids, it is a good sign that the tooth can be repaired with the nerve kept intact. On the other-hand, if the tooth reacts badly to warm or hot fluids, it suggests the tooth nerve has been compromised by the tooth abscess, which means it will likely be more costly to repair, as it may involve the removal of the nerve - root canal treatment - leaving you with a dead tooth.

Treatment:

The common treatment of tooth abscess normally involves three options:

1. One tooth abscess treatment option is the use of antibiotics, when the tooth is already dead and sealed by a dentist. The antibiotics kill the germ responsible for the tooth abscess and the body then repairs the bone and tooth, normally pretty well.
2. The second tooth abscess treatment is root canal treatment, which is the drilling out of the root canal and infected area, cleansing out the infection, and then resealing the tooth. Antibiotics appear to be rarely prescribed, as the dentist will normally paint the insides with a germ killer.
3. The third tooth abscess treatment involves extracting the tooth, cleansing the area, then allowing the wound to heal - antibiotics may be prescribed.

9. Diseases of Maxillary Sinus:

It is the inflammation of the mucous membrane of the maxillary sinus. The disease takes an acute, sub-acute or choric depending on the virulence of the organism and resistance of the host.

The bacteria may gain access from the following sources.

1. Nasal cavity: It is the most frequent route of infection following cold especially in case of children. Upper respiratory tract-infections, allergic rhinitis following measles diphtheria and whooping cough.
2. Dental diseases: Dental infection around the teeth is the second major cause of maxillary sinusitis.
   a. Acute maxillary sinusitis:
   b. Sub-acute sinusitis
   c. Chronic sinusitis

Treatment:

It is aimed at the control of an infection and removal of the causative factors. Patient is advised to maintain a good oral hygiene & a cover of antibiotics is started. If the condition is acute and nasal origin attempt is made to shrink the mucosa by spraying, some decongestant ephedrine spray Antihistaminic and steam inhalation is advised.

Caldwell-Luc operation:

The direct visual examination of the maxillary antrum is best made by cutting a window in the anterio-lateral wall of the maxillary antrum and this approach is further made use of and is combined with closure of an Oro-antral fistula procedure for obtaining better results.

Indications:

a. Removal of tooth root from the antrum that has been accidentally pushed up during course of extraction and the removal through the socket could not be achieved.
b. Removal of foreign bodies like antroliths from the sinus.
c. Chronic maxillary sinusitis where the removal of the lining of the antrum is desired.
d. For removal of cyst from the antrum.
e. For removal of any benign growth of the maxillary.
f. For control of any active haemorrhagic following trauma of the maxillary sinus.
g. For lifting the floor of the orbit in case of blow out fractures.
h. For removal of an impacted maxillary canine or third molar that is misdirected and partly erupting in the antrum.
i. This operation can be modified for simultaneous closure of the Oro-antral fistula by buccal advancement flap operation technique.

10. Temporomandibular Joint Problem:

a. Dislocation of TMJ:-
  - Acute
  - Chronic
  - Subluxation
  - Unilateral and bilateral

b. Ankylosis of TMJ:-
c. Condylar hyperplasia
d. Condylar hypoplasia

PERIODONTICS

Services:

a. Removal of calculus through scaling
b. Gingivectomy
c. Curettage
d. Treatment of halitosis & pyorrhoea,
e. Flap surgery.

Scaling:

Scaling is the process by which plaque & calculus are removed from super gingival & sub gingival tooth surfaces.

Root Planning:

It is the process by which residual embedded calculus and portions of cementum are removed from the root to produce a smooth hard, clean surface.

Gingival Curettage:

This consists of the removal of the inflamed soft tissue lateral to pocket wall.

Gingivectomy:

It is the excision of gingival by removing the pocket wall; gingivectomy provides visibility & accessibility for complete calculus removal & thorough smoothing of roots creating a favourable environment of a physiologic gingival contour.

The Periodontal Flap:

It is a section of gingival and/or mucosa surgically tissue to provide visibility of and access to the bone & root surface.

Respective Osseous Surgery:

It is defined as the procedure by which changes in the alveolar bone can be accomplished to rid it of deformities induced by the periodontal disease process or other factors such as exostosis & tooth supraeruption

Osseous surgery can be additive or subtractive osseous surgery.

OPERATIVE DENTISTRY

Conservative Dentistry: Is the art and science of the diagnosis, treatment prognosis of defects of teeth that do not require full coverage restorations for corrections.

Conservative Treatment Procedures can be categorized into three primary treatment needs.

a. Caries or decayed teeth.
b. Malformed, discoloured or fractured teeth.
c. Restoration replacement or repair

Tooth Preparation: Is defined as the mechanical alteration of a defective, injured or diseased tooth to best receive a restorative material that will re-establish a healthy state for the tooth, including aesthetic corrections, along with normal form & function.

Restorative Dental Materials are follows:

a. Silver amalgam restorations
b. Composite restorations: also called light cured restorations.
c. Glass Ionomers.
d. Direct filling gold restorations.

ENDODONTICS

Injury to the calcified structures of teeth and to the supporting tissues by noxious stimuli may cause changes in the pulp and peri-radicular tissues.

Irreversible inflammatory changes caused by severe injury can lead to necrosis of the pulp.

In such cases the diseased tooth & pulp requires root canal treatment.

RCT

Steps in root canal treatment:

a. Removal of coronal pulp
b. Biomechanical preparation of the root canal which includes cleaning & shaping.

c. Irrigation.
d. Obturation: Which involves filling of the root canal with a biocompatible substance called gutta percha.
e. Capping of the crown

Pulpotomy:

Pulpotomy is the removal of coronal pulp while preservation of the vitality of radicular pulp. (This is done when only coronal pulp is infected while radicular pulp is uninfected)

A dressing is placed over the pulp stump to protect it and promote healing.

Two most commonly used dressings contain:

- Calcium hydroxide or formocresol.

Bleaching:

Bleaching procedures is the restoration of normal colour of a tooth by decolorizing the stain with a powerful oxidizing or reducing agent.

Bleaching Agents:

Superoxol: 30% solution of hydrogen peroxide by weight & 100% by volume in pure distilled water.

Sodium per borate: Is a stable white powder, soluble in water & decomposes into sodium metaborate & H2 O2 releasing Oxygen.

PROSTHODONTICS

Replacement of teeth:

Fixed: Implants
Porcelain bridges

Removable: Complete acrylic dentures
Partial acrylic dentures
Cast partial dentures
Flexible dentures

Complete Denture

It is a dental prosthesis which replaces the entire dentition and associated structures of the maxilla and mandible.

Steps in fabrication of a complete Denture:

1. Diagnosis and treatment planning.
2. Pouring of the Diagnostic cast using dental plaster.
3. Pre-prosthetic surgery.
4. Making primary impression using impression compound.
5. Pouring primary cast using dental plaster.
6. Making secondary impression.
7. Pouring master cast.
8. Recording jaw relation.
9. Articulation.
10. Trial verification

11. Wax-up & processing the denture & finishing
12. Insertion.

Fixed denture

Can be of metallic or ceramic material

Fixed partial denture

It is a partial denture that is cemented to natural teeth or roots and which furnish the primary support to the prosthesis.

Steps: In fabrication of a fixed partial denture:

1. Diagnosis and treatment planning.
2. Crown preparation of abutment teeth.
3. Bite registration.
4. Making of impression.
5. Pouring of cast.
6. Fabrication of the partial denture.
7. Fixing or cementing of the partial denture to the prepared abutment teeth.

DENTAL IMPLANTS

A dental implant is an insert in to the jaw to support a crown or fixed or removable denture.

Materials used in dental implant:

- Metals: Titanium & its alloys
  Stainless steel
  Cobalt-chromium-molybdenum alloys
  Surface coated titanium
  Gold
  Tantalum
- Ceramics: Hydroxyapatite
  Bio-Glass
  Aluminium Oxide
- Polymers and composites
- Others: Carbons.

ORTHODONTICS

Treatment of mal/misaligned teeth

- Malocclusion
- Cross bites/Scissor bites
- Deep bites/Open bites
- Protrusion of teeth
- Retro-clined teeth
- Spacing of teeth

PEDODONTICS

Paediatric dentistry is the practices & teaching of comprehensive preventive and therapeutic oral health care of child from birth through adolescence

Professional Therapy

1. Oral prophylaxis
2. Complete rehabilitation of all carious lesions.
3. Antimicrobial therapy (Chlorhexidine gel)
4. Pit and fissure sealants
5. Topical fluoride applications
6. Diet modification
7. Dental health education
8. Nursing bottle carries
9. Rampant carries.

Home care

1. Home fluoride application
2. Sustained release fluoride tablets
3. Fluoride gel application
4. Fluoride dentifrice
5. Salivary Substitutes

ORAL PATHOLOGY

Biopsies

Oral pathology represents the confluence of basic sciences and clinical dentistry. Knowledge in this field is acquired through the adaptation of methods and disciplines of those sciences basic to dental practice like gross & microbiology anatomy, and through information and observation of pat.

DENTAL EMERGENCIES:

1. Dental Pain
2. Irreversible Pulpitis
3. Apical Periodontitis
4. Apical Abscess
5. Cellulitis
6. Dental Trauma

MEDICAL EMERGENCIES IN DENTAL PRACTICE:

1. Hypoglycaemia
2. Steroid Crisis
3. Anaphylactic Shock & Other Drug Reactions
4. Epilepsy
5. Acute Asthmatic Attack

6. Inhaled Foreign Bodies
7. Cardiac Arrest

STAFFING/MANPOWER:

1. Dental Surgeon (Dentist)
2. Dental Hygienists
3. Dental Technician/Dental Assistants
4. Dental Lab Technician

DUTIES & RESPONSIBILITIES:

A. Dental Surgeon (Dentist):

1. To diagnose and treat diseases, injuries and malfunctions of teeth, gum and oral cavity.
2. To be in proper attire and shall always wear apron and ID card.
3. To wear personal protective equipment (PPE) before starting the treatment.
4. To examine and treat the patient using all the resources available at his/her end.
5. To guide the patient about preventive dental care and good dental habits.
6. To order diagnostic measures, such as x-rays, models, etc.
7. To perform dental procedures, such as extractions, root canals, and filling cavities.
8. To do restorative (prosthodontic/orthodontic etc) work depending on his/her field of speciality.
9. To diagnose and treat primarily diseases of teeth, gums.
10. To prescribe medications for dental problems, such as pain medications or antibiotics.
11. To carry out dental work to restore a tooth or provide artificial tooth/denture.
12. To carry out oral surgery, if trained for that.

Summary:

1. Examining patients, making decisions and solving problems.
2. Documenting all relevant information. Preparing medical records.
3. Updating his/her knowledge by attending CME programs and seminars.
4. Guiding, Training, and motivating juniors.
5. To respect the privacy and dignity of patients.
6. To provide consultation to patients of other doctors whenever asked for.
7. To work following all legal and social obligations.
8. Helping the society in maintain good oral health.

B. Dental Hygienist:

Dental hygienists are mainly responsible for cleaning teeth.

1. To support dental surgeons in routine dental procedures.
2. To work under guidance and supervision of a dental surgeon in the hospital. (Can also work independently, but will not commence the treatment till specific instructions are given by dental surgeon).
3. To maintain good personal hygiene and wear prescribed dress.
4. To take phone calls and schedule appointments of this department.

5. To prepare dental chair for patients as per prescribed policies and procedures.
6. To ensure good cleanliness of the area & equipment – dental chair - and proper sterilisation of instruments.
7. To welcome patient inside the department and prepare patient for dental surgeon to carry out required procedure.
8. To perform All scaling (Oral prophylaxis) and polishing of teeth independently whether manual or with ultrasonic instruments.
9. To motivate and educate patients and community, to maintain good oral hygiene and teach correct brushing techniques for individuals in oral health camps.
10. Shall be responsible for patient's transfer in and out of the department.
11. To take dental x-rays when asked for.
12. To assist dentist during treatment. To provide chair-side assistance.
13. They are responsible for screening the patient for his/her oral health condition and recording vitals.
14. To refer patient to dental surgeon for any unusual findings or doubt, immediately.
15. They may be asked to carry out certain (basic) procedures for which they are trained such as; scaling, cleaning and polishing, extraction of a loose tooth.
16. To take dental impressions for lab work; making of denture, bridges, models and other prostheses.
17. To wash, clean and sterilise all the required instruments.
18. To ensure availability of sufficient supplies in the department. To indent and receive the supplies.
19. To maintain OPD and procedure records. Any other record required as per hospital policy has to be maintained.
20. To ensure that all information related to the patient is kept confidential.
21. To educate patients on oral hygiene and good brushing and flossing techniques.
22. To guide patients on pre and post operative precautions.
23. To assist in organising field camps.
24. To ensure proper preventive and corrective maintenance of the chair.
25. To carry out other assignments as per instruction of seniors.

C. Dental Technician (Assistant):

Dental Technicians are responsible for fabricating and repair of dentures, fabricating dental prosthetics including bridges, crowns, and dentures. Maintain dental laboratory records

1. To prepare the department ready for patient examination.
2. To be responsible for proper functioning of dental chair and other equipment of this department.
3. To sterilise dental instruments required during dental treatment.
4. To adhere to infection control policies.
5. To ensure cleanliness of the department.
6. To call patient from waiting area on schedule/turn and to make the patient comfortable on the dental chair.
7. To take dental history and monitor patient's vitals.
8. To expose and develop x-ray films.
9. To assist the dental surgeon in dental surgeries and in managing dental patients in OPD by providing chair-side assistance.
10. To work as a 'dental technician' in his absence.
11. To provide instruments to dentist during treatment.
12. To clean, wash and sterilise instruments.

13. To prepare gauze pieces, pads for day-to-day use.
14. To ensure proper supply of central medical gases (suction, compressed air and oxygen).
15. To provide material by mixing and putting in patient's mouth.
16. To keep patients' mouth clean and dry during a treatment.
17. To advise patients on oral hygiene.
18. To take impressions and cast for dental lab work.
19. To carry out minor dental procedures such as cleaning and polishing of teeth.
20. To answer phone calls.
21. To schedule appointments and to help dentist in taking patients in serial order.
22. To ensure proper billing for each patient.
23. To indent and receive dental material from the hospital stores or market.
24. To cooperate and help in maintenance/repair of equipment of this department.
25. To update all records and registers as required by the hospital.
26. To ensure confidentiality of information.
27. To keep inventory and consumption details of dental material.
28. To carry on other duties as assigned by seniors.

D. DENTAL LAB TECHNICIAN:

Basic duty is to construct and/or repair denture and dental appliances.

1. Will work under direct supervision of dental surgeon and in-charge of the dental laboratory.
2. To ensure good personal hygiene and wear prescribed dress or should be in uniform.
3. To assist dental surgeons in their day-to-day work.
4. To assist doctors during a dental surgery.
5. To carry out all work related to 'Dental Lab'.
6. To undertake the impressions and prepare dentures as required.
7. To manufacture dental prostheses like bridges, crowns, dentures as per specifications (moulds and samples) made available by the dentist.
8. To carry out all jobs required to manufacture dental prosthesis and other appliances such as preparing moulds, mixing and pouring dental material into moulds etc.
9. To work as a dental hygienist as and when required.
10. To ensure availability of supplies at all times. To indent and receive dental lab supplies. To replace expired material with fresh ones.
11. To ensure proper preventive and corrective maintenance of dental lab equipment.
12. Will be responsible for good cleanliness of the area and proper sterilisation of various instruments and articles such as impression trays, etc.
13. To maintain all records and registers as required by hospital policies and procedures.
14. To carry out other assignments as per instructions of dentist.

DENTAL RESTORATIVE MATERIALS & MEDICINES:

Zinc Oxide Eugenol	Silver Amalgam	Glass Ionomer Cement (GIC)
Calcium Hydroxide	Sodium Hypochloride	Gutta Percha (GP)
Eugenol 30-100ml.		

continued

Light Cure Composite	Ketorolac 10 mg tablet	Gum Paint (Tannic Acid)
Povidine-Iodine Germicide Gargle 20% w/v		
Glass Ionomer cement for restoration (Powder 12-15gm. With Liquid 6-9ml.)		

STANDARD OPERATING PROCEDURES:

A. Procedure for OPD:

1. Registration of each and every patient is done at central registration counter.
2. Patients are asked to wait in the waiting area.
3. The patient is guided inside the dental OPD on turn.
4. The dentist examines the patient and makes a provisional diagnosis.
5. Treatment has to be explained to the patient followed by required investigation, treatment or appointment and it should be entered in the appointment register with phone number and address of the patient.
6. Medication should be given in the prescription in neat legible handwriting.
7. Treatment should be done at the earliest and it should be neatly entered in the OPD card/ treatment register and signed by the dentist.

B. Procedure for IPD:

Procedures have been established for smooth functioning of this department.

Generally, patients are admitted for elective surgical cases, observation post surgical interventions and emergency trauma cases

1. Admission: A patient may be admitted from;
   a. From the OPD
   b. From the casualty
   c. Referred by some other healthcare facility
2. Patient Care:

   General admission procedure (completion of documents) is same as that for admission of any other surgical case.

   a. On admission all routine blood investigations are sent if not already done. E.g.
      - Routine blood investigations
      - AFB,
      - FNAC,
      - Radiological tests
      - 24 Hour urine test
   b. Orders for Medications and patient care are advised by the dental surgeon.
   c. Staff nurses on duty make sure that samples are sent and reports received.
   d. Daily rounds are taken by the Consultants.
   e. If cross reference is advised, nurse and doctor on duty make sure that concerned consultant is informed.
   f. Regular assessment of the patient is done by the doctor on duty.
   g. In case patient has to undergo an operative procedure, necessary consents are taken.
   h. PAC is carried out.

i. Blood if required, is arranged.
j. On the day of surgery patient is shifted to the operation theatre along with the ward nurse
k. Once the operative procedure is completed, the patient is shifted to the ward/ICU based on the patient condition or as decided by the anaesthetist.
l. Post operative investigations are sent by the doctor/nurse on duty.
m. Nursing care is carried out as per orders of the anaesthetist and operating surgeon.
n. Patient is discharged as per hospital protocol.

C. Procedure for Taking OPG:

1. Ask patients to remove jewellery, eyeglasses, and any metal objects that may obscure the images.
2. Instruct patients to stay very still while the x-ray is taken.
3. The patient's chin should be placed on a chin rest.
4. The jaws are held in place by biting down on a small disposable plastic guide.
5. Most OPGs are performed with the patient standing.
6. An exposure lasts a few seconds during which time the patient must remain still.
7. The film cassette is then removed and taken to a CR System.
8. Patients are advised to wear Lead aprons to avoid unnecessary exposure.

D. Procedure for Dental Chair:

BEFORE:

1. Make sure power supply is ON
2. Make sure Air and Water supply is in function [Check Air gauge after pressing Airotor pedal].
3. Movements to be checked before making patient sit for the procedure. Up/Down & Front/Back.
4. Make sure operating Light is working with High/Low Resolution.

SPITTOON:

1. Blood and saliva to be evacuated only with suction unit.
2. After each usage flush with water [Spittoon flush Button]

TUMBLER:

1. Use water from tumbler filler.

AFTER PROCEDURE:

1. Keep the chair in zero position.
2. Flush the spittoon for 1 to 2 minutes thoroughly.
3. Keep the foot control in place.
4. Switch off the Electrical system. [SWITCH OFF].

E. Procedure for RVS:

BEFORE USAGE:

1. Turn on Computer.
2. Run the Computer imaging Software application.
3. Configure the required X-ray parameter.

DURING USAGE:

1. Position the sensor at the appropriate area of the mouth.
2. The flat receptor side should face the X-ray source
3. Use of position system with paralleling technique is highly recommended.
4. After preparing the sensor for exposure, acquire an image by pressing the exposure button on the X-ray source.

F. Risk Management:

1. Be aware of the risks. Develop an understanding of those treatments and situations in dentistry that have a high probability of associated risk.
2. Develop controls to avoid or minimise the damage from risks. Remember that not all risks are clinical ones.
3. Treat patients as individuals and manage their level of expectation with case-able warnings and instructions.
4. Obtain the patient's consent to treatment.
5. Keep full, legible and accurate notes of all treatments and discussions with the patient. Update the medical history before starting a new treatment.
6. If a problem arises, contain the risk and manage the patient who has been affected in a prompt and caring manner.
7. Manage the problem that caused the damage.
8. Offer a prompt and appropriate response to any concerns raised by the patient.
9. Transfer the financial component of risk to an indemnifier like Dental Protection.
10. Regularly update your knowledge of dentistry.

STANDARDS IN DENTAL PRACTICE:

As per Indian Dental Association

Accessible, flexible and responsive services

- Standard 1 - Increase the merit of your clinic
- Standard 2 - Before the appointment
- Standard 3 - The patient's visits

Safe and effective care

- Standard 4 - Assess the patients' needs
- Standard 8 - Quality of care and treatment
- Standard 12 - Medical and other emergencies
- Standard 13 - Control of infection
- Standard 14 - Dental care environment

Effective communication and information

- Standard 5 - Deciding care and treatment
- Standard 6 - Receiving care and treatment
- Standard 9 - Expressing views
- Standard 10 - Confidentiality and information about the patient

Promoting, protecting and improving health and social well being

- Standard 7 - Ongoing care
- Standard 15 - Children, young people and vulnerable adults

Corporate leadership and accountability

- Standard 11 - The dental team and service management

PRINCIPALS OF DENTAL PRACTICE:

1. Put patients' interests first
2. Communicate effectively with patients
3. Obtain valid consent
4. Maintain, develop professional knowledge and skills
5. Have a clear and effective complaints procedure
6. Work with colleagues in a way that is in patients' best interests
7. Maintain, develop and work within your professional knowledge and skills
8. Raise concerns if patients are at risk
9. Personal behaviour must raise patients' confidence.

VARIOUS CHECKLISTS:

A. Checklist Dental Department:

SN	Check	Yes	No
1	Is the area allocated to this clinic not less than 100 sq. Ft. Per chair?		
2	Is patient consent taken before start of the treatment?		
3	Is the dental clinic having about 6 air changes per hour?		
4	Are medical records generated and stored?		
5	Is confidentiality of medical records maintained?		
6	Does dental surgeon while performing a procedure on chair-side wear proper protective garments? (Water resistant gown, face mask, gloves, safety glasses)		
7	Is history of any bleeding disorder elicited before dental extraction?		
8	Are all instruments sterilised before reuse?		
9	Are extracted teeth and other oral tissue are disposed as per 'Biomedical Waste' handling rules?		
10	Is the dental chair periodically maintained?		
11	Is Material Safety Data Sheets (MSDS) available on all hazardous substances in the department?		
12	Does the department have documented 'infection control' policy?		
13	Does the department have an alternate power back-up supply?		
14	Patient satisfaction survey is periodically undertaken?		
15	Name of the dental surgeon in-charge with qualification and registration is displayed?		
16	Timings of the OPD are displayed?		
17	Trained Chair side assistant, Dental Technician available?		
18	Minimum Dental Equipment with accessories are available?		

B. Checklist Dental Department Planning:

SN	Check	Yes	No
1	Minimum 100 sq. ft. is provided per chair in the department?		
2	Check that planning ensures visual privacy?		
3	Sign posting of Dental department is clearly done in the hospital?		
4	For ventilation purposes about 6 air changes per hour has been planned while designing HVAC services?		
5	Proper hand washing facilities (at least one) are provided?		
6	Separate or common toilet facilities are available?		
7	Firefighting facilities are planned as per norms?		
8	Room ceiling height is not less than 7′-10″.		

C. Checklist Dental Services:

SN	Check	Yes	No
1	Patient consent is taken before start of the treatment?		
2	Patient consent is also taken for treatment by a 'visiting consultant' or 'dental student' if and when applicable?		
3	Patient has identified himself/herself?		
4	Patient has identified the tooth to be extracted?		
5	Procedure to be done has been cross checked with the dental x-ray and other medical records?		
6	All required instruments are available?		
7	History of 'known allergies' documented?		
8	Verify that cavity has been properly sealed?		
9	Medical records are generated and stored?		
10	Confidentiality of medical records is maintained?		
11	Dental surgeon while performing a procedure on chair-side is in proper protective garments? (Water resistant gown, face mask, gloves, safety glasses)		
12	History of any bleeding disorder is elicited before dental extraction?		

D. Checklist Patient Satisfaction Survey:

Following points are forming part of survey format "Patient Satisfaction with Dental Services"

1. Does the hospital's dental department have an easy access?
2. How was the behaviour of the dentist and auxiliary staff?
3. Was the dentist attentive to your complaints?
4. What is the level of satisfaction with the treatment received?
5. Was the waiting time acceptable?
6. Were you seen at your number?
7. Was the equipment used for your treatment clean?
8. Are you satisfied with the time taken for the treatment?
9. Will you recommend this hospital for dental treatment to others?

E. Check List for Purchasing an Equipment:

1. The equipment meets the laid criteria: such as approval from BARC?
2. It is supplied with all the standard spares and accessories as per the PO/Quotation?
3. Training is imparted to user in its operation & maintenance?
4. Operation Manual is supplied?
5. Certificate of calibration and inspection of parts from the manufacturer?
6. Advanced maintenance tasks required are documented?
7. Take a satisfactory certificate for any existing installation from government/private hospital.
8. List of essential spares and accessories, with their part number and cost is provided?
9. Electrical safety conforms to the standards for electrical safety?
10. Warranty as per your order?
11. Contact details of manufacturer, supplier and local service agent to be provided.
12. Any Contract (AMC/CMC/On call) to be declared by the manufacturer?

F. Checklist for Infection Control:

1. Wash hands before and after wearing gloves.
2. Wash hands at other appropriate times.
3. Wear a new pair of gloves with each patient.
4. Wear protective eyewear and mask when procedure involves spatter or splashing.
5. Change the mask if wet.
6. Wear protective gowns when treating patients.
7. Infection control should be practiced as a team effort amongst all the dental staff members.
8. Staff should be immunized against infectious diseases.

KEY PERFORMANCE INDICATORS (KPI):

1. Number of new patients per month.
2. Total procedures performed per month.
3. Average number of patients per day.
4. Percentage of Cancellation or No Show after taking appointment.
5. Revenue earned per month. (Total Collection)
6. Patient satisfaction.
7. Number of unscheduled procedures.
8. Number of referred patients from other facilities.
9. Rate of patient retention.
10. Procedure success rate.
11. Misc: Medication Errors, Adverse Drug Reaction, etc.

DAILY AUDIT POINTS:

1. Cleaning of area
2. BMW Management
3. Equip. Cleaning
4. Hazard identification checklist

5. Medicine storage & labelling with open and expiry date
6. Random Check on Medicine Expiry
7. Personal hygiene of staff.
8. Checklist in Area
9. Autoclave Sets Expiry
10. Fridge and room temperature
11. Staff interview

OUTREACH PROGRAMMES:

1. School Visits
2. Camps at different Villages.

TOPICS FOR CMEs/CONFERENCES/WORKSHOPS/SEMINARS:

1. Dental Implantology
2. Discussion on Cone Beam Computed Tomography (CBCT)
3. Demonstration of Correct Brushing Techniques.

STATIONARY FORMATS:

Following registers should be maintained in a Standalone Dental Clinic. In multidisciplinary hospitals, some of these registers/documents are common.

1. Patient Registration Register
2. Cash Receipt Book
3. Inventory Register
4. Complaint cum Suggestion Register
5. MLC Record Register
6. Procedure Book

A. Agreement for outsourcing Dental Services: (Format-1)

AGREEMENT

This agreement is made and entered into as of the .... (date) by and between .... (hospital name & address) a hospital serving to the patients in .... (location) represented by its Medical Superintendent .... (name) and with Dr. .... (name) who is professional practitioner in the area of Dentistry.

In consideration, covenants and agreement herein contained, the parties agree as follows:

Section-1: Engagement

1. The Hospital herein agree to provide necessary space (state location of the area), electricity, water and also take care of maintenance of the premises for the Dr. .... for carrying on the professional Dentistry at the hospital whereas the equipment used to carry the practice would be brought in by Dr. .... and would belong to Dr. .... only.

Section-2: Payment terms

1. The payment would only depend on the inpatient and outdoor patients (OPD) of this department and shared as mutually agreed.
2. Collection from the Dental department would be shared on 30% - 70% basis i.e., 30% of the collection would go towards the hospital and 70% of the collection would go to Dr. ....
3. The cash collection will be made at the hospital reception only. The doctor will not accept any cash.
4. All consumables will be procured by Dr. .... herself.
5. Whenever a specialist is called, his payment will also be shared in the same ratio, that is, 30% (hospital) and 70 % (Dr. ....)

Section-3: Termination

1. The terms of engagements shall commence on the date of agreement and shall end when this agreement is terminated.
2. Either party may terminate this agreement at any time by giving at least three months written notice of termination to other party.

Section-4: Duties

1. Dr. .... shall devote required time that is as per hospital OPD that is from 9 AM to 1 PM only.
2. She will be on call from 6.00 pm to 8.00 pm. and will attend the hospital on requirement basis subject to patient visiting the hospital.
3. She will put all efforts to perform the services and will perform services in diligent careful thorough and professional manner consistent with good medical practice.

Section-5: Amendment

This agreement may not be amended or modified in any manner except by a written agreement signed by each of the parties hereto.

In WITNESS WHEREOF, the parties hereto executed and delivered this agreement as of the day and year first above written.

Signatures with Name & Date:	Signatures with Name & Date:
Hospital	Dr. ....

****

B. Agreement for outsourcing Dental Services: (Format-2)

This agreement is executed on the .... (date) between the .... (hospital name) through its Medical Director, Dr. .... (name & address) hereinafter called the **First Party** (this expression includes their legal heirs, assigns, agents, representatives, etc.)

AND

.... (name of second party) through Dr. .... (name & address) hereinafter called the **Second Party** (this expression includes their legal heirs, assigns, agents, representatives, etc.)

WHEREAS the First Party is a multi-speciality hospital and the Second Party presented them to provide dental services to the patients of the First Party. On the request of the Second Party the

First Party agrees to outsource the dental services to the Second Party on the following terms and conditions:

1. That the period of contract between the parties will be for a period of three years with renewable clause. The contract can be renewed with the mutual consent.
2. The First Party will provide space for setting up the Dental OPD to the Second Party and the Second Party will provide all the staff, equipment and materials for the smooth functioning of the dental OPD at .... (hospital name & address)
3. Maintenance and up-gradation of such equipment will be responsibility of second party.
4. The charge schedule will be decided mutually.
5. All interior modifications, if required will be the responsibility of the second party including Plumbing and electric work for dental chairs.
6. That the Second Party will properly look after and manage the Dental OPD with due care and caution with best of their abilities.
7. That the First Party will provide the following to the Second Party for smooth running of the Dental OPD –
   a. Space for running of Dental OPD;
   b. Reception area;
   c. OPD;
   d. Waiting area;
   e. Billing formalities;
   f. Housekeeping services;
   g. Water and electricity;
   h. Air conditioner; and
   i. Advertisement of Dental OPD.
8. That it was agreed between the parties that out of the total revenue the First Party will share 30% and 70% by the Second Party from the gross collection.
9. It is further agreed that in case of implants actual cost of implant will be deducted for calculation of gross collection.
10. That the Second Party will be whole and sole responsible for their acts and omissions and First Party will not be responsible for any negligence or deficiency in service on the part of the Second Party.
11. That the Second Party will take professional indemnity policy for doctors as well as for their staff coverage.
12. That the agreement can be terminated by either party by giving at-least two months' notice. In case the Second Party failed to fulfil the conditions of the agreement either at the time of expiry of the agreement or on termination of agreement by giving two months' notice then the Second Party will liable to pay use and occupation charges @ .... (Rs. 5,000/-) per day.
13. All disputes with respect to this agreement are subject to .... Jurisdiction.

First Party | Second Party

Signature with Name & Date | Signature with Name & Date

WITNESSES:

1.

2.

****

GUIDELINES FOR PATIENTS:

1. How to Prevent Cavities?

a. To a large extent caries may be prevented by avoiding or reducing consumption of soft and sticky foods with a high sugar content like toffees, chocolate, cakes, sweet meats or even carbonated drinks.

b. Even if these stuffs are consumed, brush your teeth properly after consuming such items.

c. Avoid sweets between meals and are only consumed (if at all) after main meals, as a dessert, because we usually consume water during the meal and also rinse our mouth after a meal.

d. Make sure that children are not left to sleep with the milk bottle in their mouths.

2. How Frequently One Should Brush Teeth?

a. Brushing twice a day in the mornings and at bed time is sufficient.

b. Brush your teeth for a period of 5 minutes, making sure that all the teeth and all their surfaces (outside, inside and biting surface) are cleaned well.

c. The brush should be a medium to soft bristle brush and usually needs to be replaced within 3 months, since the bristles become weak.

d. The teeth should be cleaned with a vertical sweeping action from the gum surface over and across the surface of the tooth. The vigorous, horizontal pull-push method of brushing which we were taught as children tends to wear away the teeth at their sides.

3. Dietary Guidelines:

The following 15 dietary guidelines provide a broad framework for appropriate action:

a. Eat variety of foods to ensure a balanced diet.

b. Ensure provision of extra food and healthcare to pregnant and lactating women.

c. Promote exclusive breastfeeding for six months and encourage breastfeeding till two years or as long as one can.

d. Feed home based semi solid foods to the infant after six months.

e. Ensure adequate and appropriate diets for children and adolescents, both in health and sickness.

f. Eat plenty of vegetables and fruits.

g. Ensure moderate use of edible oils and animal foods and very less use of ghee/butter/vanaspati.

h. Avoid overeating to prevent overweight and obesity.

i. Exercise regularly and be physically active to maintain ideal body weight.

j. Restrict salt intake to minimum.

k. Ensure the use of safe and clean foods.

l. Adopt right pre-cooking processes and appropriate cooking methods.

m. Drink plenty of water and take beverages in moderation.

n. Minimize the use of processed foods rich in salt, sugar and fats.

o. Include micronutrient-rich foods in the diets of elderly people to enable them to be fit and active.

(Source: Dietary Guidelines for Indians, National Institute of Nutrition, 2011)

BIBLIOGRAPHY, REFERENCES & ACKNOWLEDGMENTS:

1. Indian Public Health Standards (IPHS)
   Guidelines for District Hospitals (101 to 500 Bedded) Revised 2012 Directorate General of Health Services Ministry of Health & Family Welfare, Government of India

2. "Standard Operating Procedures SOP For Hospitals 2nd Edition" by Dr. Arun K. Agarwal
3. "Duties & Responsibilities of Hospital Staff" by Dr. Arun Kumar
4. "Checklists for Hospitals" by Dr. Arun K. Agarwal
5. Rajasthan Medical Services Corporation Limited, (http://rmsc.health.rajasthan.gov.in/content/dam/doitassets/Medical-and-Health-Portal/rajasthan-medical-corporation/pdf/dei.pdf)
6. Vinayak Mission's Dental College, Salem
7. Dental Council of India: Dentist Code of Ethics
8. Indian Dental Association (https://www.ida.org.in/Accreditation/Details/PracticeStandards)
9. Standard Operating Procedure Manual, Goa Dental College& Hospital, Bambolim – GOA

Chapter – 8

DEPARTMENT OF DIETETICS

INDEX

21. Directions for Patients
    a. Directions for Patients with Liver Diseases.
    b. Directions for Patients on Lactose Free Diet
    c. Directions for Patients with High Cholesterol
    d. Directions for Patients on Low Protein Diet
22. Kitchen Timings
23. Protocol/Etiquettes
24. Policies & Procedures
    a. General
    b. Main Points
    c. Food for Feeding Mothers
    d. Food for Attendants
    e. Purchase Management
    f. Procedures regarding hospital nutritional therapy:
    g. Screening For Nutritional Needs:
    h. RT Feed:
    i. Procedure for Cleaning Utensils Manually (by hand):
25. Audits
    a. Internal Audit
    b. Food Handlers Audit
    c. Audit for Food Servers
26. Key Performance Indicators
27. Quality Assurance
28. Check Lists
    a. Dietician Checklist
    b. Check List – Quality Prepared Food Items
    c. Checklist Kitchen Planning
    d. Checklist Kitchen Inspection
    e. Checklist Cafeteria
    f. Checklist Kitchen Performance
29. Stationary Formats
    a. Agreement with Contractor (2 samples)
    b. Kitchen Audit Performa
    c. Patient Diet Inquiry Format
    d. Diet Requisition
30. Topics For CMEs/Conferences:
31. Bibliography, References & Acknowledgments

INTRODUCTION:

A wise man once said, "You are what you eat". Which is why, the department of Dietetics takes extra care to look after the individual dietary requirements of patients. The team of dieticians work towards one goal, which is providing tasty, yet nutritionally balanced meals to patients as per their requirements.

Dietary services work towards maintaining or even enhancing the health of the admitted patients. Our efficient and educated dieticians provide the hygienic and nutritional food. The dietician in close coordination of treating physicians plans the diet for each patient.

The department caters to the dietary needs of the inpatients. Patient satisfaction with meals is very important. As a result, the hospital has a specialized team of dieticians, food service supervisors and an executive chef who collectively plan menus and implement quality assurance measures.

The department usually caters to more than ____ (100) patients, 50% of who are on special therapeutic diets. The food is processed hygienically with minimum handling, so as to avoid infection and is served hygienically with each dish covered individually and transported in electrically heated trolleys.

It also provides special therapeutic feeds for critically ill patients who are dependent on their diet to give them a better chance in life. Special Naso-gastric & Jejunostomy feeds are made indigenously and standardized to meet the individual needs as dictated by their medical requirements.

The kitchen for staff may be separate than patients' kitchen, if possible. We can also outsource the staff kitchen.

The hospital management should be open to the policy of running the kitchen round the clock, if conditions so demand.

The kitchen should have modern, automatic machine to decrease human handling.

The kitchen for staff may be separate than patients' kitchen, if possible. Hospital can also outsource the catering services to third party.

Before men are employed in the hospital kitchen, a Medical Officer must certify them as fit in all respects. No one will be employed in any capacity in the kitchen or in handling food who is carrier of typhoid or paratyphoid fever or who is suffering from or is under treatment for dysentery, diarrheal or other communicable diseases. A record should be maintained showing details of immunisation of kitchen staff.

Kitchen should be planned in a way that a large vehicle such as a truck can reach up to the kitchen for supply ration, vegetables and also for garbage disposal.

PLANNING:

Suggested Layout

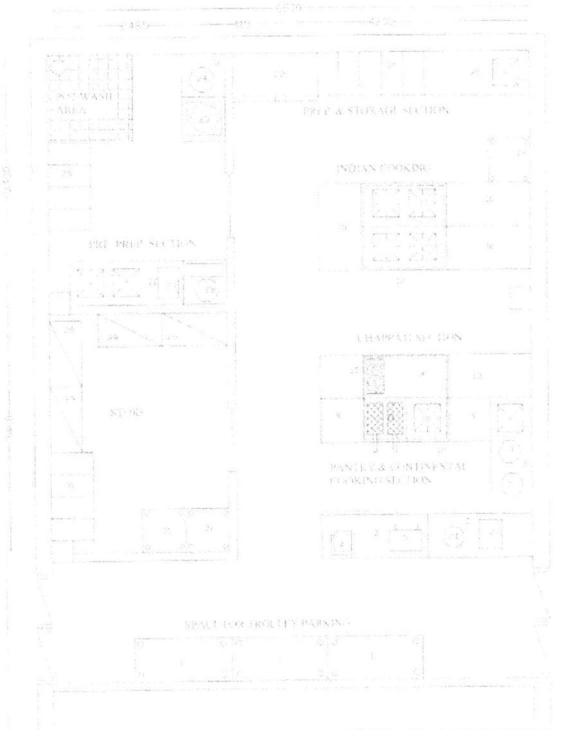

AIMS, VISION & MISSION:

1. To follow standard practices in providing Nutrition & Food Services to patients of this hospital.
2. To ensure effective, efficient and safe practices in food cooking & delivery.
3. To ensure that patients clinical and psychological demands are met.
4. To continually improve the Quality Management System.
5. To plan and provide nutritionally balanced therapeutic meals to indoor patients.
6. To Plan and provide enteral nutrition formula (Formula feed) to the indoor patients.
7. Prescribe evidence-based disease specific tailor-made Nutrition Therapy and counselling to all indoor and outdoor patients with regular follow ups.
8. Training on nutrition and therapeutic diets to healthcare professionals and catering staff.
9. Provision of Nutritional advisory services to medical professionals and administration as required.

OBJECTIVES:

1. Our prime objective is to provide clean, hygienic and healthy meal for quick recovery of patients and create world-class standards in all aspects for our valued customers.
2. To maintain good nutritional status of all patients.
3. To educate patients about how diet plays a major role in the treatment of various diseases.
4. To modify the daily diet pattern of patients to meet their requirement during various diseased condition.
5. To correct deficiencies especially in patients with prolonged hospital stay like cancer patients and critical care unit patients.
6. Diet therapy in most instances is not a remedy in itself but is a measure which supplements or makes the medical or surgical treatment more effective.

FUNCTIONS OF THE DEPARTMENT: (as per CMC Vellore)

1. Therapeutic Diet Planning and Execution
2. Food Preparation and service matching the needs of the patient
3. Providing nutritional care for in-patients
4. Providing diet consultation for both in-patients and outpatients
5. Conducting Nutrition Education and Nutrition Awareness programs for the public
6. Conducting CME (Workshops/Symposiums) on Nutrition

SERVICES OFFERED:

1. Well-equipped in-house kitchen and cafeteria
2. Fully committed to providing the highest quality nutritional care
3. Any eatable from outside is not allowed in the hospital without dietician's prior approval
4. Tailor made diet is served to all the in-patients. In-patients are under strict supervision by the staff of dietary department for their food requirement
5. Department provides Breakfast, Lunch, Evening Snacks & Dinner with the choice of beverages (Tea, Milk, Coffee, Juice) for the patients
6. Food/Snacks are also available for those who are attending the patients at our cafeteria
7. Round the clock cafeteria services for attendants and staff

8. Scheduled appointment for outpatients who need help with any diet plans that are directed by their attending consultants

OPD Service:

1. Counsels outpatients referred by the consultants
2. Provides dietary advice during preventive health check clinics/camps
3. Modifies diet to suit patient taste preference and clinical restrictions
4. Provides diet advices for the participants the antenatal wellbeing program and other relevant programs.

PROCESS FLOW:

1. Dietary Advice:

The Consultants advise diet for the patient as per the nutritional requirement of patient and also according to the ailment of the patient.

2. Calculation of No. of Diet:

The Nutritional Assessment is done by the dietician according to the advice of the doctor after taking in consideration the dietary needs of the patient on the basis of their condition then diet sheets are prepared by the dietician that is given to the Kitchen Supervisor.

3. Preparation of Food:

The food is prepared by the cook under supervision (Kitchen Supervisor) in a hygienic environment wearing gloves, caps and kitchen gown in case the kitchen is in-house. Otherwise, random checks are done by our kitchen supervisor.

4. Quality Check of Cooked Food:

a. The quality of the food is first checked by the cook
b. After cook, quality of food is checked for ***ORGANOLEPTIC*** tests by appointed authorities (Dietician or ICN) daily before serving these includes smell, appearance and taste.
c. External surveillance for raw materials.
d. If adverse reports come action is taken against vendor/supplier by dietician/hospital authorities.
e. A visit to out sourced kitchen is done by dietician and ICN once in three months.

5. Distribution of Cooked Food:

The Kitchen Supervisor with service boys distributes the food to the admitted patients at the definite time with the intimation of concerned nurse.

6. Feedback on Cooked Food:

Feedback is taken from the IPD patient by the concerned nurse and is reported to head.

7. Cessation of Dietary Services to patient:

When discharge or referral is advised to the patient the concerned nurse update the dietician and informs the concerned person at the kitchen to stop the dietary services of the patient.

8. Health check-up of cooks

a. Hospital has staff health screening policy before recruitment in kitchen.
b. Annually Health check-up of all the workers of dietary department is done.
c. Following tests are to carried out;
   Stool test for cyst and ova.
   - Haemoglobin.
   - Routine Urine test
   - Routine Blood test.
   - Serology
d. Hospital ensures that staff is immunized for Hepatitis B

EQUIPMENT:

List of Suggested Equipment

S.N.	Description	Size in mm	Qty.
Store			
1	Storage Bin	600 x 600 x 600	3
3	Storage Rack	900 x 450 x 1800	8
Trolley Section			
4	Platform Trolley	900 x 600 x 1000	2
5	Hot Food Service Trolley	900 x 600 x 1200	5
6	Tray rack trolley	900 x 600 x 1200	5
Prep Area			
7	Work Table w/sink	1050 x 750 x 850 + 150	1
8	Wet Masala Grinder	10 ltr	1
9	Potato Peeler	10 kg	1
10	Pantry Mixer	25 ltr	1
11	Work Table w/sink	1500 x 750 x 850 + 150	1
12	Veg Cutting Machine	Local	1
13	Work Table	1500 x 750 x 850+150	1
14	U/c Ref.	1500 x 600 x 850+150	1
15	Work Table	1500 x 600 x 850+150	1
16	Salad Counter Ref.	1500 x 600 x 850+150	1
Bulk Cooking Area			
17	Chinese Range	1200 x 750 x 850+450	1
18	Work Table	1200 x 750 x 850+150	1
19	Bulk Cooker	100 Ltr.	1
20	Work Table w/sink	1500 x 600 x 850+150	1
21	Wall Shelf	1500 x 300	1
22	Work Table	1500 x 600 x 850+150	1

S.N.	Description	Size in mm	Qty.
23	Wall Shelf	1500 x 300	1
24	Stock Pot Range	750 x 750 x 600	4
25	Exhaust Hood	3600 x 900	3
Cooking Area			
26	Four Burner Gas Range w/oven	900 x 900 x 850+150	1
27	Work Table w/sink	900 x 750 x 850+150	1
28	Idli Steamer	54 idli	1
29	Hot Plate With griddle	1200 x 750 x 850+150	1
30	Deep Fat Fryer	600 x 750 x 850+150	1
31	Work Table w/sink	1500 x 600 x 850+150	1
32	Chapati rolling Table w/Sink	1650 x 600 x 850+150	1
33	Chapati Plate w/Puffer	1800 x 750 x 850+150	2
34	Chapati Collection Table	900 x 750 x 850+150	1
35	Exhaust Hood	4650 x 900	1
Pot Wash Area			
36	Pot Rack	900 x 450 x 1800	4
Pickup Area			
37	Bain Marie	1500 x 600+300 x 850	2
38	Four door Refrigerator	1200 x 750 x 2100	2
Pantry			
39	Work Counter with Storage underneath	1500 x 750 x 850+150	1
40	Blender	Counter Top	1
41	Salamander	Wall Mounted	1
42	Tea Water Boiler	25 ltr	1
43	Milk Warmer	15 ltr	1
44	Work Table w/sink	1200 x 750 x 850+150	1
45	Sandwich Counter	1500 x 750 x 850+150	1
46	Work Table	1200 x 750 x 850+150	1
47	Sandwich Griller	Single	1
48	Pickup Counter	1800 x 600 x 850+450	1
Service Area			
49	Bain Marie	1800 x 600+300 x 850	2
50	Cutlery Table	600 x 600+300 x 850	1
51	Glass Rack	900 x 450 x 1800	1
52	Water Cooler	100 Ltr.	1
53	Bussing Trolley	900 x 600 x 1000	2
54	Hand Wash Sink	600 x 600 x 850	1

S.N.	Description	Size in mm	Qty.
Dish Wash Area			
55	Dirty Dish Landing Table	1200 x 600 x 850	1
56	Two Pre wash Sink Unit	1800 x 600 x 850+150	1
57	Dish Washer (AP 1000)	Imported	1
58	Clean Dish Table	1200 x 600 x 850+150	1
59	Clean Dish Rack	900 x 450 x 1800	1
60	walk in cooler	8ft x 8ft x 8ft	1
61	insect killer		5
62	Air curtain	5ft x 5ft	4

STAFFING/MANPOWER:

1. Diet Consultant (Dietician)
2. Kitchen Manager
3. Cook
4. Bearers/Waiters
5. Helper

DUTIES & RESPONSIBILITIES:

A. Kitchen Managers:

1. Will be overall responsible for dietary services of the hospital.
2. Will organise and manage employees who are directly or indirectly responsible for food services in the hospital.
3. Will prepare roaster of kitchen staff for round the clock functioning of the services.
4. Will ensure proper maintenance and repair of kitchen equipment.
5. Will assist hospital administration in hiring and firing of kitchen employees.
6. They may be given additional responsibility of budgeting and preparing payroll.
7. Will be responsible that staff is in uniform and will monitor their turn out and discipline.
8. Will supervise food preparation, its quality and quantity.
9. Will taste the food before serving to patients and staff.
10. Will ensure proper storage of raw materials and cooked food.
11. Will also supervise food distribution to patients.
12. Will periodically check admissions and discharges for managing meals for all new and old patients.
13. Will ensure that patients get diet as prescribed by the consultant and/or dietician.
14. Will coordinate with dietician in menu planning for staff canteen.
15. Will be responsible for proper running of staff canteen.
16. Will ensure that unauthorised persons don't take meals.
17. Will ensure minimum or no wastage. Remember "You may afford wastage; hospital may afford but the nation cannot".
18. Will ensure proper cleaning and washing of utensils.

19. Will ensure hygienic conditions of the food preparation area and staff dining hall.
20. Will respond and resolve patients' complaints and queries.
21. Will be responsible for indenting, purchasing rations and vegetables for the hospital kitchen.
22. Will document inventory (inventory management) and consumption details.
23. Will carry out physical verification of stack every month.
24. Will ensure periodical medical check-up of kitchen staff.
25. Will comply with all safety regulations.
26. Will ensure that all licenses are up-to-date and are displayed.

Summary:

1. Employee management.
2. Inventory control and purchasing.
3. Supervision of normal cooking and that off therapeutic diets.

B. Duties of a Dietician-1:

1. To oversee the food preparation.
2. To visit admitted patients twice a day and recording their dietary habits & history. Ensure that good and hygienic food is served to patients by asking specific questions during interaction with patients.
3. To identify nutritional status and nutritional needs of a patient.
4. To respond quickly to a patient's complaint cum suggestions.
5. To check food quality by eating food herself before being served to patients.
6. To inspect every meal cooked before being served to patients.
7. The dietician will also supervise whether the "daily diet" is properly carried from the kitchen to the wards.
8. To maintain daily record of quality of food served.
9. Will note remarks in the 'Kitchen Report Book'.
10. To plan their (patients) diet and prepare 'Diet Slips' to be given to the kitchen.
11. To change diet plan of a patient as per his/her medical condition.
12. To verify about food allergies a patient may have.
13. Advising kitchen on how to prepare a particular diet for each and every patient.
14. To exercise supervision over preparation of therapeutic diets.
15. To keep a record of type of diets given to each patient.
16. To prepare diet for 'intravenous feeding' or 'tube feeding'.
17. To ensure that all chargeable diets are entered in 'Charge Sheet'/'Activity Sheet' in the patient file.
18. Counselling patients and their relatives about the type of diet for patient post discharge.
19. To provide relevant diet chart to each discharged patient.
20. To conduct OPD for advice on diet to outpatients. Handing over 'Diet Charts' when required.
21. To provide nutritional counselling to OPD & IPD patients.
22. To maintain duty roaster of kitchen staff.
23. To ensure that material purchase bills are paid only after her due verification.
24. To participate in various training programs.
25. To help in developing/improving Standard Operating Procedures for this department.
26. To arrange meetings and seminars to promote good eating habits.

27. To perform duties of In-Charge Food Services in his/her absence.
28. Will ensure the practices of the "Baby Breast Feeding" are observed.

Summary of Duties

The dietician will be the advisor on problems of nutrition and dietetics and will in that capacity carry out the following duties:

1. Drawing up standard diet sheets, in consultation with medical staff for special therapeutic diets like, diabetic, low salt, low fat, gastric, reducing etc.
2. Exercising supervision over preparation of such special diets.
3. Calculation of individual diet required for in-patients.
4. Compilation of weekly menus for patients.
5. Providing recipes for special dishes.
6. General training and detailed instructions of diet cooks.
7. Visiting wards to interview and advise patients regarding their diets and to discuss dietetic problems with ward sister.
8. Advising the supplying department regarding the nutritive values and suitability of items to be procured, keeping in mind the need for economy.
9. Participation in training programs.
10. Dietary surveys as desired by medical staff.

C. Duties of a Dietician-2:

a. **FOR IPD Work:**

1. Will always be in prescribed dress while on duty.
2. Will get a list of admitted patients every day in the morning.
3. Will take morning and afternoon rounds of each patient to discuss about quality & quantity of food, patients' preferences to adjust their diet accordingly.
4. Will be responsible for nutritional care of patients.
5. Will chalk out the diet plan for each patient after nutritional assessment according to their diagnosis and clinicians' instructions.
6. Will regularly evaluate their meal plans and will change on need basis.
7. It will be her/his duty to prepare "Diet Requisition Slips" for the whole day for each patient and supply it to the kitchen. A record of all such instructions should be maintained.
8. Patients who are 'NPO' (Nil orally) or on 'Liquid Diet' or on RT feed should be clearly highlighted.
9. Patients on therapeutic diet should be clearly mentioned on diet requisition slips.
10. In the absence of the dietician, ward nurse will raise the "Diet Requisition Slips".
11. Dietician will follow hospital policies and procedures.
12. Will help in drafting and updating Standard Operating Procedures (SOPs) for this department.
13. On discharge, every patient should be given a customised diet chart by the dietician.
14. If diet is chargeable in the hospital, it is the duty of the dietician to enter diet details in the patient's case sheet under 'Activity Sheet'/Charge Sheet.

b. **For OPD Work:**

1. Will conduct OPD in one of the OPD chambers for the benefit of walk-in patients looking for diet counselling.

2. Patient may also be referred to her from their (clinicians) OPD for dietary consultation.
3. In OPD consultation, the dietician can also take help of printed diet charts.

c. **General:**

1. Will supervise cleanliness of the kitchen and cafeteria.
2. Will attend to grievances of patients and visitors.
3. Will be responsible for proper cooking of food for patients as well as for staff (cafeteria).
4. Will randomly supervise the cooking.
5. Will guide cooks in their cooking. Can have training sessions of cooks.
6. Will be responsible for procuring quality raw materials.
7. Will check quality of the food by eating a portion herself.
8. Will provide recipes for special dishes.
9. Will compile of weekly menus for patients.
10. Will cross check all purchase bills and contractor's bill, if the canteen is outsourced.
11. The timings of dietician(s) should be set such as to cover supervision of all the three major meals. Otherwise, there must be one dietician available round the clock.
12. They will be asked to give group talks in camps or conferences on good eating habits.
(http://www.indianrailways.gov.in/railwayboard/uploads/codesmanual/MMVol-I/Chapter2.pdf) (Retrieved on 17 May 2018)

D. Cooks:

General Duties:

1. Cooks will observe personal hygiene very strictly & keep their nails short and will wash their hand with soap and water before starting work.
2. Smoking is strictly NO in the kitchen. Hospital as such is a no smoking zone.
3. They will ensure enough supply of dusters and other consumables for washing and cleaning of utensils and kitchen area.
4. They will always keep cooking utensils clean and free from grease.
5. They will ensure proper disposal of kitchen waste.
6. Will observe safe and sanitary food preparation practices.
7. Will be responsible for safe custody of kitchen equipment and utensils.

Specific Duties:

1. Primary duty is to cook food in a hygienic manner.
2. Will be preparing regular and therapeutic diet following instructions from the dieticians.
3. Will open and close the kitchen as per working hours.
4. Will be in proper dress and head gear and apron over and above the prescribed dress.
5. Will observe high standard of personal hygiene.
6. Will be working in rotational duties, if the kitchen services are provided round the clock by the hospital.
7. Will always wash hands before handling anything for cooking.
8. Will peel, cut and cook as per standard methods of cooking.
9. Will not put any peeled, cut items on floor.
10. Will cook both vegetarian and non-vegetarian food.
11. Will maintain sanitation and safety standards of work areas.
12. Will maintain the kitchen clean and tidy.

13. Will indent and receive the day's supply.
14. Will operate equipment available in the hospital kitchen.
15. Will be responsible for care and maintenance of those equipment.
16. Will ensure the quality of the raw material before cooking.
17. Will prepare other beverages as per instructions of the dietician.
18. Will be responsible for proper storage of cooked food till its distribution to keep protected from dust, flies and insects.
19. Will also cook special diets (therapeutic diets) as per instructions of dietician and/or doctors.
20. Will also cook meals for patients on demand.
21. Will avoid wastage and will observe economy during cooking.
22. Will maintain cooking and serving schedule for patients and cafeteria.
23. Will clean the utensils when separate washer (*masalchi*)/helpers are absent or is not available.
24. Will be responsible for proper maintenance and security of kitchen equipment.
25. Will be responsible for proper disposal of leftovers and other wastes.
26. Will ensure judicious use of electricity.
27. Will not allow entry to any unauthorised person.
28. Will ensure that all the kitchen workers are not sick and will report any illness to nursing superintendent/dietician immediately.
29. Will ensure periodical medical examination of all staff.
30. Will ensure compliance with regulatory agencies.
31. Will perform other duties as assigned by seniors.

E. Duties of a Bearer (Food Server):

1. Will be punctual and in proper dress while on duty.
2. Will observe high standards of personal hygiene.
3. Will be very polite while dealing with patients and their attendants.
4. Will clean ration and cut vegetables to the satisfaction of the cook.
5. Will do dusting and other cleaning in the kitchen.
6. Will serve food to patients in wards and other visitors in the dining hall.
7. Will bring back used food trays, cutlery and crockery from patient rooms and/or dining hall.
8. Will wash and dry all used utensils to the satisfaction of his/her seniors.
9. Will wash and clean all work tops.
10. Will bring required/indented items from the hospital stores.
11. Should be able to prepare/cook basic diet in emergency situations and will carry out duties of a cook if no cook is available.
12. Will ensure that correct diet is served to specific patients.
13. Will load and unload the supplies.
14. Will help the cook in all his work.
15. Will carry out other orders of the seniors.

F. Kitchen Attendants:

1. Should be able to read diet charts issued by the dietician for each patient.
2. Will set up the food tray for each patient as per instructions.

3. Will serve the food to visitors sitting in the cafeteria.
4. May also be asked to serve food to patients.
5. Collect all utensils/food trays from the cafeteria tables/patient rooms.
6. Will wash all used utensils and cutlery.
7. Will properly wash food cooking vessels.
8. Will clean tables and cooking area. Will also clean other kitchen areas using prescribed solutions and detergents.
9. Will observe all infection control methods as hospital manual.
10. Will dispose kitchen waste properly at designated place only.
11. Will maintain a clean, hygienic environment inside the kitchen.
12. Will sweep and mop the floors of the kitchen.
13. At times they will also help in basic food preparations.
14. Will do other errands as per instruction of seniors.

ORDERS FOR KITCHEN:

1. Before the employment of kitchen staff, the dietician will make sure that they are fit in all respects.
2. No one will be employed in any capacity in the kitchen or in handling food who is carrier of typhoid or paratyphoid fever or who is suffering from or is under treatment for dysentery, diarrhoea or other communicable diseases.
3. Soap and clean towel will be available at all times near every wash basin.
4. All kitchen staff will keep their nails clipped short and will invariably wash their hands using soap and nailbrush before handling food and after visiting bathrooms.
5. Personnel employed in cooking food will be dressed in authorised uniforms. Aprons and caps will always be worn while at work and these will be kept clean at all times.
6. Smoking is prohibited in the kitchen.
7. The head cook will ensure that there is always adequate supply of clean dusters for drying dishes and cooking utensils. After the last meal each day, these dusters will be boiled in water containing washing soda, rinsed and hung up to dry.
8. All pots and pans used in cooking or serving food will be freed from grease, cleaned and dried after the last meal and arranged in shelves on their sides with their interior exposed to view.
9. The kitchen sinks, tables, chopping blocks, pastry slabs, mincing machines, knives, forks, spoons and all other utensils and appliances will be kept as clean as possible when in use and will be thoroughly cleaned after the last meal. Any item not in use will be kept in an orderly manner on shelves provided for the purpose.
10. The kitchen should be provided with fly proof doors and windows to prevent flies getting into it. Care will be taken that the fly-proof doors and windows are kept closed at all times and in good state of repairs.
11. Food scraps vegetable peelings and such other refuse will not be thrown on the floor but deposited in covered refuse bins provided for the purpose. The cutting up of meat (if permitted by hospital policies) and pastry will be carried out only in blocks/slabs provided.
12. All plates, thalis and tumblers used for eating and drinking will be washed, rinsed.
13. The floors of the kitchen complex will be scrubbed and washed daily and the excess of water dried.
14. Any defects in the cooking rang and other apparatus used in the kitchen will be attended to and set right promptly by the contractor if the kitchen services are outsourced.

QUALITY CHECKS:

1. **Quality Check**:
   Quality check of food is done by dietician every day when diet is supplied.
2. **Food preservation**:
   Kitchen staff always ensures that they have preserved the small quantity of food for at least 24 hours which was served to patients or attendants.
3. **Kitchen visit report**:
   The visit report is prepared once in three months shall be submitted to Hospital Administrator.

SERVICE STANDARDS:

1. The patient diet is served in accordance with the diet specified by the dietician.
2. A dietician specified ingredients and time frame is followed while serving the RT feeds.
3. Caps are mandatory for all the service and cooking staff.
4. The service staffs knock on the door and wishes the guest and the patient while entering their rooms.
5. Service staffs follow social hand washing practices.

SAFETY ASPECTS:

1. Shoes are worn by the all staff to prevent any accident.
2. The floor of the kitchen is cleaned after every service to avoid any mishappening due to slipping.
3. The caps, masks and gloves are mandatory to avoid any infection and maintain hygiene standards.
4. The garbage bins are cleaned and the garbage bags disposed regularly to avoid any food contamination from spreading.
5. A strict schedule is followed with the pest control department to avoid any type of rodent or pest infestation.
6. Fire extinguishers are installed in the kitchen to avert any kind of fire mishappening.
7. A strict protocol is maintained for medical examination prior to joining the organization.

DOS AND DON'TS:

A. Do's

1. Kitchen cleaning is done after every service.
2. Equipment is cleaned after every usage.
3. Kitchen cleaning is an ongoing process.
4. Patient food is checked by kitchen supervisor and dietician before service.
5. The tray layout for every order is checked before dispatch of the order.
6. Nails to be well clipped and hands clean.
7. Hands to be washed every time before going for patient service and after coming back.
8. Food is served in a timely manner to preserve the nutritive value.
9. Cook wears apron while on duty and kitchen staff wears authorized uniform that is kept clean all the time.

B. Don'ts

1. Smoking is strictly prohibited in the area.
2. Chewing of tobacco is prohibited in the area.

3. Any of the staff suffering from infectious disease is not allowed to work.
4. Cook with long and uncovered hair is not allowed to work.
5. Arguing with the guest is not allowed The Guest Is Always Right.
6. There should be no uncovered cuts and wounds.

PERSONAL HYGIENE:

1. Bath before coming on duty.
2. Wear complete uniform.
3. Shave daily.
4. Trim your Beard/Moustaches.
5. Wear clean socks.
6. Wear ironed uniform.
7. Clean your teeth daily.
8. Take care of body odour.
9. Wash your hands on regular intervals, especially after using toilet, after sneezing and coughing.
10. Comb your hair.
11. Cut your nails and clean it regularly
12. Always wear cap and cover your hair.
13. Avoid smoking, chewing and drinking on duty.
14. Avoid spitting in work area.
15. In case your fingers have cuts, boils etc contact the doctor.
16. Avoid sneezing and coughing on food.
17. Do not reuse the disposable gloves.
18. Use disposable gloves while dispensing food.
19. Avoid wearing jewellery in food area.

PATIENT ROOM SERVICE:

1. Food is packed in tightly packed container and transported to the area from kitchen.
2. All the clean trays are brought to the table.
3. Each tray is set up by using crockery, cutlery glassware as per the meal service requirement e.g., Tea/Breakfast/Lunch/Dinner
4. Tray layout of the food is checked & food tasting is done by the dietician.
5. Transportation of food to be distributed is done on electrically heated trolleys.
6. While dispensing patient meal in the area, the trays are checked against the dietician diet sheet by nursing staff once again and then the tray is served to the patient.
7. The clearance is done within one hour of service.

MEAL SERVICE TIMINGS:

SN	Meals	Timings
1.	Bed Tea	06:30 am -07:00 am
2.	Breakfast	08:30 am- 09:00 am

SN	Meals	Timings
3.	Lunch	12:00 Noon -01:00 pm
4.	Evening Tea	03:00 pm -03:30 pm
5.	Soup	05:00 pm -05:30 pm
6.	Dinner	07:00 pm-07:30 pm

DISH WASHING:

1. After the clearance the soiled trays, cutlery, crockery, glassware etc. are brought back to the kitchen.
2. The trays are washed by using the soap solution and water to remove any kind of stains.
3. From the Cutlery/Crockery the leftovers are first crumbed out and dropped into the garbage bin.
4. Crockery/Cutlery is washed using the sink.

TYPES OF DIETS:

1. Normal diet
2. Salt restricted diet
3. Low fat diet
4. High Protein diet
5. Diabetic diet
6. Bland diet
7. Paediatrics diet

DIRECTIONS FOR PATIENTS:

A. Directions For Patients with Liver Diseases:

Foods to be avoided:

Fried foods and preparations, dry fruits and nuts, pickles, spices, seasoned foods, ghee, butter, eggs yolk, meat, cold drinks, cakes, pastries, whole milk and whole milk products, alcoholic drinks

Foods to be taken in prescribed amounts:

All cereals and cereal products, oils, skimmed milk and milk products

B. Directions For Patients on Lactose Free Diet:

Food to be avoided:

Milk & Milk beverages like Milk, Shakes, Butter Milk, Tea, and Coffee with Milk. Condensed or Skimmed Milk. Cheese, Khoa, sweets containing Milk, Paneer, Cream, Butter. Cakes, Biscuits, Pastries containing Milk. Ice-Creams, Kulfi, Deserts & Milk Puddings, Custards, Chocolates, Milk Toffees

C. Directions for Patients with High Cholesterol:

Foods to be avoided:

Ghee, butter, fried preparations, coconut oil, dried fruits and nuts (except Almonds). Whole milk and concentrated milk preparations like Burfi etc, Cream, and Processed Cheese. Pork, organ meats like Liver,

Kidney, Brain, Red Meat, and all types of processed meats like Bacon, Ham, Sausages, Egg yolk. Cold drinks, salted foods and preparations, Pickles, Oil, Bakery products as Cakes, Pastries etc. Chutneys, canned foods

Foods to be taken in prescribed amounts:

Cereal and Cereal products, Pulses, Legumes, Sprouts, Roasted Black Chana, Root Vegetables - like potato, Sweet Potato, Arbi, Yam etc. Lean meat, Fish, Egg white, Sugar, Jaggery, Jam/Honey, Vegetable oils such as Sunflower oil, Soya oil, Mustard oil and Olive oil

Free foods:

Raw and green leafy vegetables, clear soups, lemon, thin buttermilk (Lassi), cottage cheese, fruits, garlic, ginger, salad.

Special instructions:

Use whole grain cereals and pulses. Take regular physical exercise like walking in the morning, Avoid exercise immediately after meal. Avoid rich fatty and heavy meals at any one time. Take frequent but small meals. In case of hypertension, avoid salt and foods containing baking powder, baking soda, green leafy vegetables, and processed food items. Prefer baking, boiling, roasting and steaming instead of frying foods.

D. Directions for Patients on Low Protein Diet

Foods to be avoided:

Extra Pulses, Beans & Legumes, Dried Fruits & Nuts, Extra Milk & Milk Products, Meat, Fish & Poultry Products. Avoid salt & salty preparations, Pickles, Cold Drinks, Processed food items, Tinned foods, Green leafy Vegetables and bakery products in case of Sodium Restriction. Avoid Fruits, Fruit Juices, Green Leafy vegetables, Salads, Soups in case of Potassium restriction

Foods allowed:

VEGETABLES: Ghia, Petha, Tinda, Tori, Potatoes, Carrots, Radish, Lauki, Arbi., Cucumber.

FRUITS: Apple, Anar, Papaya, Amrud, Nashpati

Besides the following fruits and vegetables can be eaten after washing them repeatedly 2-3 times and discarding away their water e.g., Cabbage and Carrots, Onion, Radish (White), Karela, Baigan, Cauliflower, Ladies finger, Pumpkin, Water Melon, Anar, Ripe Tomato

KITCHEN TIMINGS:

Timings will be from 8.00 am to 8.00 p.m. or round the clock, if possible.

Tea will be served from 7.00 am to 10 p.m.

PROTOCOL/ETIQUETTES:

1. All kitchen staff shall be in prescribed dress, put an apron and head cap while on duty. Additionally, Hair nets should be used by female staff.
2. All staff handling food must wear gloves.
3. The arrangement of work stations in the kitchen should be such that there is no contamination of cooked food from raw food.
4. There should be no interchange of personnel working on raw food and those on cooked food.
5. Personnel handling and serving the food are trained to observe universal precautions to protect themselves.

6. Personnel are also trained in following aspects.
    a. The mainstay in preventing spread of disease with an oro-faecal mode of transmission is the proper washing of hands.
    b. Hand washing should cover exposed portions of arms and hands with special attention to fingernails and areas between fingers.
    c. Finger nails should always be kept up to acceptable length
    d. Clothing should be free from obvious dirt and food spills.
    e. All food is prepared and served into covered containers and set into trays in the main kitchen and then sent to patient care areas. This activity is supervised by trained personnel.
7. Hot and cold food is transported in such a manner that appropriate temperatures will be maintained during transportation. For this purpose, kitchen is provided with hot food trolleys.
8. Kitchen staff should not keep any used utensils and crockery unclean. They will make sure that these items are cleaned as soon as those arrive at washing zone of the kitchen.
9. Similarly, all the utensils used to cook should always be washed properly at the end of the day.
10. All the kitchen equipment, appliances, kitchen shelves and canteen furniture should be cleaned every day before closing the kitchen.
11. There should be adequate supply of cleaning detergents and dusters.
12. There should be a bulk store by the side of the kitchen from where they can take the consumables as required.
13. All the food articles should be kept covered and special precautions to control pests
14. Pests control activities should be done on regular basis.
15. Food returned to the kitchen is discarded into black bags. Mouths of bags are tied before disposal
16. The wastes should always be kept in closed bin and should be disposed as per waste management policy.
17. Waste is carried out of kitchen three times daily
18. Housekeeping is done according to the set procedures of the department

POLICIES & PROCEDURES:

Even kitchen services are outsourced these days. It is not unwise to do so, provided the agreement clause gives sufficient powers to hospital management for timely intervention, if thighs go bad. The dietician should always be recruited by the hospital and more so, if the services are outsourced. It enables the management to have good control over the quality of patients' meals and kitchen cleanliness.

If the kitchen is run on contract, contractor may be allowed to charge from the patient directly on daily basis, or the contractor enters the type of diet supplied, in the patient's case sheet (charge sheet), and total bill is cleared at the time of discharge.

1. There should be a policy to serve only vegetarian diet in the hospital. Though there are different schools of thoughts.
2. Meals serving time to patients and staff dining time should be prominently displayed at the main reception and also in the dining area. The patients' meal serving time and pick up time along with other necessary information should be displayed in each ward and patient room.
3. The hospital should normally provide (a) Regular diet (b) Semi solid diet and (c) Liquid diet. All diets will be of high protein content.
4. Tube feeding diets should also be prepared for patients on naso-gastric feedings (RT Feed).
5. Diet should also be prepared with 'Low Sodium", "Low Cholesterol", and "Low Protein" content.

6. Hospital dietician should also provide counselling to the OPD patients and there should be a regular OPD for this purpose at least once a week or as frequently as possible by the dietician.
7. Kitchen employees should be put to medical examination before recruitment, even if the Kitchen is being run 'On Contract". These employees will also be regularly screened for being carrier of communicable diseases, Dysentery or Diarrhoea, and worm infestations etc.
8. Their personal hygiene should also be periodically checked such as long nails, long hair etc. All kitchen staff will keep their nails clipped short and should invariably wash their hand after attending natural calls and before handling food in the kitchen.
9. All kitchen staff must put an apron while on duty and should be in authorized dress which must be kept clean all time.
10. Kitchen is a place for making food for sick. The toilets etc of the kitchen should not be used for staff other than those on duty.
11. Smoking is not allowed in the kitchen.
12. Kitchen staff should not keep any used utensils and crockery unclean. They will make sure that these items are cleaned as soon as those arrive at the kitchen.
13. Similarly, all the utensils used to cook the meals should always be washed properly at the end of day every day.
14. All the kitchen equipment, appliances, kitchen shelves and canteen furniture should be cleaned every day before closing the kitchen
15. There should be adequate supply of cleaning detergents and dusters.
16. There should be a bulk store by the side of the kitchen. The kitchen should be issued material every day for one day's consumption only.
17. All the food articles should be kept covered and special precautions should be taken to control flies, mosquitoes and cockroaches.
18. Doors of the kitchen should be provided with air curtains and all windows should have fly proof net.
19. The refuse and wastes should always be kept in a closed bin and should be disposed as soon as possible.
20. The kitchen should be cleaned, washed and scrubbed daily.
21. The food prepared for the distribution to patients, is to be checked daily by hospital managers. Two or three officers should be on rotation for this purpose and not that only one officer carries out checking every day. The report of such inspection should be noted down in a register for record purposes.
22. As usual for inventory taking of all other hospital departments, the Physical Verification of the kitchen's inventory should be carried out periodically by people assigned by the Hospital Administrator/MS/MD.
23. Ward nurse should inform the kitchen immediately after admission, in writing, (Diet Requisition) so that the next due meals can be served to him.
24. The ward sister will maintain a daily account of diets served to patients. It also helps in paying bill of the Kitchen contractor (if it is outsourced).
25. A register should be kept at the bulk store to show the daily withdrawals and purchases for audit purposes.
26. Ration for the kitchen should be purchased in bulk but perishable items should be purchased on daily basis.
27. Hospital Administrator should be the overall in-charge of the kitchen, even if it is outsourced. It should be his duty to see that high quality raw material is purchased and food served to patients and visitors in most hygienic manner.

28. Supplementary Feeding:
    Whenever additional than served food is required by a patient, the charge nurse;
    a. Should consult the doctor, whether it can be given or not as per his medical condition
    b. She will than inform the food service department about the particular requirement.
    c. It should be the duty of the kitchen to serve the additional requirements.
29. If kitchen is being run by the hospital, it should keep a check on breakage and loss of various durable items. If such item is found missing at the time of physical verification, the administrative officers will try to find out the reasons for shortage and the person responsible for it.

    If the loss is due to normal wear and tear, and the item has lived its life, the culprit may be slightly fined and reprimanded. But is loss due to negligence of the staff, that person or all such staff should be fined to recover the present cost of that item.

    If the loss is due to breakage and it is unintentional, fine should not be levied and staff should only be reprimanded.

    In this department, most of the crockery and cutlery are of breakable nature; some amount should be allocated towards this head to meet unintentional losses.

MAIN POINTS:

1. All kitchen staff must put an apron and cap while on duty and should be in prescribed dress which must be kept clean all time. Hair nets should be used by female staff.
2. Staff handling food should wear gloves.
3. The arrangement of work stations in the kitchen should be such that there is no contamination of cooked food from raw food.
4. There should be no interchange of personnel working on raw food and those on cooked food.
5. Personnel handling and serving the food are trained to observe universal precautions to protect themselves.
6. Hand washing should cover exposed portions of arms and hands with special attention to fingernails and areas between fingers.
7. Finger nails of all kitchen staff should always be short and clean.
8. All food is prepared and served into covered containers and set into trays in the main kitchen and then sent to patient care areas.
9. Hot and cold food is transported in such a manner that appropriate temperatures will be maintained during transportation
10. All the food articles should be kept covered.
11. Pest control (rodents, cockroaches and flies) measures should be regularly taken.
12. Food returned to the kitchen is discarded into black bags. Bags are tied properly before disposal.

FOOD FOR FEEDING MOTHERS:

a. If a bed or room has been allotted to the Feeding Mother and if she is willing to take food from the Hospital then Hospital Kitchen provides it free of cost.
b. If the mother has not opted for any bed or room, the food can still be provided from the hospital kitchen of chargeable basis.

FOOD FOR ATTENDANTS:

a. Food is served to attendants on demand after advance payment.
b. Food from outside is not allowed in patient areas.

c. If any visitor/attendant/feeding mother want to eat their own home cooked food brought from outside the hospital, they can have it in the cafeteria of the hospital.
d. On special consideration if outside food is to be brought inside the hospital, special 'Food Passes' are issued for security to allow such entry.

PURCHASE MANAGEMENT: (In short)

a. Purchasing of raw material for canteen is under the canteen contractor, if the services are outsourced.
b. Ration for the kitchen should be purchased in bulk but perishable items should be purchased on daily basis
c. Purchases are ordered to suppliers in written, on the approved rate as per requirements.
d. Stock is updated 2 days before, if any item is about to finish before time.
e. Quantity checks of all materials purchased are done by contractor while the quality check is done by dieticians.

A. Procedures Regarding Hospital Nutritional Therapy:

1. To ensure that each patient gets diet as per their nutritional needs based on their therapeutic, physiological and metabolic requirements.
2. To provide health education to patients about their nutritional requirements.
3. The dietician & attending consultant shall be responsible for ensuring it.
4. All new admissions are informed to the dieticians. In addition, they are also required to find out about new admissions on the start of their daily routine.
5. Nutritional assessment is carried out by the dietician before ordering any diet.
6. Assessment is done considering their illness, height, weight, metabolic condition.
7. The plan is discussed with the treating doctor by the dietician.
8. The diet chart is prepared by the dietician and a copy is given to the kitchen (service provider) and one copy is attached to the patient's file.
9. If the patient is not able to take the required diet by mouth (orally), RT feeding is done in consultation with the consultant.
10. Special diets are prepared for patients on RT feed and with special needs.
11. Patients are reassessed as and when required and diet plan modified accordingly.
12. If the patient is bringing food from home, family members responsible for food are taught about the patient's nutritional needs and various types of food allowed with emphasis on foods that are not allowed.

B. Screening For Nutritional Needs:

Procedure:

1. **Dietary advice:**

   The doctor/dietician advise diet for the patient as per the nutritional requirement of patient and also according to the ailment of the patient.
2. **Calculation of No. of Diet:**

   The concerned nurses at the IPD calculate the meal requirement of the patient in the diet register as per the types and send it to the kitchen in-charge or the outsourced agency which prepares food for the patients.
3. **Preparation of Food:**

   The food is prepared by the cook in the kitchen at some other place in a hygienic environment wearing gloves, caps and kitchen gown.

4. **Quality Check of Cooked Food:**
   a. The quality of the food is first checked by the cook.
   b. After cook, quality of food is checked for Organoleptic tests by appointed authorities daily before serving. This includes smell, appearance, and taste.
   c. External surveillance for raw materials.
   d. If adverse reports come action is taken against vendor/supplier after consulting the patients, concerned Nursing in-charge and dietician prepares monthly report and submits it to the administrator.
5. **Distribution of Cooked Food:**
   The service Boys distributes the food to the admitted patients at the definite time with the intimation of concerned nurse.
6. **Feedback on Cooked Food:**
   Feedback is taken from the IPD patient and reported to the nurses.
7. **Cessation of Dietary Services to patient:**
   When discharge or referral is advised to the patient the concerned nurse update the dietician and informs the concerned person at the kitchen to stop the dietary services of the patient.
8. **Health check-up of cooks:**
   Hospital has staff health screening policy before recruitment in kitchen. Health check-up of All the Worker of dietary department is done in every 3 months. It includes;
   a. Stool test for cyst and ova.
   b. Haemoglobin.
   c. Routine Urine test
   d. Routine Blood test.
9. **Hospital ensure**s that staff is immunised for following things;
   Typhoid and cholera, Hepatitis A, B, C, AND MMR,

C. RT FEED:

Following patients may require Ryle's Tube Feeding:

1. Multisystem Trauma
   a. Patients anticipated requiring > 48 hrs of mechanical ventilation.
   b. Non-intubated patients with altered mental status or closed head injury that precludes oral intake.
   c. Patients with an open abdomen should not receive enteral feeds until confirmation otherwise from primary surgical team.
2. Burn Patients
   a. Adults (15-59 years of age) with > 19% TBSA burns. Adults >59 years of age with >14% TBSA
   b. Paediatric (under 15 years of age) with >14% TBSA
   c. Intubated patients anticipated to require > 48 hrs of mechanical ventilation.
3. Surgical/Neurology/Neuro Surgery Patients
   All necrotizing fasciitis patients admitted to the ICU.
   a. Patients anticipated being on 'NPO' orders for more than 5 days or with severe malnutrition on admission.
   b. Pre-operative patients with malnutrition and altered mental status. d. All patients less than 15 years of age should be carefully evaluated for the need for early nutrition support.

4. MICU Patients

   All patients receive enteral feeds <48 hours after admission with exception of the following:

   a. Expected to be NPO less than 3 days.
   b. Acute pancreatitis unless decision is made for post-ligament of Treitz feeding tube placement.
   c. Ongoing GI bleeding.
   d. Bowel obstruction.
   e. Need for continued NPO status due to procedures.

5. Medicine Wards

   a. Patients expected to be NPO for any reason for more than 5 days unless they have a contraindication to enteral feedings such as those above, provided they give consent.
   b. Special attention paid to patients who are nutritionally compromised at admission (cachexia, albumin<2.5, ESLD, ESRD, HIV, chronic infection, etc.).

Notes:

1. All tubes not being used for continuous enteral feeds should be flushed with 30 cc (for adults) or 5-10 cc (for paediatric patients) sterilized water every 4 hrs to ensure patency.
2. All tubes should be marked at the skin entrance to allow monitoring for migration of the tube. Tube position should be monitored by the nursing staff q Shift.

RT Tube Feeding Protocol:

Rate of Administration: depends on different infusion techniques

a. Continuous method is to feed via an infusion pump or gravity flow 50 ml/hour.
b. Cyclic method has off and on periods in 24 hours e.g., 8 hours on and 16 hours off.
c. Interrupted method is a regular period of interruption in 24 hours e.g., 4 hours on and 4 hours off.
d. Bolus method where large volumes are given in a short time e.g., 200 cc in a minimum of 10 minutes time.

D. Procedure for Cleaning Utensils Manually (by hand):

1. First all the utensils containing any left overs should be scraped properly with a spatula.
2. Then the utensils should be put in tub of plain hot water
3. Then the utensils should be put in first sink filled with soap and hot water.
   a. Fill the sink with hot water.
   b. Soak pots and pans
   c. Add the soap: Add soap to the sink and stir it around with your hands to make a uniform solution with lots of bubbles.)
4. In the second sink utensils are washed with hot water
5. Then the dishes are rinsed finally another hot stream of water
6. The dishes are to be stacked in a vertical dish rack and allowed to air dry, or they can be dried with clean dish towels and stored in their proper cabinets
7. Wash the cups/glasses/spoons/plates/bowls/trays separately.
8. The thermos should not be soaked in water but they should be cleaned individually with soap and water and once a week they should be rinsed with vinegar or salt solution for at least half an hour.

AUDITS:

A. Internal Audit:

Internal Audit

Name of Auditor: ....

Date of Audit: ....

Audit Checklist for Kitchen/Canteen		
SN	**Check**	**Remark Yes/No**
1	License for canteen available?	
2	Layout of the kitchen?	
3	Food is prepared, handled, stored and distributed safely o Storage of raw materials especially pest?	
4	control, dry storage, cold storage o Washing facility o Unidirectional/ non-cross-over of flow of activities (clean/dirty) o Hygiene and cleanliness o Food handlers use personal protective gear?	
5	Maintenance plan of machinery	
6	Any usage of domestic gas cylinders?	
7	Fire-fighting equipment available?	
8	Is the staff aware about the fire safety methods?	
9	Electrical safety practices been done?	
10	Staff awareness on safety practices?	
11	Health status of employees – Immunization for Typhoid and Hepatitis A/Stool culture and sensitivity?	
12	Adherence to MRP/Hospital agreed rates?	
13	Monitoring of T & C in case this activity is outsourced?	
Signature of Auditor:		

B. Food Handlers Audit:

Food Handlers Audit Points

SN	Audit Points	Remark
1	Social hand washing?	
2	Wearing Cap, mask, gloves, and slippers?	
3	Clothes are neat & clean?	
4	Kitchen cleaning after service?	
5	Well clipped nails and clean hands?	
6	Kitchen floor clean and dry?	
7	Disposal of waste as per existing BMW rules?	
8	Properly storage of food items?	

SN	Audit Points	Remark
9	Trim beard/moustaches?	
10	Any cut and skin infection on hands?	
11	Medical screening of employee done?	

Remarks:

Signature of the observer:

C. Audit of Food Servers (Waiters)

SN	Check	Remark Yes/No
1	Did the waiter knock or ring the bell and waited for 20 seconds before opening the door patient's room.	
2	Did the waiter greet and introduced himself to the patient	
3	Did the waiter provide information regarding the meal and also about various services of pantry. (Ex: food can be reheated; attendant meal can be served etc.)	
4	Did the person taking order mentioned about the approximate time taken for delivering the order	
5	Timing of distribution of various meals as per schedule	
6	Timely clearing of utensils	
7	Wearing gloves and caps	
Checked by Auditor Signature:		

KEY PERFORMANCE INDICATORS:

1. Serving of Wrong Diet: (Percentage or Incidence):
   For example, instead of diabetic diet to a patient of diabetes, normal diet was given to patient.
   Description: Root cause analysis (RCA) should be done and corrective & preventive actions (CAPA) should be taken.
2. Patients Satisfaction Level on Hospital Food Services.
3. Percentage of patients whose Nutritional Screening is done by the dietician.
4. Usages of Hospital dietary services by patients.

QUALITY ASSURANCE:

1. **Quality Check:**
   Quality check is done under supervision of the appointed at every time the diet is supplied.
2. **Food preservation**:
   Kitchen staff always ensures that they have preserved the small quality of food for 24 hours at least, which was served to patients or attendants.
3. **Kitchen/Diet Report**:
   The diet report on monthly basis shall be submitted to MS office up to 5th of every following month.

CHECK LISTS:

A. Dietician Checklist

S.N.	Parameters	Remark
1	IPD on 2nd floor & 1st Floor?	
2	IPD in ICU?	
3	Patient round taken in the morning?	
4	Any night issue regarding diet?	
5	Any adverse opinion about food from patients?	
6	Nutritional Assessment done for all patients?	
7	Food Quality checked and is satisfactory?	
8	Kitchen cleaning done?	
9	Cooks are in proper uniform.	
10	Staff nails, hair is short?	
11	Staff vaccination is up to date?	
12	Any staff having diarrhoea?	
13	Room no. of Patents on "Nil Orally" (NPO)	
14	All meals served on time. Any delay, please report.	
15	Number of patients on RT	
19	Coming after leave/weekly off, pending work taken care?	
20	Remarks	

B. Check List – Quality Prepared Food Items

A surprise check is done by dietician, manager and in-charge whether the cooks are preparing food according to pre-planned menu and adhering to recipe given by dietician.

Checklist

Date: .... Time: ....

SN	Checked Item Name	Appearance	Consistency	Taste	Item Prepared by	Remarks
1						
2						
3						

C. Checklist Kitchen Planning:

Checklist Kitchen Planning

SN	Check	Yes	No	Remark
1	Ideally located on ground floor?			
2	It is away from normal hospital traffic?			
3	It has access to vehicle bringing provision (ration) and vegetables?			

SN	Check	Yes	No	Remark
4	The kitchen area is divided in; • Administrative area. • Cooking area • Provision (ration) store • Cold room or refrigeration room • Wash area • Dining hall/Cafeteria			
5	Area provided to this department is adequate? • For a hospital of 100 - 200 beds; 20 sq. ft per bed • Up to 400 beds; 16 sq. ft per bed • More than 400 beds; it may be 15 sq. ft per bed			
6	Equipment (automatic, semi-automatic or manual) are planned as per load – number of meals to be cooked in each shift or per day.			
7	Cooking gas cylinders are placed outside the main cooking area (Cooking stoves)?			
8	Is it having proper water supply and drainage system?			
9	Kitchen is planned for different types of therapeutic diets. • General Diet • Liquid Diet • Semi Solid Diet • Low cholesterol diet. • Diabetic diet • Nephrotic Diet • Etc.			
10	Fire detection and firefighting arrangements meet the legal requirements?			
11	Proper signage is provided in local as well as in English language?			
12	Sufficient utensils and cookware are provided?			
13	All equipment is under AMC			
14	Hand washing facilities are available?			
15	Separate routes are planned for clean and dirty items, cooked and uncooked food and trolleys?			

D. Checklist Kitchen Inspection:

Checklist Kitchen Inspection

SN	Check	Yes	No	Remark
1	Kitchen should be inspected daily.			
2	Dry provision received is stored in clean hygienic containers in a clean store room?			
3	Pest control methods are seriously adopted?			
4	Kitchen is free from Pests and insects? Rodents' droppings are not seen during inspection.			
5	An electric 'Fly Killer' is put inside the kitchen?			

SN	Check	Yes	No	Remark
6	All windows and ventilators are covered with 'Mosquito Mesh'?			
7	All containers/bins are stored in shelves at least 6 inches above the finished floor level?			
8	Containers are labelled and dated?			
9	Food articles are stored at recommended temperatures?			
10	Work counters are clean and surfaces are easy to wash?			
11	All equipment is clean and maintained?			
12	There is no water overflow.			
13	Basins and sinks are working properly that is 'not blocked'?			
14	Proper ventilation has been provided for smoke to go out? (Smoke Chimney is provided)			
15	Kitchen waste is stored in closed bins and is disposed at least twice a day?			
16	All utensils and crockery are washed clean?			
17	Kitchen is washed and floor scrubbed every night?			
18	Kitchen staff is observing basic hygiene practices?			
19	All personnel are in clean uniforms?			
20	Cooking staff wash hands before starting their work. Hand wash is done in between every time a new work is undertaken?			
21	Toilets are located a little away from the main kitchen?			
22	Kitchen equipment are regularly inspected and always kept in working order?			
23	Cooking gas manifold is located away from main cooking area? (away from naked flame)			
24	Rubber tubing connecting gas supply to burners is in good condition?			
25	Staffs have regular medical check-up? Sick employees (suffering with Diarrhoea, Cold etc) are not coming to duty in kitchen?			
26	Employees with infectious disease are not allowed to work temporarily?			

E. Checklist Cafeteria:

Checklist Cafeteria

SN	Check	Yes	No	Remark
1	Area housekeeping is good?			
2	All tables & chairs are clean?			
3	Dust bins are available?			
4	Area temperature is appropriate?			
5	Area lighting is appropriate?			
6	There are no cobwebs on corners and ceiling?			
7	Drinking water is available?			
8	Wash basin is working and there are no leaking taps?			
9	Toilet facilities are available? Toilets are clean and dry?			

F. Checklist Kitchen Performance:

Checklist Kitchen Performance

1. How many cases of food poisoning are reported during a given period?
   More cases, bad performance.
2. How many complaints from patients and/or staff, received in a given period?
   More complaints; kitchen services are not at par.
3. Check the amount of wastage and also pilferage every day. It reflects on kitchen management.
4. Incidences of pests and rodents in the kitchen.
5. Incidences of new admissions not getting their first meal.
6. Incidences of patients getting an un-prescribed diet.
7. Patients' satisfaction survey reports.

STATIONARY FORMATS:

A. Agreement with Contractor, if Services are Outsourced:

AGREEMENT (may be on a stamp paper)

This agreement is made this day __________ (date) between ___________________ (hospital name & address), here after called the principal.

AND

Mr. ______ (Name of the contractor) S/o _______ (father's name) R/o ________________ (address) here after called the contractor.

The contractor which expression shall include all their executors and assignees on the **First Part** and _______ (Name of the hospital) through its Medical Superintendent (Dr. ....) hereinafter called the **Second Part**.

And whereas the contractor has applied for execution of contract to be engaged as contractor to run the patients' mess. Contractor has been awarded contact of the same in the premises of the hospital on the contract basis. Now therefore, the terms and conditions for running the patients mess and Canteens on contract basis will be as under:

1. The hospital shall provide rent free premises for running of the patients' mess and canteen fitted with water, electricity/power connection, light fitting with bulbs, fans, exhaust fan, telephone etc. The bulbs etc shall have to be replaced and maintained by the contractor at their own cost during the contract period and the hospital/second party, will provide all these electrical fixtures like exhaust fans, bulbs etc. with complete fitting in the beginning of the contract. The contractor shall not ask for additional during the period of the agreement.
2. Be it clearly understood that the contractor will pay service charges @ Rs. ..../- (Rs. ......only) per month for first year, Rs. 000.00/- (Rs. ......only) in second year and Rs. 000.00/- (Rs. ... only) in third year and will vacate the premises immediately on the termination of contract.
3. A refundable security of Rs. 000.00/- (Rs. ... only) will be deposited by the contractor which will be refunded after expiry/termination of the contract within a period of 3 months after the expiry of the contract.
4. It is the responsibility of the contractor to get all fittings, fixtures and other appliance etc. properly cleaned, overhauled as and when required at their own cost, and ensure that everything is in perfect working condition at all times.

5. That any damage caused to the water, electricity, power fans, light fittings, other fixtures or to the building etc. by the contractor and/or by their staff employees, the contractor will make the payments to the hospital for the entire loss.
6. One of the contractors/his representatives will be personally available every day in their working area.
7. The contractor shall use utensils, crockery and cutlery of good standard as approved by the hospital management.
8. The preparation of food and other eatables would be strictly in accordance with the provision of the prevention of food and adulteration Act.
9. The contractor further agrees to inspect all dishes before service and to post and employ suitable staff. The contractors also give and bind themselves to give an undertaking/declaration to the proper authority of prevention of food adulteration Act, about the proper, fair and due compliance/adherence of the provisions. The hospital or its employees will not be liable for any violation of such provisions.
10. The management of the hospital reserves the right to appoint any officer to inspect the quality of the items of food prepared in the patient's mess and the canteen, the contractors shall have to carry out the instructions given by such officer or any authorized person of the management. Non-compliance of the instruction shall be treated as breach of this contract for which penalty as deemed fit and suitable by the management may be imposed or even this contact may also be terminated before its maturity.
11. The contractor is liable for statutory dues and P.F. & ESI for the Canteen Staff.
12. The contractors shall be fully responsible for maintaining discipline and decorum, peace, good behaviour, dealings, appearance and presentation manner of their employees/workers in the patient's mess and canteens.
13. The contractors shall supply uniform including shoes to the service boys with the prior approval and suggestion by the management. The contractors hereby agree to serve the following meals at the given rates to the patients: -
    A. DELUXE/PRIVATE ROOMS: @ Rs. 000/- per day

Bed Tea:	Tea with two Biscuits
Breakfast:	Cornflakes or Porridge with milk, Two Butter Toast/Sandwich (Jam, Slice)
Mid-Day:	Soup
Lunch:	Cooked Vegetable, Dal, Salad, Rice, Curd, Four Chapatti, Pappad, Fruits
Evening Tea:	Tea with four Biscuits
Dinner:	Two Vegetable, Dal, Salad, Four Chapatti, Sweet Dish
Semi-Solid Diet:	Khichri, Curd, Dal, Salty Dalia, Sweet Dish, Soup as per doctor orders.
Liquid Diet:	Milk, Juice, Soup, Limca, Frooti, Tea two hourly as per hospital orders

    B. ECONOMY AND GENERAL/WARDS: At the rate of Rs. 00/- per day

Bed Tea:	Tea with Two Biscuits
Breakfast:	Porridge with milk, Two Butter Toast/Sandwich (Jam, Slice) & Tea
Lunch:	Vegetable, Dal, Salad, Rice, Curd, Four Chapattis
Evening Tea:	Tea with two Biscuits
Dinner:	Vegetable, Dal, Salad, Rice, Four Chapattis
Semi-Solid Diet:	Khichri, Curd, Dal, Salty Dalia, Sweet Dish, Soup
Liquid Diet:	Milk, Juice, Soup, Limca, Frooti, Tea two hourly as per hospital rules

14. The contractor shall use the patient's mess/canteen premises only for the purpose of mess and not for any other business commercial purpose.
15. In the event of any breach of terms of contract of non-compliance or violation of any provision of any law as applicable for running the patient's mess/canteen; the management of hospital can

terminate this contract, and the contractor shall wind up the mess/canteen and handover the vacant premises within 30 days to the management in good working condition.

Otherwise also the agreement can be terminated by either party by giving three months prior notice in writing without giving any cause and reason thereof. In such case the security amount shall be refunded within three months of termination of this agreement.

16. In case of dispute between the parties, the matter will be referred to the sole arbitrator, the Director of the ________ (Name of the hospital), who's decision shall be final and binding on the parties.
17. The legal jurisdiction of any dispute will be ....

The validity of this contract will be three years from ____________ to _________ and shall stand terminate on _________ by afflux of time unless and until the agreement is extended in writing with mutual consent.

In witness whereof both the parties append their signatures in token of having accepted the above terms and condition on the day, month and year mentioned above.

Contractor: - Mr. _______ (name) (Hospital Authorised Representative)

_____ Hospital name

****

B. Agreement – Format-2 (Legal)

AGREEMENT

This agreement is executed on this the day of between the .... (Hospital name) through its Medical Director, Dr. ...., R/O .... (Address) hereinafter called the **First Party** (this expression includes their legal heirs, assigns, agents, representatives, etc.)

AND

Name the company .... Address .... Represented by Mr .... hereinafter called the **Second Party** (this expression includes their legal heirs, assigns, agents, representatives, etc.)

WHEREAS the First Party is a multi-specialty hospital and the Second Party presented them to provide Canteen to the patients of the First Party. On the request of the Second Party the First Party agrees to outsource the cafeteria services to the Second Party on the Following terms and conditions:

1. Mr. .... will represent the First Party and Mr. .... will represent the Second Party.
2. That the Second Party will be responsible for setting up the cafeteria in the space provided by the First Party. For managing the Cafeteria at the First Party the Second Party will provide the following items for smooth running of the cafeteria;
   a. Tea & Coffee Vending Machine: Second Party will be responsible for payment of the same to the vendor
   b. Hot display Showcase
   c. Cold display Showcase
   d. Water Dispenser
   e. Their own storage shelves
3. The timings for running the cafeteria will be 7 am-10 pm.
4. That the Second Party shall use the side premises for the sale of pre-cooked, ready to serve meals, refreshments, tea and snacks to the attendants, Family & Visitors of patients and employees of the First Party. There shall be discounted rates of food for the Employees of the First Party.
5. That the First Party will provide the following to the Second Party for running the cafeteria;

a. Space for running the cafeteria
b. Pantry for cooking of food
c. Storage space
d. The cost of electricity energy consumed in the cafeteria premises will be borne by Fist Party

6. The following items will be provided by the First Party to the Second Party;
   a. Fridge: 1 Qty
   b. Phone: 1 Qty
   c. Table (5) and Chairs (20)
   d. Water Facility

   It is solely the responsibility of the Second Party to maintain the above-mentioned things. Cost of repair of any damage will be borne by Second Party.
7. The 2nd Party shall be responsible for:
   a. Maintaining hygienic standards of food, utensils and the place. The food shall be covered.
   b. The proper upkeep of the canteen premises and shall ensure that the same is kept clean and well maintained in all respects to the satisfaction of the Hospital management
   c. Providing uniform to the cafeteria staff.
   d. Maintaining confidentiality of all the information pertaining to this hospital and its patients.
   e. Patients will only be served cafeteria food after consultation with Dietician.
   f. The Second Party will be responsible for patient room service, tray clearance from patients' room if the food is served from cafeteria. For Patient Room Service, cafeteria staff will be given training by the Second Party.
   g. All refreshment, Tea, snacks, aerated water, etc sold at the canteen shall be of standard quality and quantity. In-charge appointed for the purpose aforesaid shall supervise the catering and other arrangements in the canteen including the cleanliness and sanitation thereof and the caterer shall comply with all direction, issued by the said In-charge. Bills and Invoices to be maintained and submitted to the management by the Contractor.
   h. A list showing the rates of eatable items chargeable shall be prominently displayed in the said premises and the said canteen will be kept open for all 365 days of years including Sunday & Holidays round the clock, without any interruption.
   i. No request for revision of rates in respect of items to be sold in the canteen shall be considered for a period of one year from the date of the Agreement.
   j. Caterer/Contractor should employ adequate number of Waiters (Not below the age of 18 years).
   k. The caterer shall also abide all labour laws which are in force in the state. He will ensure record of all salaries; PF & ESI & minimum wages rules have to be observed strictly. The first party will not be responsible for any proceedings or prosecution initiated against the second party. The second party will be responsible for all penalties, fines levied by the authorities with respect to labour and other activities with respect to the functioning of the cafeteria.
   l. The caterer shall not exhibit any sign board, name plate or advertisement within or outside the said canteen premises.
   m. The caterer/Second Party shall provide proper uniform in a year to all servants working in the cafeteria labour.
   n. The First Party shall under no circumstance be liable to the caterer for any theft or other loss or damage to the equipment or any other property of any kind whatsoever and howsoever arising out of this agreement. You shall be responsible for repair and rectification of your equipment and ensure that cafeteria services do not suffer on any day because of this.

o. The caterer shall pay facility charges of Rs 000/- per month & the 20% over and above the revenue of Rs … Lakhs per month to the Second Party. The amount shall be paid by 15th of the following month.

p. This catering agreement shall remain in force for a period of two years and shall be extended at the option of the Hospital for such period as the management may desire. The Agreement may be terminated by either party by giving to the other, one calendar month's written notice which shall expire on the last day of any calendar months.

q. In case, the contract is terminated in the manner provided, the Second Party shall hand over peaceful possession of the premises entrusted to him including fixtures, utensils, furniture and any other articles in good condition and shall also compensate reasonably for any other damage/loss done to the property including the premises, fixtures, etc.

r. Use of kerosene or domestic LPG Cylinder in the cafeteria premises shall not be permitted.

s. The Second Party shall be required to enter into an agreement within 15 days of the acceptance of the proposal.

t. The Second Party should keep the cafeteria clean and neat and shall not keep any unwanted inflammable material in the canteen.

u. The Second Party shall make all necessary arrangement to procure the essential items for sale on time. The Second Party is to ensure that the eatables served are not degraded and shall not use the leftover of the previous day.

v. Visits or inspections by any statutory body of the Central/State Government (Food Department or any other) as regards quality of food or its ingredients, will have to be dealt with by the Second Party himself and in this aspect the First Party and its Administrations shall remain indemnified by the Second Party and materials in the eatables being sold is entirely of the Second Party.

w. The disputes are subject to …………… Jurisdiction.

x. Photo, Address and Police Verification report of each bonafide worker working in the canteen should be provided.

FIRST PARTY SECOND PARTY

****

C. Kitchen Audit Performa:

AUDIT REPORT OF KITCHEN

AS PER ISO 9001:2008, ISO 14001:2004 & OHSAS 18001

Date of Audit: ……………

Auditors: a) ………………

Auditees: a) …………………

The following non-conformities/observations are made during the audit:

S.N.	Observations	Remarks
1.	Staffs are aware of Quality policies and objectives?	
1	SOPs to be reviewed for adequacy & submitted in new format.	
2	HIRA/environmental analysis to be reviewed.	
3	List of records/activities to be maintained in the department.	
4	Key indicators for process performance to be maintained in the department. Trend analysis to be maintained	

D. Patient's Diet Inquiry Performa:

Patient's Inquiry Performa

Pt's Name .... Age/Sex ....

Room No. .... Date ....

Diagnosis .... Diet Recommended ....

1	Are you	□ Veg	□ Non-Veg	□ Both
2	If Non-Veg, how many times in a week you would like to take non-Veg	□ Once	□ Twice	□ More
3	At what time, you want your morning tea?	□ 6:30 am	□ 7:00 am	□ ??
4	At what time, you want your breakfast?	□ 8:00 am	□ 8:30 am	
5	What type of food do you like?	□ Bland	□ Normal	□ Spicy
6	Any special Liking			

E. Diet Requisition Format:

Hospital Name & Address

Diet Requisition Format

Date: ....

Pt's Name: .... Age/Sex: ....

Room No.: .... Date of Admission (DOA): ....

Diagnosis: .... Allergy: ....

Diet Recommended: .... (NPO/Only Liquids/Semi Solid/Soft/Normal/Special Feed)

TOPICS FOR CMEs/CONFERENCES:

1. Therapeutic Nutrition for Diabetes and ESRD
2. Recent advances in the arena of Obesity and diabetes
3. Medical Nutrition therapy in Surgical patients
4. Malnutrition in Children
5. Nutrition in Cardiac Health

BIBLIOGRAPHY, REFERENCES & ACKNOWLEDGMENTS:

1. "Standard Operating Procedures SOP For Hospitals 2nd Edition" by Dr. Arun K. Agarwal
2. "Duties & Responsibilities of Hospital Staff" by Dr. Arun Kumar
3. "Checklists for Hospitals" by Dr. Arun K. Agarwal
4. Stationary Formats. By Dr. Arun K. Agarwal
5. Hospital Manual. DGHS, Ministry of Health & Family Welfare, GOI
6. NABH Guide Book to Accreditation Standards for Hospitals.

Chapter – 9

DEPARTMENT OF EMERGENCY

INDEX

   f. Admission Procedure
   g. Referral Procedure
   h. Triage Guidelines
   i. Managing Brought Dead
   j. Patient's/Relative's refusal for admission
   k. Discharge of MLC Patient
   l. Death on Arrival
   m. Handling of Death & Release of Dead Body
   n. Issuing of Death Certificate
   o. MLC Protocol
   p. Minor Surgical & Other Procedures
21. Crowd Management at Emergency Department
22. Crash Cart
23. List of Medico Legal Cases
24. Key Performance Indicators
25. Quality Indicators
26. KPI Capturing Documents
27. Audits
28. Checklists
   a. Checklist Monitoring of Emergency Services
   b. Checklist Emergency Department
29. Stationary Formats
   a. Master Register Casualty
   b. Police Information Book
   c. Medico Legal Report Format
   d. Format for LAMA/DAMA/DOR
30. Glasgow Coma Scale
31. Bibliography, References & Acknowledgments

INTRODUCTION:

It is now mandatory to provide treatment to patients entering emergency departments (Supreme Court of India; Parmanand Katara vs. Union of India AIR 1989 SC 2039). Failure to comply is considered as an act of negligence.

The core principle of Emergency Medicine: "Treat first that kills first."

Emergency Medicine is an emerging specialty which deals with critical illness or injuries that require immediate intervention.

Every case is of highest priority in our hospital. Adhering to the highest standards of medical supervision and safety, we are dedicated to provide the finest of treatment and care to emergency and trauma patients.

a. Emergency department of the hospital works round the clock seven days in a week. Anybody can approach this department for urgent medical care. This department has been set up to provide immediate attention to seriously ill patients.

b. Critically ill or injured patients with life-threatening conditions are immediately taken under the care of a team of specialized emergency doctors, and the patient is evaluated, resuscitated and stabilized as per protocols.
c. It is well equipped to respond to any accident and emergency situation and provide critical care to trauma patients in order to ensure faster recovery. It has a direct and easy access from outside.
d. The ambulances have fully equipped mobile ICUs with advanced cardiac life support systems.
e. Medico-Legal Services are also provided thru this department.
f. An efficient and fool proof communication system should he available. There should be efficient communication system within the department and from department to the various intensive care areas of the hospital and also to contact consultants or senior doctors on matters pertaining to better patient care. These can be telephones, intercoms, paging system or public announcement system.

DESCRIPTION:

Emergency medicine doctors assess and treat patients in the Emergency department, regardless of their illness. Their main focus is to stabilise patients as quickly as possible and determine the next best step. ER physicians treat patients from all walks of life and all ages.

LOCATION:

The Emergency Department of this hospital is located at the main entrance of the hospital. It is easily approachable from main road. "Emergency" display signboards are mounted on strategic locations for guiding a patient.

PLANNING:

Main points in planning:

1. For resuscitation, an area of at least 3m x 4m should be allocated per bed space.
2. It is advisable to have ICU near the emergency area.
3. The resuscitation area & patient hold in the casualty could be combined and it is not advisable to have these across a common lobby area.
4. There should be provision for observation beds in this area.
5. There should be provision for dirty utility and toilets.
6. There should be provision for doctor duty cum examination room.
7. Doctor on duty may or may not have an attached toilet.
8. The nurse station in emergency area should have an unrestricted view of resuscitation and observation beds.
9. Emergency area should not have rooms but only cubicles made by curtain partitions.

Points in Detail:

1. The emergency wing should be planned to keep in mind easy accessibility and quick response.
2. Emergency service provision through adequately trained human resources for health should be available round-the-clock.
3. It should preferably have a distinct entry independent of OPD main entry so that minimum time is lost in attending to cases that need resuscitation and also to others requiring emergency

management. There should be easy approach and access for ambulances with adequate space for the free passage of vehicles and a covered area for alighting patients.

4. Stretchers, wheelchairs, and trolleys should be available at the entrance of the emergency at a designated area.
5. Lay out should be such that it follows the functional flow for clinical management of the patient.
6. Signage of emergency should be displayed at the entry of the hospital with additional signage at key points.
7. The Emergency should have a dedicated triage and four clinical management zones (red, yellow, green, black). The triage area should have dedicated space with wall-mounted multipara monitors and medical gases outlets.
8. Duty rooms for doctors/nurses/allied health professionals should be available.
9. Sufficient separate waiting areas and public amenities for patients and relatives should be available and located in such a way that it does not disturb the effective functioning of the emergency department.
10. The emergency area should have close linkages with the emergency OT, procedure room, dressing room, plaster room, lab and radiology services, and critical care areas (HDU/ICU). There should be ready access to vital diagnostic services.
11. All the points should be checked every fortnight for their functionality and a record for this should be available with the emergency in charge.
12. The hospital should also designate a nodal officer, preferably the casualty/emergency in charge who will ensure that all required actions are taken to implement the disaster management plan for managing unforeseen incidences.
13. Regular monitoring must be done to ensure availability of buffer stock of various consumables and their periodic replenishment, training of various stakeholders such as doctors, allied health professionals, and security personnel, mock drills including inter-departmental drills, adequate human resources for health, and rapidly available ambulance services.

Checklist for Emergency Department Planning:

SN	Check	Yes	No
1	Each bed has a floor area of 3-meter x 4 metes? Minimum required is 113 square feet that is 10.5 square meter. Minimum space between two beds should be about eight feet.		
2	The triage is a ward with curtain cubicles?		
3	The department functions round the clock, 365 days a year?		
4	Each bed can be visually assessed (viewed) from nurse station? (Nurse station provided uninterrupted view of all admitted patients.		
5	The corridors of movement of men & material of this department are not crisscrossing with other corridors?		
6	The department has a separate dedicated entrance with access to public/private transport?		
7	The department is located on ground floor?		
8	Safety and security have been taken care while planning this department?		
9	Separate amenities are provided?		
10	The department has visible bilingual postings of signage in local language and English?		
11	Standard fire detection and firefighting equipment are available?		

SN	Check	Yes	No
12	Department is having central supply of medical gases?		
13	Department has adequate electrical sockets on each bed?		
14	Doors allow passage of beds?		
15	Hand washing facilities are available?		
16	A security post is located near this department?		
17	CCTV cameras are installed? (not in patient care areas)		
18	Pharmacy is located nearby?		

AIMS, VISION & MISSION:

1. To provide high quality affordable medical care to provide immediate relief to patients with medical and surgical emergencies.
2. To ensure fastest response time in accidents and various emergencies.
3. To provide swift and versatile emergency care to the patients, in line with the international standards, with the aim to make significant prognostic impact.
4. To have a good teamwork between various specialties.
5. To provide highest level of quality of patient care and services.
6. To provide unrestricted access to appropriate emergency medical care.
7. Provides 24 x 7 Ambulance services.
8. To provide appropriate and expedient evaluation, management, and treatment of patients.
9. To ensure availability of resources in the Emergency Department to accommodate each patient from the time of arrival through evaluation, decision making, treatment, and disposition.
10. To provide medical and surgical care to patients arriving at the hospital in need of immediate care.

Vision:

1. Ultimate goal of the Department is to provide high-quality medical care to patients who are in need of immediate care.

OBJECTIVES:

1. To provide emergency medical and nursing care to patients brought into the emergency ward.
2. To standardize clinical protocols in the department.
3. To liaise with the Police in case of medico-legal cases.
4. To be prepared to handle any emergency on any scale, e.g., mass casualties, accident cases, food poisoning, etc.
5. To manage Day Care admissions.
6. To manage Procedure Room cases.

GOAL:

- The goal is to establish efficient and effective Casualty and Trauma Care services to reduce disability, morbidity and mortality in hospitals by providing right treatment at right time, right place, with right resources, science, sympathy and speed.

POLICY:

1. Emergency care has to be provided to all patients seeking emergency medical services irrespective of caste, creed or paying capacity. Hospital Staff shall be well qualified and trained in emergency care policy/procedures.
2. Emergency care has to be provided by emergency department on 24 X 7 bases. Admission or discharge to home or transfer to another organization from emergency department is recorded.
3. All patient vital signs & complaints are recorded.
4. Depending upon the situation required treatment is started by Resident officer/Casualty Medical Officer.
5. Resuscitation/Treatment is started as per the requirement.
6. Required investigations are done.
7. Clinical consultant is informed & details of line of medical management will be recorded.
8. After stabilizing the patient, the patient shall be shifted to respective ward.

SCOPE OF SERVICES:

a. To treat and manage all types of critically ill patients visiting this department whether during OPD hours or outside OPD hours.
b. Manage patients who come for procedures on OPD/IPD/day care basis, e.g., endoscopy, plastering, CLW suturing, etc.
c. To provide services round the clock, 7 days a week.
d. To provide ambulance services on 24 x 7 basis.
e. To manage Medico-Legal Cases.
f. To refer the patient to a suitable healthcare facility if required services are not available here.
g. Treating all other patient on outdoor basis, when regular OPD is closed.
h. To admit a patient in this hospital at any time of day or night.

SERVICES PROVIDED:

1. Medical evaluation, diagnosis, recommended treatment and disposition of the emergency patient, as well as the direction and coordination of all other care provided to the patient.
2. Minor surgical procedures: removal of superficial foreign bodies, superficial wound suturing.
3. Airway Management -non-Invasive and Invasive Ventilation.
4. CPR
5. Burn dressing, wound debridement/washout, incision and drainage of superficial abscess.
6. Cardioversion and Defibrillation.
7. Temporary Cardiac Pacing Facilities.
8. Intercostal Tube Insertion.
9. Central Line Insertion.
10. Adult, Paediatric and Neonatal Resuscitation.

INFRASTRUCTURE:

The department of Emergency/Casualty of this hospital has been provided with;

1. Triage area for 3 patients
2. Three 'Day Care Beds'

3. One Minor OT for procedures such as suturing, I & D, etc.
4. One Plaster room for POP application

Each bed is provided with central supply of medical gases and all necessary monitoring and life support systems.

EQUIPMENT:

1. General Equipment:

Vital Sign Monitors	Ventilators
Portable X-Ray Machine	12 Channel ECG Machine
Transport Ventilator	Transport Monitor
Nebuliser	Pulse Oximeter
Laryngoscope- Adult & Paediatric	Proctoscope
Suction Machine, Electric	Syringe Pumps
Ambu Bags, Adult, Paedia & Neonate	Ophthalmoscope
Defibrillator	Torch, Thermometer
BP Apparatus, Stethoscope	Glucometer
Weighing Machines, Adult & Neonate	Airways
ET Tubes (Assorted)	Foleys & Plain Catheters
Splints, Assorted	

2. Equipment in Minor OT:

Operation Table cum Plaster Table	Anaesthesia Workstation
Operation Shadowless Lights	Spot Light

3. Items Required in Injection/Dressing Room:

Item	Qty		Item	Qty
Instruments:				
Artery Forceps, 5″	4		B.P. Handle, No. 3 & 4	2 each
Cheatle Forceps	2		Dissecting Forceps, Plain, 5″	2
Dissecting Forceps, Tooth, 5″	2		Needle Holder, Mayo Hegar	1
Scissors, Mayo	2		Scissors, Stitch removal	2
Scissors, Tailor	1		Container, Cheatle Forceps	1
Sponge Holder	2		Kidney Tray, 6″/8″	2
Bowl, 3″	4		Basin, 8″/10″	2
Consumables:				
Acriflavin			Betadine Lotion	
Hydrogen Per oxide			Mag-Sulf	
Normal Saline			Savlon	

Item	Qty	Item	Qty
Spirit		Tincture Benzoin	
Skin Ointment – assorted		Needle, Disposable, assorted	
Syringes, disposable, assorted		Surgical Blades, No. 3 & 4	
Gloves, Surgical, assorted		Apron, Plastic	
Cotton, Gauge, Bandage			

ESSENTIAL MEDICINES EMERGENCY DEPARTMENT:

Following is the major requirement of drugs and consumables for an emergency department.

Injection Diazepam, 5 mg/ml, 2 ml/ampoule	Injection Atropine, 0.6 mg/ml, 1 ml/ampoule
Injection Morphine Sulphate, 10 mg/ml.	Injection Diclofenac Acid, 25 mg/ml.
Injection Paracetamol, 150 mg/ml.	Injection Paracetamol, 150 mg/ml.
Injection Tramadol, 50 mg/ml.	Injection Fentanyl, 50 microgram/ml.
Injection Adrenaline, 1 mg/ml, 1 ml/ampoule	Injection Hydrocortisone Sodium Succinate, 100 mg.
Injection Pheniramine Maleate, 22.75 mg/ml.	Injection Calcium Gluconate, 100 mg/ml.
Injection Phenytoin Sodium, 25 mg/ml.	Injection Frusemide, 10 mg/ml, 2 ml/ampoule
Injection Promethazine hydrochloride) 25 mg/ml, 2 ml/ampoule	Injection Deriphylline
Injection Lignocaine, 2% w/v/vial, 30 ml/vial	Injection Dopamine, 40 mg/ml, 20 ml/vial
Injection Soda Bicarbonate, 5% w/v, 10 ml/ampoule	Injection Anti Snake Venum
Injection Sterile Water	Lignocaine Jelly
IV Fluid: RL, NS, DNS, Dextrose 20%	

FUNCTIONS:

1. Emergency Care
2. Care in Transit
3. Transfer of needy patients to a suitable healthcare facility

PROCESS FLOW:

1. As soon as the patient comes to emergency necessary treatment is provided by medical officer.
2. Medical officer directs the patient/relative to registration counter for registration formalities.
3. In case of MLC Medical officer informs the detail to the concerned police station & to patient's relatives.
4. On confirmation of admission the patient is shifted to respective wards or department after stabilisation.
5. If the patient requires any urgent radiology/pathology investigation the needful shall be done before shifting the patient to ward.
6. Any such investigation done at emergency is entered to the proper registers and the ward is informed to avoid duplication.
7. Any patient who requires isolation due to any infection or immuno compromised state is informed to the ward before bed arrangement

STAFFING/MANPOWER:

1. The department is under supervision of a senior most EMO who is designated as In-charge.
2. A duty roaster is prepared out of total number of EMO(s), and it is ensured that at least one EMO is always present in this department.
3. Duty roaster of staff nurses and emergency technicians ensures that at least 3 nursing/technician staff is always available in this department in every shift.
4. It is managed by doctors and nurses well versed in providing emergency care. They are well trained in 'Basic Life Support' and 'Advanced Life Support' activities.
5. Other roasters ensure that two GDAs and two HKs are available here to provide support to emergency services.
6. Consultants of all specialities by rotation remain 'On Call' outside their OPD hours.
7. If a consultant is available in the hospital, in the OPD or anywhere because of any reason, he may be called to emergency department, if his services are required.
8. Care givers from other departments may also be called when necessary.

ORGANOGRAM:

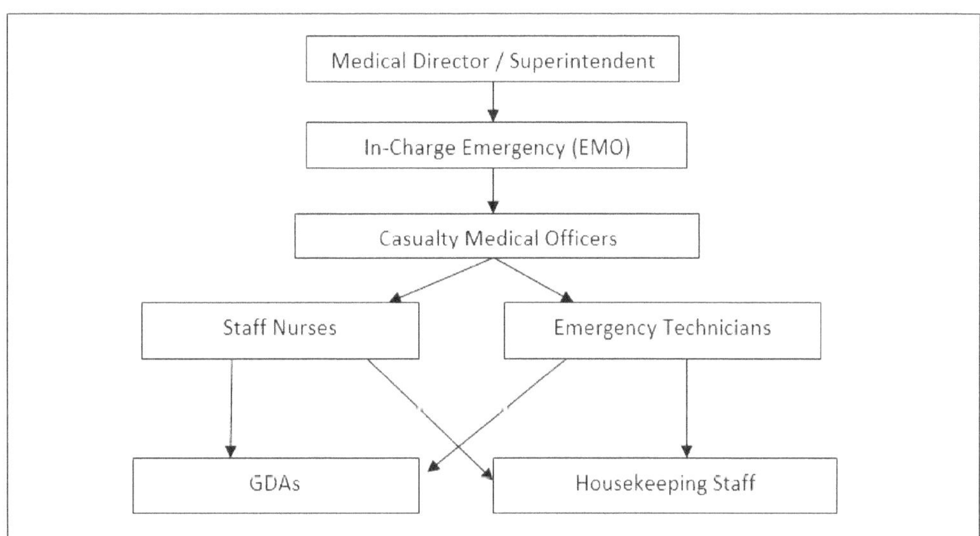

The staff posted in the emergency will work on shift basis.

1. Casualty Medical Officers
2. Emergency Technicians
3. Staff Nurses
4. General Duty Assistants
5. Housekeeping Staff

Staff Allocation:

Personnel	Morning	Night
CMO	1 on duty 1 on call	1 on duty 1 on call

	General	Morning	Evening	Night
Nurse In-charge	1	-	-	-
Staff Nurse	-	3	3	2
Ambulance driver	-	2	2	2
Ambulance attendant	-	1	1	1
GDA	-	1	1	1
Housekeeper	-	1	1	1

Responsibility Matrix:

SN	Activity	Person Initiating/Attending the Activity	Person Supervising
1	Receiving the patient	Nurse/security/Housekeeping	Nurse/CMO
2	Medico legal case	Staff nurses/CMO/Sr. Nurse	CMO/Nurse
3	Surgical emergency	Staff nurses/CMO	Surgeon on call/CMO
4	Medical emergency	Staff nurses/CMO	Physician on call/CMO
5	Paediatric emergency	Staff nurses/CMO	Consultant/CMO
6	Information to Consultant	Staff nurse/CMO	Consultant/CMO
7	ICU admission from casualty	Staff nurse/CMO	Consultant/CMO
8	Death	CMO	CMO/Consultant
9	Medical orders	Staff nurse/CMO	Consultant
10	Carrying out procedures	Staff nurse/CMO	Nurse/Consultant
11	Blood transfusion	Staff nurse/CMO	CMO/BB Officer
12	Patient brought in dead	Staff nurse/CMO	CMO/MS/NS
13	Indenting medicines	Staff nurses	nurse
14	Requesting for diagnostics	CMO	Consultant/CMO
15	Dangerous drugs Cupboard	Staff nurses	Nurse
16	Key handling.	Staff nurses	Nurse
17	Transfer out of patient	Staff Nurse/CMO	CMO/Consultant/Nurse
18	Daily inventory	Staff nurses	nurse
19	Nurses Records	Staff Nurses	Nurses
20	Equipment management	Staff nurses	Biomedical eng/nurse/MS
21	Nursing procedures	Staff nurses	Executive nurse
22	Infection control in ward/OT/ Procedure Room	Staff nurses	nurse/HICC
23	Waste disposal	Staff nurses/Housekeeping staff	nurse/Supervisor
24	Medical Records	CMO/consultant	CMO/Dir. Nursing/MRD
26	Complaints	Staff nurses	Nurse/NS/PRO
27	CMO Duty Schedule	Casualty In-charge	
28	Ambulance driver – duty schedule	Manager Admin	Manager Admin
29	Housekeeping staff	Supervisor house keeping	Supervisor house keeping
30	Morgue	Staff Nurse	Nurse/NS

DUTIES & RESPONSIBILITIES:

Medical Officer on duty will be responsible for the clinical management of the patient in the emergency room. He will also be responsible for general administration and control of other staff, cleanliness, equipment maintenance, etc.

A. Casualty Medical Officer:

1. Will be punctual in duty and will be in prescribed dress.
2. Will carry our all duties of a Resident Medical Officer (RMO).
3. Will be on rotational duties.
4. Will ensure appropriate staffing of this department round the clock.
5. Will be responsible for discipline, performance and turnout of all junior staff posted in this department.
6. Will ensure that the department is fully operational and ready to meet any emergency at any time of day and night.
7. Will ensure prompt attention, reception and transportation to emergency department.
8. Will be responsible for stabilising any incoming emergency without waiting for other formalities to be completed.
9. Should reassure relatives accompanying the patients but inform them of seriousness of illness/injury in each case.
10. Will examine and start treatment (assessing & managing) of all incoming patients. Later on, treatment plan may be changed as per consultant's advice.
11. The relative/friend of the patient should be asked to go to main reception to complete the formalities as laid down in admissions.
12. Will ensure safe custody of valuables of an unconscious or dead patient.
13. To ensure correct referral of the patient depending on his/her diagnosis.
14. Will be responsible for conducting all investigations as deemed fit by him or as ordered by the specialist.
15. Will ensure that all medicines and injections are always available as per the check-list.
16. Will be responsible for replenishing all used stock.
17. Will ensure that crash cart is fully loaded at all times.
18. Will ensure that near expiry and expired medicines are replaced immediately.
19. Will ensure that resuscitation equipment is available and functional at all times.
20. Will ensure proper maintenance of equipment placed in this department.
21. Will ensure that these life saving devices (monitors, defibrillators, ECG machines) are always on charge (plugged into electrical sockets).
22. Will be responsible for monitoring day care admissions and minor OT.
23. Will assist other doctors in carrying out procedures in minor OT.
24. Will be responsible for complete and correct documentation of all cases specially so in medico-legal cases.
25. Will ensure that police have been informed in all MLC and brought dead cases.
26. Will be responsible for completing Injury Register (MLC Report).
27. Formalities for police information and medico-legal examination (MLC) should be completed on the authorised forms.
28. Will ensure that abbreviations are used neither on prescription nor on other records.
29. Will be responsible for issuing various certificates such as 'Death Certificate', 'Medical Certificate' etc.

B. Emergency Technician:

1. These persons provide critical care in the department of casualty. They may be required to accompany ambulance on emergency duty. In addition to providing emergency medical care, they also provide normal nursing care.
2. Will be performing all duties of a staff nurse.
3. Will be responsible for providing efficient and immediate care to the sick and injured brought to emergency department.
4. Will be doing a on the spot assessment and will ensure a proper course of treatment even before a consultant arrives.
5. Will be responsible for taking patients from this hospital to other health care facility and vice versa, if required.
6. Will administer first aid life support care to all patients brought in casualty.
7. Will assist doctors during examination and procedures.
8. Will be operating equipment placed in this department for emergency care such as ECG machine, defibrillator, monitors, syringe pumps etc.
9. Will be performing emergency procedures such as stomach wash, catheterisation etc.
10. Ensure a clear airway, maintain breathing and blood pressure. Will place appropriate splint for immobilisation of the patient.
11. You will be responsible for continuous monitoring of vital parameters of a critical patient till he is under your care.
12. You will carry out CPR (cardio-pulmonary resuscitation) in emergency situations without waiting for any senior to come.
13. Will be responsible for proper inventory management.
14. Will be responsible for replenishment of used stocks. Will indent and receive the supplies.
15. Will maintain and update all records and registers as required by hospital policies and procedures.
16. Will dispose all waste including biomedical waste as per norms.

C. Emergency Nurses:

In addition to basic nursing care, responsibilities of emergency ward nurses include (but are not limited to) following;

1. To be punctual on duty and in prescribed dress/uniform.
2. Will be responsible for carrying out all duties specified for a 'Staff Nurse'.
3. They should be able to respond at a moment's notice.
4. To triage all patients.
5. To ensure basic life support needs and stabilise the patient as soon as possible.
6. To inform the concerned doctor after stabilising for further instructions.
7. They should be trained and able to carry out CPR.
8. To ensure that the department is fully functional to meet an emergency round the clock.
9. To ensure all equipment are in working order. She will check all equipment at the start of her shift.
10. She will be overall responsible and will be in-charge of equipment and consumables placed in this department.
11. To ensure that crash cart is fully loaded. She will ensure that all expired or near expiry drugs are replaced.
12. She should be able to recognise life-threatening conditions and should give priority in attending such patients.
13. She will be very careful while handling medico-legal cases.

14. To ensure that police information is sent about all MLCs.
15. To ensure that injury report (MLC report) is completed as per format.
16. She will ensure completion of formalities in 'Brought Dead' cases.
17. To ensure that abbreviations, short forms are not used while writing prescription or other medical documents.
18. She will assist in carrying out special procedures here such as intubation, catheterisation, stomach wash at bedside. She should also be able to carry out such procedures. Independently.
19. Other routine jobs are;
    a. Admission and discharge/transfer of a patient.
    b. Recording of patient's vital more frequently.
    c. Arrange for investigations, sample collection, sending to labs and getting back results on urgent basis.
    d. Give medication and treatment as prescribed by the doctor.
    e. Carrying out procedures as per her skill and knowledge.
    f. Cleaning and dressing of wounds including stitching of wounds.
20. To ensure completion of all records and registers as per hospital polices.
21. To report to seniors immediately about any loss or damage.
22. To maintain barrier nursing and prevent cross infection.
23. To carry out any other assignment given by seniors.

D. Security Guard:

He is responsible for;

1. Polite, tactful, sympathetic, courteous service under all circumstances.
2. Duty as per roster prepared by Security Officer/CMO In-charge casualty.
3. Regulating the flow of patients or their attendants.
4. Security of the area under his charge and is answerable to CMO Casualty for any untoward incidence.

PATIENT FLOW & PROCEDURE:

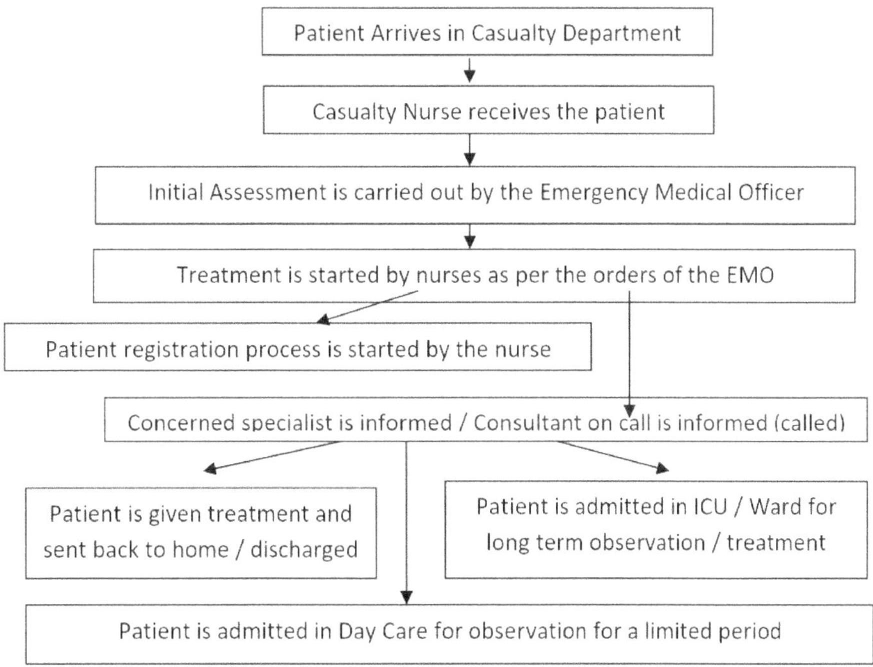

STANDARD OPERATING PROCEDURES:

1. Patients Requiring Ambulatory Treatment:

Such patients are gives required treatment and sent back with appropriate advice on follow ups.

If such patients require to be referred to a specialist OPD, suitable instructions are given.

2. Patients Requiring Short Term Observation:

Such patients are kept in 'day care' and monitored continuously along with suitable treatment. Investigations are carried out and are discharged/sent to OPD or admitted as per advice of the attending consultant.

3. Patients Requiring Hospitalisation:

Patients who require indoor treatment are admitted.

4. Patients Requiring Transfer to Other Healthcare Facilities:

It may be due to non-availability of beds or required facilities in this hospital.

In all such cases, it must be ensured that proper first aid has been given and the reason of transfer is explained to the patient and relatives.

5. General Procedure:

1. Patient is brought in the emergency by Ambulance of any other mode of transport.
2. Main gate security has either already informed the Emergency Team or the security at Emergency informs the Emergency Team.
3. The patient is received on wheel chair/stretcher by GDAs including security personnel. All shall extend help in transporting the patient to the Emergency bed/trolley.
4. Patient is immediately attended by the staff including duty doctor and first priority is to settle the patient.
5. Once the patient is settled, detailed history is taken and physical examination is carried out.
6. Valuables of the patient are handed over to attendants.
7. The patient may be having minor, moderate or major problem.
8. For minor ailments, the patient is given required treatment, medicines are prescribed by the EMO himself and the patient is sent back to home after asking him to come in the regular OPD to consult the specialist.
9. For other cases the concerned specialist is called. He then decides for limited observation (patient is shifted to Observation Bed/Day Care) or for admission in the hospital.
10. Investigations, if ordered by the EMO or the specialist are carried out in this department only and immediately.
11. For Laboratory investigations, the lab technician (or the nursing staff) collects the sample on bed side itself.
12. For radiological investigations, the patient is gently transferred to radiology department, if that investigation cannot be carried out at bedside.
13. If/till the patient is not admitted, billing is done on OPD basis and attendants are asked to approach front desk to settle the bill.
14. If the patient is admitted and IPD file is prepared, hospital expenses are written on the 'Activity Sheet' of the file and entered in the computer software (HIS).

15. Reports of investigations are sent to patient's bedside.
16. Remember the ABC of managing an emergency:
    - AIRWAY:
      Ensure clear airway clear airway: remove any debris/vomitus/foreign body from the mouth.
    - Breathing
      Check for respiration.
      If patient is not breathing, start Ambu Bag and mouth to mouth ventilation.
      Start oxygen inhalation at the rate of 6 lit/min if adults and 2 lit/min in children.
    - Circulation
      Check pulse and BP
      Put an IV line.

    Give head low position if BP is less than 90 mm Hg.
17. Summary:
    a. All patients visiting emergency department for medical evaluation or treatment will receive care by qualified personnel in a timely manner consistent with the acuteness of their illness.
    b. It is the policy of the hospital to attend patients visiting this department immediately.
    c. The initial assessment by nurses and doctors is done immediately.
    d. There are standing instructions that all patients are examined and attended by doctors without delay.
    e. Specialists of respective specialty are called when needed & they attend to the patient immediately, if they are available inside the hospital. Otherwise, they are immediately contacted by cell phones and asked to attend the emergency.
    f. Initial assessment and treatment of the patient starts without waiting for completion of any paperwork (documentation, consent, payment, etc).
    g. In case of DEATH: Following flow is the sequence of activities.
       - Inform Duty Doctor immediately & Counsel the relatives
       - Send the bill (if any) to the billing counter
       - Ask relatives to clear the bill
       - Remove all tubing's from the body
       - Respectfully wrap the body in mortuary sheets
       - Prepare Death Summary/Certificate
       - Hand over relevant papers to relatives after payment
       - Ask relatives to arrange for transport or arrange hospital transport
       - Ask relatives to take the body if it is not a Medico Legal Case.

6. Admission Procedure:

1. If the patient is critically ill, he is shifted directly to ICU after initial stabilisation.
2. Normal admission procedures of; taking consent, financial counselling, preparation of IPD file and payment is handled at front desk.
3. Attendants of the patient are guided to proceed to front desk for completing admission formalities.
4. If it is a surgical case requiring urgent procedure, the patient is prepared in the emergency itself (depending on the time available) and then shifted to the OT under care of required specialist.
5. From the OT after the procedure patient is moved to either ICU or to chosen room.

6. Normal admission procedure is as below:
   a. All admissions are done in separate counselling rooms/cabins away from general public.
   b. Admitting executive checks the written admission orders of the concerned doctor.
   c. A "General Consent Form" is given to the patient and all points are explained verbally also.
   d. Availability of various categories of rooms is explained along with its charges.
   e. A rough estimate is provided to the patient about the total expenses including/excluding medicines based on his selection of type of room.
   f. A proper photo ID of the patient is collected.
   g. Entry is done in computer software. Here an IPD/MRD number is generated.
   h. Sticker sheet is printed containing admission details for onward use in the ward.
   i. Advance is collected as per policy/hospital charge schedule.
   j. Following documents are put in an "IPD File" and the patient is sent to respective ward/bed along with a hospital GDA.

      (General Consent Form, Photo copy of the patient's ID, Payment receipt, Medical Insurance papers, Old/Present Treatment papers, Referral slip- if any and other papers required/ collected from the patient at that time)
   k. Behaviour of admission staff is always courteous and helpful in all circumstances.

7. Referral Procedure:

1. In case a patient who comes to emergency department of this hospital requires services which are not in the scope of services this hospital, he is stabilised and then referred to higher centre or to eth facility of his choice.
2. Preferable SOP for transfer of a patient to other healthcare facility is as below:
   a. Prior to transfer, the MO in-charge of treatment informs and takes approval of the other hospital about shifting of the patient there and confirms the availability of desired facility and bed.
   b. If the request is received from other hospital for shifting the patient on patient's request, it is immediately approved.
   c. Simultaneously the hospital's ambulance is readied and loaded with required equipment and medicines.
   d. The other hospital is also requested to send their ambulance. It is preferred to shift the patient in other hospital's ambulance.
   e. Patient is stabilised (securing air-way, IV lines, etc) within the capabilities of *ABC hospital* before transfer in order to minimise the risks during transfer.
   f. Risks during transfer, if any, are explained to patient and attendants.
   g. Transfer is done with the knowledge of treating doctor. The treating doctor will talk (in person or on phone) and explain the medical condition to medical attendants of other facility, if possible.
   h. Necessary papers (transfer summary containing all the treatment, interventions done at this hospital, Diagnostic tests reports in original – photocopy is to be retained by *ABC Hospital*,
   i. Patient is accompanied with a doctor, nurse, medical attendant as per the condition of the patient of this hospital or other facility.
   j. Even stable patients are transferred to other facility from ABC Hospital, in case of non-availability of bed, facilities or on patient's request.
   k. CONSENT is always taken for all Inter Hospital transfers.

8. Triage Guidelines:

Catg	Definition	Colour	Treatment
P1	Life threatening	Red	Immediate
P2	Urgent	Yellow	Observation
P3	Minor	Green	Wait
P4	Dead	Black	Dead

1. Triage is the process of assessment of a patient on arrival to the ED to determine the priority for medical care based on the clinical urgency of the patient's presenting condition. Triage enables prioritisation of limited resources to obtain the maximum clinical utility for all patients presenting to the ED.
2. The purpose of this policy is to outline the key components of triage of patients representing to Emergency Departments in *ABC Hospital* including the role, key responsibilities and the processes that support efficient and safe triage.

   There are four categories of triage. Beds in Triage are marked with the colour coded plates.

   a. RED: First Priority, Most Urgent, Life Threatening shock or hypoxia is present or imminent, but patient can be stabilised if given immediate care, shall probably survive.

      Following cases are put under this category;

      - Compromised airway Page
      - Respiratory arrest or severe respiratory distress or SpO2 < 90
      - Cardiac arrest
      - Hypotension (BP < 90 mm Hg) • Trauma patient who is unresponsive or requires immediate fluid resuscitation
      - Overdose with a respiratory rate of 6.
      - Severe bradycardia or tachycardia with signs of hypo-perfusion.
      - Chest pain, pale, diaphoretic, blood pressure 70/palpable.
      - Anaphylactic reaction.
      - Baby that is flaccid.
      - Hypoglycaemia with a change in mental status.

   b. Yellow: Second Priority, Urgent, Injuries have systemic implications or effects, but patient is not yet in life threatening shock or hypoxia, although systemic decline shall ensure, given appropriate care, patient seems able to withstand a 45-to-60-minute wait without risk.

      Following cases are put under this category;

      - Following diagnosis with stable blood pressure. Tachycardia/dyspnoea may or may not be present
      - Acute abdominal pain
      - Gastro-intestinal bleeding
      - Acute arterial occlusion
      - Fever in immuno-compromised patients
      - Testicular torsion
      - Acute renal failure
      - Ectopic pregnancy
      - Spontaneous abortion
      - Rule out meningitis
      - Acute Cerebro-vascular accident

- Vomiting/diarrhoea in children
- Acute asthmatic attack
- Pleural effusion
- Spontaneous pneumothorax
- Road traffic accident with transient loss of consciousness.

c. GREEN: Third Priority, Non-urgent, Injuries are localised and without immediate systemic implications, with a minimum of care, patient generally does not deteriorate for up to several hours. Following cases are put under this category;

- Pregnancy with Bleeding PV
- Acute Gastroenteritis
- Minor Trauma

d. Black: Dead, no distinction can be made between clinical and biologic death in a mass casualty incident, and any unresponsive patient who has no spontaneous ventilation or circulation is classified as dead.

9. Managing Brought in Dead:

1. A patient shall be declared 'Brought in Dead', if on examination;
   a. Patient is not breathing.
   b. Bothe pupils are dilated and are non-reactive to light.
   c. No Pulse, No Heart Beat.
   d. ECG is taken immediately – it is a straight line.
2. CPR is to be carried out immediately.
3. If there is no response, the patient is declared 'Brought in Dead'.
4. Registration is done in the Emergency register and case sheet is prepared documenting initial examination details, CPR details and the flat ECG is attached with it.
5. If the body is not immediately taken by relatives, it is shifted to mortuary.
6. If needed, police have to be informed and then body is handed over to police personnel.
7. A certificate mentioning that the patient was brought in dead may be issued.
8. Now all case papers are filed and sent to MRD for further storage.

10. Patient's/Relative's Refusal for Admission:

1. After examining the patient, if the C.M.O. determines the necessity of admitting the patient, he will make the same known to the relatives.
2. If the patient/relatives insist on not being admitted, the C.M.O. will again inform them of the gravity of the patient's condition, and take the patient's/relative's signature on the case sheet and will write - "Discharged against medical advice" OR "Discharged on Request".
3. In cases of DAMA, private ambulance services, if requested, shall be provided for shifting the patient to another hospital.
4. The 'Treatment Summary', along with reports, may be given to the patient, if requested.

11. Discharge of MLC Patient:

1. The C.M.O./R.M.O. inform the police about the discharge of the patient.
2. The Staff Nurse/C.M.O./R.M.O. writes on the case paper "Patient is discharged" with the signature of the C.M.O./Consultant/R.M.O.

3. The Staff Nurse ensures that the patient waits until the Police see the patient.
4. She ensures that the Police signs on the case file before the patient leaves the Hospital.
5. The relatives will wait till the Police arrive and collect the Panchnama.

12. Death on Arrival:

If a patient has sudden Cardio-Respiratory arrest on arrival at the Emergency Room, the patient has to be resuscitated as per ACLS protocols. Once death is confirmed the case should be treated as death on arrival, and necessary documentation should be done. MO should go into the detailed history of the patient and arrive at the probable cause of death. On the basis of this, death certificate should be issued and arrangements for release of the body are undertaken.

13. Handling of Death & Release of Dead Body:

a. All deaths in ABC Hospital are handled with utmost care.
b. Counselling is done of next of kin. Behaviour of all concerned staff should be helping and sympathetic.
c. All help is extended to the next of kin in shifting the body from the hospital.
d. Required certificate is issued and acknowledgment of receipt of body is obtained on the case papers. All case papers are filed and sent to MRD.

14. Issuing of Death Certificate:

1. All certificates are to be issued on proper forms with serial numbers.
2. If a patient dies before admission but after receiving him in the emergency, the local police should be informed as in a case of MLC. Death certificate may be issued as usual.
3. No duplicate death certificate can be issued without proper investigations.
4. In case of death of any patient in the hospital after admission, the hospital may issue a certificate to the next of kin at their request. The cause of death should be indicated in the certificate wherever it is known and in case the cause of death in not known, the circumstances under which the patient died should be mentioned in the certificate.
5. The next of kin is defined as: -
   i. For minor children it would be the parents or guardians.
   ii. For married persons – spouse, children if they are major, parents, brother or sister.
   iii. For legal purposes the next of kin is defined as above but in case none of these survive or are present, uncle or distant relative may be considered as next of kin.
6. The doctor who has seen the patient last and entered so in the case sheet would issue the certificate. This certificate should be signed by the duty doctor. The certificate will be in triplicate; one copy of the certificate should be kept in the hospital in the patient's case sheet (IPD File), second copy should be sent to the Govt. authorities if required & the original should be given to the relatives of the deceased (Next of kin) after getting the signature of the next of kin, on the hospital copy.
7. Death certificate shall not be issued by a medical officer (duty doctor) without contacting attending clinician.

15. MLC Protocol

1. The duty doctor decides about a case being medico-legal or not. It is as per the case. Conclusion of medico legal case is made based on patient's condition being due to unnatural cause of injury, etc.

2. All case papers of such patient are marked in bold or STAMPED as "MLC" in red ink.
3. "Police Information" is sent on a prescribed format. Treatment is started simultaneously without any delay. If local Police Station is not responding, information should be passed on at telephone number "100"
4. Details of injury are noted down in the MLC register (mandatory).
5. Following cases are treated as MLC;
   a. All Poisonings
   b. All Disaster Patients
   c. All Married ladies in first seven year after marriage
   d. And any type of injury or any other suspicion in them.
   e. All Suicides, Suicide attempts
   f. All Accidents (RSA)
   g. All Homicides
   h. Burns (unless it is obviously a minor with no suspicious situation)
   i. Below 18 years unmarried patient for MTP, police should be informed.
   j. Married patient below age of 16 years for MTP, police should be informed.
   k. Alleged sexual assault
   l. Unidentified patient
   m. Drowning
   n. Weapon injury
   o. If unsure
   p. If bought dead with improper history creating suspicion of an offense
      i. Any Suspicion of foul play
      ii. If Married lady; in first 7 years of Marriage,
      iii. Age below 50 years and No History of illness or any Treatment Record.
   q. Any other case not falling under the above categories but has legal implications.

      All case papers are kept secured as details are required to be submitted in Court of law.
6. During noting of the history, use the word "Alleged" and details of person giving history are to be recorded.
7. If the MLC report has already been prepared in some other hospital, MLC number of this patient of that hospital shall be recorded.

Don'ts for MLC

1. Do not take consent to mark a case MLC. It is your decision.
2. Do not heed to the request/order from any one asking you not to mark it MLC.
3. Do not overwrite on MLC sheets. If you want to correct any word cut it once, counter sign it and write the change next to it or above it.
4. Do not give your result/opinion on MLC cases immediately after finishing the task. It is always better to write K.U.O. OR opinion reserved.
5. Do not discuss the case with anyone other than one close authorized relative after taking the consent from the patient.
6. Do not discuss the patient's condition with press when they come to your asking about the condition of the patient. Refer them to the spoke person/MS.
7. Do not leave any column blank in the MLC sheet/police intimation sheet.
8. Do not leave work related to MLC unattended on half done.

9. Do not hand over MLC documents to the relatives or the patient.
10. Do not hand over body to the relatives (in case of death).

16. Minor Surgical and Other Procedures:

Following procedures are carried out in the emergency department of the ABC Hospital.

These procedures are either carried out at bedside or in the adjoining Minor OT.

1. **Incision & Drainage (I & D):**
   Only minor procedures are undertaken here which do not require deep sedation/general anaesthesia.
2. **POP Bandage:**
   For cases with simple fractures (not compound fractures), the consultant or duty doctors may apply cast or full plaster in this department itself. Carry out Reductions of dislocations.
3. Dressings & Small suturing.
4. Other procedures which do not require general anaesthesia.
5. Universal safety and infection control precautions shall always be followed.

CROWD MANAGEMENT AT EMERGENCY DEPARTMENT:

1. Managing the crowd at emergency department is most difficult and important issue in any hospital.
2. Patients are brought either by relatives or by police and in both cases are generally accompanied with many well-wishers.
3. As presence of many people around the patient hinders the treatment procedure, it is very important to keep them away from the patient for proper and urgent treatment of the patient.
4. As soon as the patient arrives, the security guard tries to counsel the relatives and tries to convenience them that to wait outside, so that treatment can be given in a better manner.
5. He has to ensure that after leaving the patient inside the department with the doctor and staff of the hospital, attendant must come out of the department.
6. Attending staff of the hospital shall also persuade relatives to wait outside.
7. Security guard should note down the registration number of the vehicle by which the patient has been brought to the hospital.

CRASH CART:

List of Items on Crash Cart & its Checklist:

M = Morning E = Evening N = Night

		DATE	....		
	NAME OF THE ITEM	**SHIFT**	**M**	**E**	**N**
Top Most Shelf		Stock			
1	Defibrillator	1			
2	Tissue Roll	1			
3	ECG Electrodes & Jelly	1 Pkt.			
Middle Shelf					
1	Knee Hammer, Torch,	1 Each			
2	Tuning Fork (256 HZ)	1			

		DATE	....		
	NAME OF THE ITEM	**SHIFT**	**M**	**E**	**N**
3	Measuring Tape	1			
4	Stethoscope	1			
5	B. P. Apparatus with various cuffs	1 set			
6	Spirit swab container	1			
7	Thermometer with container	1			
Bottom Shelf					
1	IV 25% Dextrose 100 ML	3			
2	IV NS 100 ML	3			
3	IV DNS 500 ML	2			
4	IV Dextrose 5% 500 ML	2			
5	IV Dextrose 10% 500 ML	2			
6	IV R.L. 500 ML	2			
7	IV Mannitol 100 ML	2			
8	IV NS 500 ML	2			
Coloured Bin No. 1					
1	Inj. Betaloc	4			
2	Inj. Digoxin	2			
3	Inj. Cordarone	3			
4	Inj. Calmpose	5			
Coloured Bin No. 2					
1	Inj. Deriphylline	5			
2	Inj. Decadron	5			
3	Inj. Dopamine	5			
4	Inj. Dobutamine	1			
Coloured Bin No. 3					
1	Inj. Fortwin + INJ. Phenergan	5+5			
2	Inj. Eptoin	5			
3	Inj. Magnesium Sulphate 25%	1			
4	Inj. Emeset	5			
Coloured Bin No. 4					
1	INJ. KCL	5			
2	INJ. 2% Xylocaine	2			
3	INJ. VPL	3			
4	INJ. Adenocor	2			
5	INJ. 2% Xylocard	1			
Coloured Bin No. 5					
1	Inj. Noradrenaline [VESCUE]	5			
2	Inj. Rantac	5			
3	Inj. Aminophylline	5			

		DATE	....		
	NAME OF THE ITEM	**SHIFT**	**M**	**E**	**N**
Coloured Bin No. 6					
1	Inj. Sodabicarb	5			
2	Inj. Effcorlin	5			
3	Inj. Avil	5			
4	D/W 10 ML	10			
First Left Drawer					
1	Tab. Sorbitrate 5 MG	1 Strip			
2	Tab. Ecosprin/Disprin 75 MG	1 Strip			
3	Tab. Clopilet 75 MG	1 Strip			
4	Cap. Depin 5 MG	1 Strip			
5	Tab. Betaloc 25 MG	1 Strip			
6	Skin Ointments (Neosporin, Betadine)				
7	Savlon, Tr. Benzoin, Spirit, H2O2				
Second Left Drawer					
1	INJ. 25% Dextrose	5			
2	INJ. 50% Dextrose	5			
3	INJ. Cal. Gluconate	5			
4	INJ. Adrenaline	15			
5	INJ. Atropine	15			
6	INJ. Fulsed 1 ML	2			
7	INJ. N.T. G.	5			
8	INJ. Lasix	5			
Third Left Drawer					
1	Certofix Duo V-715	1			
2	Certofix Trio V-720	1			
3	Mucus Extractor	1			
4	Nasal Prongs (Adult, Paedia)	1 Each			
5	Oxygen Face Masks (Adult, Paedia)	1 Each			
First Right Drawer					
1	DIS. Syringes All Sizes	5 Each			
2	D/S Insulin	5			
3	DIS. Needles All Sizes	5 Each			
Second Right Drawer					
1	IV Set	5			
2	Microset	5			
3	Blood Transfusion Set	2			
4	Vein-O-Line (10, 50, 100, 150 CM)	2 Each			
5	Dosi Flow	2			

		DATE	....		
	NAME OF THE ITEM	**SHIFT**	**M**	**E**	**N**
6	Scalp Vein # 21, 24	1 Each			
7	Spinal Needle # 23, 25	1			
8	Venflon # 18, 20, 22, 24	2 Each			
9	Tourniquet Band	1			
10	Tegaderm (Small)	5			
Third Right Drawer					
1	Gloves # 6, 6.5, 7, 7.5	2 Each			
2	Ryle's Tubes # 8, 10, 12, 14, 16	1 Each			
3	Foley's Catheter s # 8, 12, 14, 16, 18	1 each			
4	Urosac	2			
5	Endotracheal Tubes # 2.5, 3, 3.5, 4, 4.5, 5, 5.5, 6, 6.5, 7, 7.5, 8, 8.5, 9, 9.5	1 each			
6	Airway # 00, 0, 1, 2, 3, 4	1 each			
7	Suction Catheter # 6, 8, 10, 12, 14, 16	1 each			
CHECKED BY: (SIGNATURE)					

LIST OF MEDICO LEGAL CASES

1. All Poisonings.
2. All Disaster Patients.
3. All Married ladies in first seven years of marriage with any type of injury or any other suspicious history in them.
4. All Suicides or Suicide attempts.
5. All Accidents.
6. All Homicides.
7. Burns (unless it is obviously a minor with no suspicious situation).
8. Below 18 years unmarried patient for MTP, police should be informed.
9. Married patient below age of 16 years for MTP, police should be informed.
10. Sudden death within 24 hours of admission if reason not known.
11. Alleged sexual assault.
12. Unidentified patient.
13. Drowning.
14. Weapon injury.
15. If unsure.
16. If bought dead
    a. Any Suspicion of foul play.
    b. If married lady first 7 years of Marriage.
    c. Age below 50 years with no history of illness or any treatment record.
    d. Record Status of Brought Dead.

KEY PERFORMANCE INDICATORS:

Parameters for Quality Assurance:

a. Accuracy of maintenance of Patient Records.
b. Time taken to provide emergency care.
c. Training of staff in ED.
d. Hospital Infection rate due to emergency care.
e. Availability of trained staff

Quality Indicators are;

1. Return to ER within 72 hrs of similar presenting complaints
2. Time taken for Initial Assessment
3. No. of sentinel events reported, collected and analysed within the defined time frame.
4. % of medication Errors,
5. % of admissions with Adverse drug Reaction,
6. % of medication Charts with error prone abbreviations:

There can be many more Quality Indicators:

1. Patients seen and discharged within X hours (hospital to determine their standard)
2. Patients admitted from ED
3. Time to treatment
4. Patient satisfaction
5. Standard of care treatment
6. Correct diagnosis
7. ED occupancy/crowding
8. Time to treatment
9. ED LOS (length of stay)/wait
10. ED returns
11. Left Without Being Seen
12. Time to diagnosis
13. Effectiveness
14. Mortality
15. Time to pain management
16. Rate of complaints
17. Provider satisfaction
18. Waiting time
19. Time diagnostics to treatment
20. Time to diagnosis
21. Patient participation in own care
22. Satisfaction: pain control Satisfaction: hygiene
23. Triage vs. time to see provider
24. Staff safety

KPI CAPTURING DOCUMENTS:

Indicator: % of medication Errors, % of admissions with Adverse drug Reaction, % of medication Charts with error prone abbreviations													
Sn	**Date**	**Patient Name**	**UHID No.**	**Diagnosis**	**Department Name**	**Medication Errors Reported**	**Dispensing Errors Reported**	**Prescription Errors Reported**	**Adverse Drug Reaction Reported**	**Reason For Adverse Drug Reaction**	**Medication Chart with Error Prone Abbreviations**	**Signature Of Nursing Staff**
Note: Separate registers can be maintained for each indicator.												

AUDITS:

Internal Audit

Name of Auditor:

Date of Audit

Audit Checklist for Emergency Room and Ambulance

SN	Audit Points	Yes/No
1	Are the documented policies/procedure/protocols for emergency care present?	
2	Are the procedures for handling MLC cases (like capturing identification marks and police intimation) followed?	
3	Are the emergency care/admission/discharge documented?	
4	Whether a documented triage policy present?	
5	Is the triage policy followed by the staff? (ask for demo)	
6	Whether disaster management Kit available, up to date and regularly documented?	
7	Is the staff trained in CPR – BLS/ACLS?	
8	Patient admission/time for admission request completion	
9	Whether the policy for managing non availability of beds present?	
10	Is the policy for management of patient during non-availability of beds followed by the staff?	
11	Is the policy for admission criteria for ICU documented and followed by the staff?	
12	Are the various signposting and directional signage's (bilingual) from approach road present?	
13	Is the department easily accessible?	
14	Is the flow of patients to the department unobstructed?	
15	Are the transfer notes for the case been recorded and given to?	

SN	Audit Points	Yes/No
16	Are the initial assessments and re-assessment of patients done according to policy?	
17	Is the staff aware about assessment policy?	
18	Is the Informed consent for administration of moderate sedation is obtained?	
19	Is the Emergency drug management done?	
20	Does the documented policy exist for prescription of medicines?	
21	Is the medication administration policy followed?	
22	Is the staff aware about the methodology of medication administration?	
23	Are the medication administered documented and duly named, signed, dated and timed by the concerned doctors?	
24	Patient interview	
25	Is the hand washing facility available?	
26	Is the Segregation of bio-medical waste done?	
27	Does adequate parking space available for Ambulances?	
28	Does the ambulance have proper communication system?	
29	Is the check list of ambulance for drugs and equipment daily followed and documented?	
30	Does the ambulance have adequate equipment in working order?	
31	Are the personnel trained on BLS/ACLS?	
32	Are the following Statutory requirements fulfilled? o RC book o License of driver (s) o Insurance o Emission check	

Comments:

Signature of the Auditor:

CHECK LISTS:

1. Checklist Monitoring of Emergency Services:

SN	Question/Observation	Remarks
1	Is the level of cleanliness satisfactory?	
2	Are signs & posting displayed clearly?	
3	Are the furniture & equipment available?	
4	Allocated staff is present on duty?	
5	The staffs are in prescribed uniform?	
6	Is the patient received properly?	
7	Do the patients wait less than 10 minutes?	
8	Is resuscitation in case of need done immediately?	
9	Is history taken & examination done properly?	
10	Are the necessary investigation done?	
11	Are the urgent investigation done within 1 hour?	
12	Is the patient send to the proper place for further treatment?	

2. Checklist Emergency Department:

		Date"		Date:	
SN	**Check**	**8 am**	**4 pm**	**8 am**	**4 pm**
1	Central Oxygen available in all outlets?				
2	Central Suction available in all outlets?				
	Oxygen in Portable cylinder full?				
4	Crash cart is loaded?				
5	BP, Stethoscope, etc. working?				
6	Vaccines are available?				
7	Linen is available?				
8	Stretcher, Wheel chair available?				
9	Monitors are working?				
10	Monitor accessories are available?				
11	Defibrillator is working?				
12	Syringe pumps working?				
13	ECG machine working?				
14	Ventilator is checked?				
15	Check Dressing Trolley?				
16	Instruments Set are available?				

STATIONARY FORMATS:

Following forms and registers should be maintained in this department:

1. Master Register
2. CSSD Register
3. Police Information Book
4. Daily Inventory Register.
5. Crash Cart Register
6. Hand over Register
7. MLR (Medico Legal Report) Register
8. Death Certificate Book
9. Patient Referral Forms
10. Investigation Requisition Forms
11. Medical Certificate Book
12. Patient Case Sheet Papers (IPD File)

1. Master Register/Casualty Register:

Casualty Register

Date	Time	Pt. Name	Age/Sex	Address/Tel No.	Attendant Name & Tel No.	Presenting Complaint/Condition at Time of Arrival	Treatment Given	Transferred To	Time of Transfer	Condition at Transfer	MLC No.	Consultant	Remark	CMO Sign

Note: Landscape Printing OR Both Right & left side is used

2. Police Information Book:

Hospital Name & Address

MEDICO-LEGAL CASE (MLC)- POLICE INFORMATION

(Prepare in triplicate and obtain signatures of the receiving officer)

Time .... AM/PM

Date ....

To;

The SHO

Thana: ....

A Patient with the following particulars has come/been brought to the emergency/OPD and is being treated/discharged/has expired. This is for your information and necessary action please.

Name ....

Father's/Husband's Name ....

Age .... Sex .... CR (UHID) No. ....

Date and time of admission ....

Location of Incident: .... Time & Date of Incident: ....

Diagnosis .... (RSA, Medico-legal, Injuries, Poisoning, Burns, BD etc)

Signature of Medical Officer: .... Name: ....

****

Time .... AM/PM Signature of Receiving Police Officer

Date .... Name ....

3. MLR (Medico Legal Report) Format:

Now a day's MLR is filled online in many states.

The register is in Landscape Format

Hospital Name & Address

Injury Report Register

CR No.: ....

Name: .... Son of........................ Aged: .... Sex: ....

Resident of: .... Police Station: ....

Name of relative or friend: .... Date & time of examination: ....

<table>
<tr><td>Date and Time of arrival: ....
No. and Name of constable: ....
Police Station: ....
Date of admission: ....
Date of Discharge: ....
Date and hour of report sent to police:</td><td rowspan="2">Particulars Of Injuries/Symptoms in Case of Poisoning</td></tr>
<tr><td rowspan="2">Space for particulars as to further reference to the case date of giving evidence in the Court. Dispatch of articles said to contain poison etc.
Identification marks</td></tr>
<tr><td>1. Nature of injuries: ....
(Simple/grievous/dangerous)
2. The kind of weapon used or poison in suspected case of poisoning:
3. Probable duration of injuries:</td></tr>
</table>

Guidelines: - It is on a long register in landscape format, printed in triplicate. One copy for police, 2nd for court & 3rd for hospital records

Page-2 (back of P-1) Lay out for marking of the injuries.

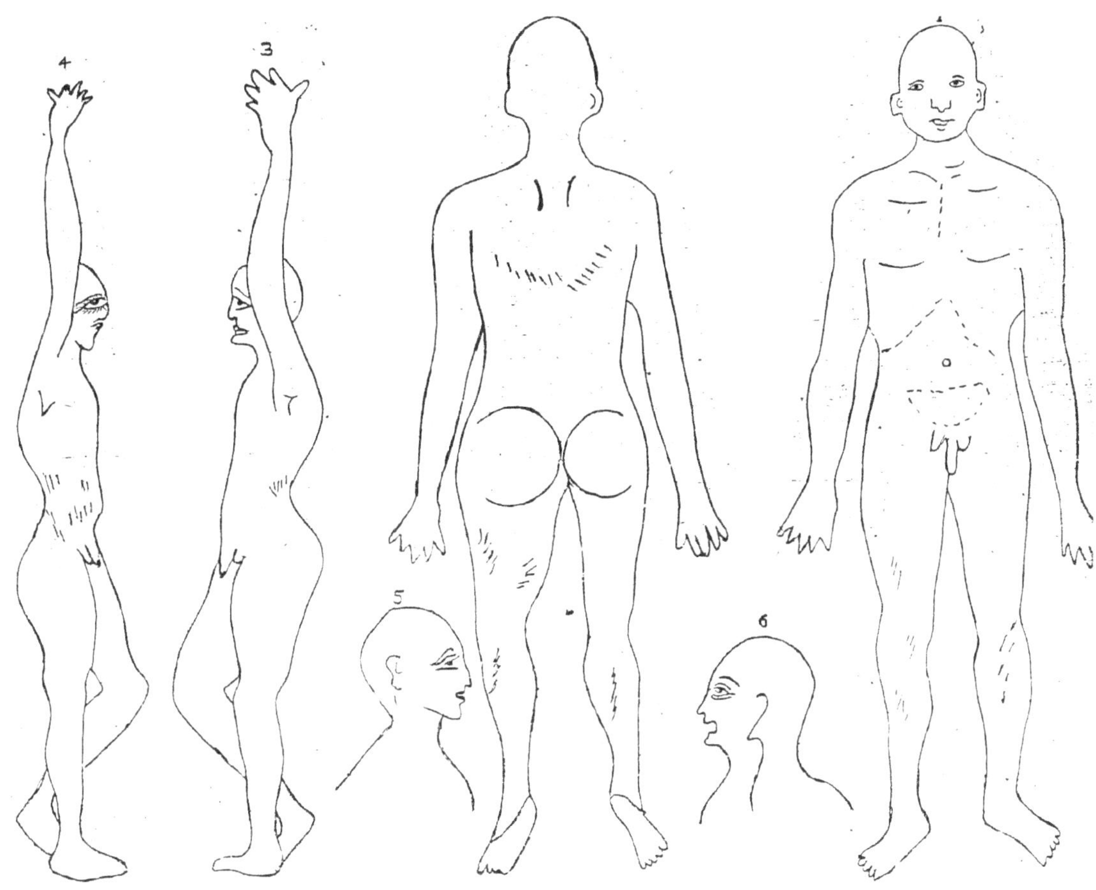

4. Format for LAMA/DAMA/DOR:

Hospital Name & Address

LEFT AGAINST MEDICAL ADVICE/DISCHARGE ON REQUEST

Patient Name: .... Age/Sex: ....

Hospital Registration No.: .... Treating Doctor (Doctor I/C): ....

I... S/D/W/of.. do hereby certify that I/my patient .... S/D/W/ of... is being treated at this Hospital under care of Dr................. ...and his team.

Due to my personal reasons, I am not able to continue further treatment, although I have been explained by the doctor, the nature of illness, need for continued hospitalization & treatment & the risks of discharge at this stage.

I have been given the options of second opinion & referral to another hospital of my, my patient's choice.

I undertake that I alone shall be responsible for my decision for myself/my patient to leave against the medical advice/discharge on request and the hospital shall not be held responsible for adverse consequences, if any.

Patient Signature: .... Name: .... Date: ....

Witness Signature: .... Name: .... Date: ....

Relationship: ....

Doctor Signature: .... Name: .... Date: ....

If patient is not competent to give consent, relative to give the same:

Relative Signature: .... Name: .... Date: ....

Address: ....

Relationship: ....

Reason for patient's incompetency to give consent: ....

GLASGOW COMA SCALE

1. **EYE OPENING (E 1 to 4)**

   E1=No Eye Opening
   E2=Eye Opening to Pain (DPS)
   E3=Eye Opening to Command
   E4=Spontaneous Eye Opening

2. **Motor Response (M 1 To 6)**

   M1=No Movement
   M2=Deceleration (Extension to Pain)
   M3=Abnormal Flexion
   M4=Normal Flexion
   M5=Localises to Pain
   M6=Normal Movement

3. **Verbal Response (V 1 To 5)**

   V1=No Verbal Response
   V2=Incomprehensible Sounds
   V3=Inappropriate Words
   V4=Disorientated to Time, Place and Person
   V5=Normal Speech

BIBLIOGRAPHY, REFERENCES & ACKNOWLEDGMENTS:

1. Indian Public Health Standards (IPHS)
   Guidelines for District Hospitals (101 to 500 Bedded) Revised 2012 Directorate General of Health Services Ministry of Health & Family Welfare, Government of India
2. "Standard Operating Procedures SOP For Hospitals 2nd Edition" by Dr. Arun K. Agarwal
3. "Duties & Responsibilities of Hospital Staff" by Dr. Arun Kumar
4. "Checklists for Hospitals" by Dr. Arun K. Agarwal
5. Stationary Formats. By Dr. Arun K. Agarwal
6. Hospital Manual. DGHS, Ministry of Health & Family Welfare, GOI

Chapter – 10

HOSPITAL EMERGENCY CODES

INDEX

   k. Types Of Fire Extinguisher:
   l. Installation Of Fire Alarm & Fire Fighting System
   m. Hydrant System: (Specifications)
   n. Pumping System
   o. Sprinkler System
   p. Fire Alarm System
   q. Difference between wireless & wired Fire Alarm System
8. Code Pink
   a. Definition
   b. Introduction
   c. Purpose
   d. SOP
      i. Area In-charge will
      ii. In-charges of other wards
      iii. OPD and Emergency
      iv. Security
      v. Hospital Administrator
   e. Calling Code Pink Off
   f. Procedure After "All Over"
9. Code Orange
   a. Introduction
   b. Definition
   c. Types
   d. Hazmat kit
   e. SOPs
   f. ETO Spill Management
   g. Mercury Spill Management
   h. List of Hazardous Material
10. Code Violet
    a. Definition
    b. Purpose
    c. Code Violet Situations
    d. Procedure (SOP)
    e. Prevention Of Such Incidences
11. Code Yellow
    a. Definition
    b. Types of Disasters
    c. Steps
    d. Procedure
12. Disaster Management Manual
13. Cod Black
    a. Definition
    b. Types

c. Important
d. Procedure
e. Action by the Individual on Detection
f. Action by Security Officer

14. Bibliography, References & Acknowledgments

INTRODUCTION:

Hospitals in India use code names to alert its staff to an emergency.

Announcement of an emergency by code names does not create panic among other patients and visitors. Simultaneously it allows trained hospital personnel to respond quickly and appropriately to various events.

Hospital Emergency Codes are coded messages often announced over a public address system of a hospital to alert staff to various classes of on-site emergencies.

The use of codes is intended to convey essential information quickly and with minimal misunderstanding to staff while preventing stress and panic among visitors to the hospital.

These codes are communicated through a Public Address System which is available in almost all hospitals.

The announcement also tells the location of emergency. Hospital personnel are trained to respond to all codes used in the hospital.

OBJECTIVE:

1. To prepare healthcare workers to deal with disaster if any, effectively
2. Safety of patient, HCW, Visitors etc

SCOPE:

- Hospital wide

EMERGENCY CODES IN INDIA:

1. Code Blue:
   Individual disaster/Cardiac arrest
2. Code Red:
   Fire
3. Code Pink:
   Baby Missing/Abduction
4. Code Orange:
   Hazardous Spill/HAZMAT
5. Code Violet:
   Violence
6. Code Yellow:
   External Disaster
7. Code Black:
   Bomb Threat

CODE ACTIVATION:

In case of an emergency, public call emergency number.

To activate a code in the Hospital;

1. Dial Hospital Emergency number/Main Reception.
2. Tell the operator the code to be activated and the location of the code.
3. Ensure that the operator clearly understands your massage.
4. After end of the vent, call the operator again to announce "All Clear"

FREQUENCY OF MOCK DRILLS:

1. Mock drills shall be conducted every month,
2. In-charges shall conduct mock drill in their department every month for training of their staff

CODE BLUE

Code Blue means someone is experiencing a life-threatening medical emergency.

Code Blue is one of the emergency procedure codes for cardiopulmonary arrests and life-threatening emergencies in areas of the hospital. A Code Blue is the term used to alert the Code Blue team (resuscitation team) to an area where a person has had a cardiac/respiratory arrest.

All staff members near the location of the code may need to go to the patient. Each employee of the resuscitation team has a pre-assigned role in the event of a Code Blue.

Code Blue is for **Cardiac arrest/Respiratory failure, Medical emergency**.

What happens in a code blue?

Any hospital staff who finds a patient who isn't breathing, has no pulse or is unresponsive will immediately call a code blue. Simultaneously staff will try to resuscitate the patient if they are trained in these techniques, while waiting for help to arrive.

The Resuscitation Team members are especially trained in advanced cardiac life support techniques.

How serious is a code blue?

Code Blue is serious as the person (patient or anybody else) is in cardiac or respiratory arrest and needs immediate, lifesaving care.

How it is activated?

Dial **EMERGENCY NUMBER** and advise the operator to announce a **"CODE BLUE",** along with the location of the code (which floor/which room). This should be announced **THREE times** in rapid succession.

The following personnel will respond:

1. Available attending Physician from Emergency or ICU
2. Trained Staff Nurse, Patient attendant and housekeeping staff
3. The ACLS/BLS trained staff will lead the resuscitation team until the attending physician arrives.
4. In each department there should be at least one ACLS or BLS trained (as per facility)
5. In Emergency Department max staff must be ACLS trained (as per facility)

General Principles of Code Blue:

CPR is an integral part of management of cardiac arrest. It is started as soon as possible and is continued uninterrupted till desired results are obtained. If even after 20 minutes of CPR, the collapsed person has not responded, then only he is declared dead and CPR is stopped.

Old school of thought says that if heart stops beating for more than 6 to 10 minutes, then the brain would be dead. But now a day the research suggests that CPR should be carried out even if the heart has stopped for more than 20 minutes.

After ensuring the safety of the patient, staff will be responsible for further management of the collapsed patient.

It involves;

1. Prevention of further injury
2. Checking response to verbal and tactile stimuli
3. Care of airway, breathing and circulation
4. Control of bleeding
5. Protection from the environment
6. Maintenance of normal body temperature
7. Protection of bony prominences from hard objects
8. Reassurance and continued observation of the collapsed patient.

Requirements for Providing CPR:

1. At least one Crash Cart should be available at each patient floor/area loaded with all necessary lifesaving drugs and equipment. It is to be inspected daily and used only at the time of crash of a patient.
2. Code blue team is constituted to provide resuscitation in all patient areas. The team members are trained in Advanced Cardiac Life Support and Basic Life Support.
3. The hospital has a Code Blue Committee which is responsible for training, assessing of its members. It can make changes, amendments in CPR plans.
4. All events of code blue are recorded and end result analysed.
5. Corrective and Preventive actions are planned based on the analysis of all the events in the hospital in the Code Blue Committee meeting.
6. In the Hospital all staffs related to patient care are trained in BLS and staff of critical areas, code blue team is trained in ACLS.

Process Flow:

1. First Clinical staff who discovers the need for CPR:
   a. Ensure the area is safe & free from any obstacles.
   b. Will shout and shake the patient and try to arouse him.
   c. Will call for help by announcing Code Blue.
   d. Will start CPR and will continue till the "Resuscitation Team" arrives.
2. Second Staff who is present:
   a. Will activate "Code Blue".
   b. Will bring the Crash Cart near the site.
   c. Will arrange all necessary drugs.
   d. Will assist the first person till the team arrives.

3. Arrival of Team Blue: Duties are listed below.
4. Post Resuscitation:
5. Documentation:

CRASH CART:

The hospital has provided one crash cart in each department.

The Crash cart is always equipped/loaded with required medicines and other paraphernalia.

List of medicines available in the cart is pasted on its drawers.

List of major items on Crash Cart is as below:

a. Cardiac Monitor
b. Defibrillator
c. Ambu Bags
d. Laryngoscopes
e. Intubation aids.
f. Emergency Medicines.
g. Oxygen gas Cylinder
h. Consumables like: ET Tubes, IV canula, IV Sets, Syringes & Needles. IV Fluids

CODE BLUE TEAM:

1. The hospital should constitute three 'Code Blue Team' and one of it must be available round the clock in the hospital.
2. This is a team of trained professionals who can competently provide life saving measures to a patient under medical emergency.
3. Every hospital should modify team members as per availability in the hospital.
4. This team handles any medical emergency situation arising anywhere in the hospital.

SN	Name/Designation	Remarks
1	Anaesthetist	
2	ICU In-charge	
3	Resident Doctor	
4	Nurses trained in CPR	
5	Ward Attendant	

Responsibilities of Code Blue Team:

1. Duty Doctor: will be responsible for
   - Airway Management
   - Drug Administration
   - Patient Analysis and management
2. Ward RMO: is responsible for
   - Chest compression
   - Will be team Captain in the absence of the ICU Doctor

3. Nurse/ICU Nurse In-charge: is responsible for
   - ECG (leads and electrode placement)
   - I/V Access
   - Drug Administration
   - Blood sample
   - Defibrillator
   - Glucometer
4. Assigned Nurse of patient:
   - To give complete history of patient
   - Give compressions till Code Blue Team arrives
   - Additional assistance to the members of the Code Blue team
   - Arrange Crash Cart immediately
5. Security Supervisor
   - To clear the passage
   - Request attendants (if present in the room) to wait outside till the event is over
   - To ensure the availability of stretcher at the site
   - To cordon the area
   - To ensure that lift is available and is on standby on the floor of Code Blue Event
6. Front Office:
   - Announcing the code in a prescribed manner.
   - Informing all code blue team members on phone also.
7. Other specialists available in the hospital will reach the site.

   The Code Blue Team is free to seek help from other staff in managing the patient.

   Team shall not leave the site till ordered by the team captain.

STANDARD OPERATING PROCEDURE (SOP):

1. First responder/medical/nursing/paramedical personnel shall check the responsiveness of the patient by speaking loudly and trying to rouse them by shaking his shoulder.
2. If there is no response send/call/shout for help before starting any resuscitation measures.
3. A code blue medical emergency shall be anticipated if patient is unresponsive, meaning he is not breathing or his heart has stopped beating, or both, in which case nearby medical/nursing personnel shall be summoned immediately.
4. Nursing/medical personnel on site initiates CPR as per BLS protocols.
5. Dial 'Front Office' numbers immediately and he/she should be intimated with word 'Code Blue' followed by place of occurrence. For e.g., "Code blue – room no. XXX, in XXX Floor" or "Code blue – imaging department waiting room"
6. The reception staff will announce code blue on internal hospital communication system by 3 consecutive times and also inform code blue team members through phone. e.g., "Code blue – room no. 202, Second Floor" or "Code blue – imaging department waiting room,
7. Initiate basic life support until the code blue team can respond by the first responder.
8. Code blue team members shall NOT use the lift.
9. Code blue team shall reach the site as early as possible but not later than 2 minutes.
10. Emergency crash cart, intubation tray, defibrillator is all pushed into the area.
11. Place the patient on hard surface in supine position and rescuer also in correct position.

12. If patient requires CPR start cardiac massage (chest compressions) should be started with the rate of 100 compressions/min and depth should be at least 5 cm or 2 inches.
13. Ratio of cardiac massage and external ventilation should be 5:1.
14. Ensures the safety of self and the victim.
15. Make sure that airway is cleared by proper position (Hyperextension of head & neck) and artificial dentures are removed.
16. At least Initiate mouth-to-mouth breathing if breathing not restored
17. Ensure the closing of nostrils of victim with thumb and index finger and enclosing his mouth with rescuers mouth to maintain the airtight seal for effective ventilation of lungs.
18. Repeat the procedure 12-20 times at the rate of 1 inflation every 3-5 secs.
19. Ensure the inflation of lungs corresponds to the respiration of the victim.
20. If victim is pulse less, give cardiac compression following initial four rapid breaths to maintain circulation.
21. Ensure the establishment of respiration and circulation: constriction of pupils, regular pulse, normal B.P, normal skin colour& rhythmic respiration.
22. Observe for any complications: Sternal and rib fracture pneumothorax.
23. Patient is to be taken in to advance cardiac life care area and mechanical support is provided as soon as possible.
24. Fill the code blue form after provision of resuscitation effort and send it to Code Blue Committee

TECHNICAL PROCEDURE:

CPR can be carried out by one person or two persons. Though the procedure is same for all patients, there is slight difference in infants and children.

STEPS IN CPR:

a. One person CPR:

Step 1: Assess responsiveness of the patient by yelling his name near the victim, and gently/ vigorously shaking the shoulders.

1. If there is response from the patient, shout for help, even if no one is in sight.
2. If the victim is lying face down on the bed, roll him back down. Place a firm board below his back if possible.

Step 2: Try to keep airway open.

1. Use head tilt/chin lift manoeuvre
2. Place hand on the patient's forehead, and pull backwards to tilt the head.
3. Support the lower jaw by placing the index finger and middle finger under the bony part of the jaw. – Try not to press soft tissues
4. If neck injury is suspected, do not move the neck.

Step 3: Clear the airway:

1. If liquid or semi liquid is visible in the airway, wipe it out.
2. If a foreign body is visible or his tongue has fallen back in the airway, take it out with the index finger.
3. Leave dentures in place unless they are loose, and cannot be kept in place.
4. Assess breathing by placing your cheek in front of the victim's mouth.
5. Look for chest movements
6. Listen to breathing sounds

7. Feel for expired air by putting your ears near patient's nostrils.

Step 4: If the patient is not breathing:

1. Maintain airway.
2. Give mouth-to-mouth breathing.
3. Give adequate interval in between two air flows.

Step 5: Assess Circulation: Check for carotid pulse.

1. Feel for carotid pulse, at the side nearest to you.
2. If pulse is not present, announce Code Blue and start CPR.
3. Put you're both hands interlocked together on patient's chest and start chest compressions.
4. Maximum pressure should be achieved with least efforts.
5. Release the pressure to allow blood flow into the heart.
6. Give about 30 compressions per minute.
7. Open the mouth and give two forced breaths.
8. After 4 such cycles reassess for self-breathing by the patient (spontaneous breathing).
9. Check for carotid pulse.

b. Two person CPR:

If two persons are available, CPR is done in the same way but one person takes charge of keeping ventilation (mouth-to-mouth breathing, etc) and second person takes charge of chest compression.

Summary of Procedure:

1. Start by placing the heel of one hand at the centre of the person's chest and interlock your fingers. With arms straightened, press down hard and fast, letting the chest come back up fully each time.
2. Fast means around 2 times every second and hard means that the chest needs to go down by about 2 inches.
3. Compressions – 30 compressions at 2 inches deep, 100-120 per minute.
4. If the rescuer is trained in CPR, they should give 2 rescue breaths, otherwise, continue with compressions
5. Rescue breaths begin by tilting the victim's head back and lifting the chin slightly to open the airway, then pinching the nostrils closed and giving 2 normal breaths, watching the victim's chest rise and fall.
6. However, if that is not possible just keep going with 'hand-only' continuous chest compressions. Don't stop until either a health professional takes over, or the person is definitely breathing normally.
7. If required, we can add another step 'D' i.e., for Defibrillator, which is about delivering a shock to restart the heartbeat.

POST-EVENT ANALYSIS:

1. A post-event analysis of all cardio-pulmonary resuscitations is done by a multidisciplinary committee:
2. Post event, by team members of CODE BLUE Committee shall analyse all the recorded events.
3. Committee may call in the actual team or involve the consultant-in-charge in the evaluation of the event.
4. Analysis is made to see if all laid down protocols were followed or not.
5. Explanations are sought from the Code Blue team for any deviations, omissions or new commissions.
6. The time lag on performing the necessary procedures is taken into stock and if inappropriate then cause analysis is done.

7. The usage of drugs, adequate dosages and appropriateness of use along with important inclusions and omissions are noted and discussed.
8. The final outcome is noted and a statement is made about the proper course and outcome of the CPR procedure.

Aspects to be analysed:

1. Was the Response Time of the CPR committee according to set protocol?
2. Did all the members report at the time of call?
3. Was the announcement of Code Blue audible to all team members?
4. Was the CPR Initial Assessment correctly done?
5. Was the CPR protocol performed according to set guidelines?
6. Was the outcome of the CPR satisfactory?
7. Was the emergency medication and crash cart available with the CPR team on time?
8. Was there any equipment failure that hindered in smooth CPR implementation?

CAPA:

1. Corrective and preventive measures are taken based on the post-event analysis:
2. Analysis reports by multidisciplinary committee or all Code Blue events shall be presented and discussed in the periodic Code Blue Committee meetings for planning preventive steps.
3. Corrective and preventive measures based on findings and recommendations are discussed with all members of the resuscitation team and further updates and trainings are conducted as per the need.

DOCUMENTATION:

- Event Recording Form
- Event analysis record
- MOM of code blue committee.

1. The events during a cardio-pulmonary resuscitation are recorded.
2. All the events during CPR are recorded.
   a. To facilitate accurate and complete documentation of Code occurrence and action taken.
   b. To provide a record for review and evaluation of CPR and advanced life support measures.
3. This starts by documenting the time of initiation and termination of CPR efforts.
4. All medications used with the quantity and strength are documented.
5. All steps are documented including use of defibrillator and time taken/time delays in following a laid down step in protocol.
6. An entry as to who all were present in the Code Blue team and other members present is made.
7. CPR Form shall be maintained by the Nursing Supervisor.
8. Signatures of the recorder and the Team Leader are required for the completion of the log. This affirms that all documented interventions were ordered.

Audit Form – Code Blue/CPR Evaluation Form

Code Blue Announcement Date & Time: ....

Announced By: .... Location of Code Blue: ....

Team Arrival Time: ....

Code Blue Team Members:

1. Physician
2. Anaesthetist
3. Medical Officer
4. Nurse Supervisor

Patient Profile:

1. Name, Age/Sex: .... OPD/IPD Number: ....
2. Ward/Unit/Location: ....
3. Diagnosis: ....

Code Blue/CPR Assessment:

Pulse Rate: .... Carotid Pulse: yes/no BP: ....

ECG: Rate/Rhythm

Airway: Obstructed? Any foreign body?/Secretions/etc?

Breathing: Yes/No Respiration Rate: .... SpO2: ....

Any Disability: ....

Code Blue/CPR Team Interventions:

Secured By: ....

Circulation: IV Line/IV Fluids

Drugs

Airway: Ambu/Oral/Nasal/ET Tube

Breathing: Oxygen Ventilator

Outcome:

Transferred to (ward): Time

Explained to (relatives): Yes/No Time

Valuables handed over to: Name Yes/No Time

Comments:

Team Members all arrived: Yes/No

Delayed/Absent

Any other Problem:

1. Supplies/Equipment
2. Etc.

Physician Name: ....

Signature: .... Date: .... Time: ....

Nursing Supervisor Name: ....

Signature: .... Date: .... Time: ....

****

Code Blue Audit Tools

Attribute:

1. Did the team respond in time?
2. Was assessment DOCUMENTED?
3. Was assessment doubtful?
4. Was Quality of CPR satisfactory?
5. Was IV access established immediately (IF NOT EXISTING ALREADY)?
6. Were medication orders followed properly?
7. Was all equipment in a functional state?

More Tools:

8. Was the Assessment done correctly and in time?
9. Was the Response of the CPR team according to set protocol?
10. Were compressions started immediately after call for help?
11. Was airway clearance achieved without delay?
12. Was Rate of compression, depth, and no interruption protocol observed during compressions?
13. Was ventilation rate optimal?
14. Were any problems identified during defibrillation? *(If applicable)
15. Was IV access established without delay/previously established?
16. Was there any confusion observed regarding roles and knowledge?
17. Was appropriate Medication Given to Patient?
18. Were too many team members present?
19. Was all required equipment available and functioned well without hindrance?
20. Was documentation appropriately done?

****

Code Blue Audit

Post Event Analysis

CPR Post Event Analysis by CPR Committee

CPR Committee Held on:

CPR Committee Members for Review:

IPD No.:

Date of CPR:

SN	Aspects to be Analysed	Aspects Taken Care		Remark
		Yes	No	
1	Was the Response Time of the CPR committee according to set protocol?			
2	Did all the members report at the time of call?			
3	Was the announcement of Code Blue audible to all team members?			
4	Was the CPR Initial Assessment correctly done?			
5	Was the CPR protocol performed according to set guidelines?			

SN	Aspects to be Analysed	Aspects Taken Care		Remark
		Yes	No	
6	Was the outcome of the CPR satisfactory?			
7	Was the emergency medication and crash cart available with the CPR team on time?			
8	Was there any equipment failure that hindered in smooth CPR implementation?			

Corrective and Preventing Action Taken:

Signature of CPR Committee Chairman:

****

Code Blue Audit Report - Incident

Mr/Ms. ____________________________, __________ year old lady/man, with IPD No: ___________ went into cardiac arrest on bed no ______________ on_________________ (date & year).

Immediate medical intervention was given with CPR and DC shock.

An audit was done and inputs were taken from the respective staff:

History:

Pt was admitted on ____________________ under Dr. __________________

She/he was nondiabetic/Diabetic with complain of: ____ ______________________

Findings and Opinions:

****

Post Event Analysis/Checklist:

SN	Events	Answer	Remark
1	Was the Assessment done Correctly and in time?	Yes/No	
2	Was the Response of the CPR team according to set protocol?		
3	Did all the members report at the time of call?		
4	Were compressions started immediately after call for help? Rate being 100/minute?		
5	Was airway clearance achieved without delay?		
6	Were any problems identified during defibrillation? *(If applicable)		
7	Was IV access established without delay/previously established?		
8	Were all required equipment/medicines available and functioned well without hindrance?		
9	Was documentation appropriately done?		

CODE BLUE COMMITTEE:

1. Meets every 6 month or on need basis.
2. Members: as below

SN	Name/Designation	Role in the Committee
1	Medical Superintendent	Chairman
2	HOD Anaesthesia	Convenor
3	HOD Cardiology/Physician	Member
4	Quality Manager	Member

Scope/Responsibilities:

1. To monitor and track response to all Code Blue cases in the hospital.
2. To develop policy on prevention, management, and control of cases of cardiac arrest and related emergencies within the hospital.
3. To work for improving response time and easy access to emergency medical equipment including crash cart.
4. To decide upon the composition and responsibilities of each member of the Code Blue team.
5. To ensure effective resuscitation in such cases.
6. Recommend special training initiatives for the Code Blue team members.
7. To ensure availability of required resources. (Men & Material)
8. To ensure availability of all emergency drugs in crash carts at all times.
9. To organise & supervise Mock Drills.
10. To carry out post-event analysis of all cardiac arrests in this hospital. To analyse and evaluate all episodes of Cardiac Arrest in the hospital by a multi-disciplinary committee and to formulate preventive measures based upon this analysis
11. To advise and supervise corrective and preventive measures to be taken based on the post-event analysis

Procedure:

1. Circular for a meeting is prepared and circulated by the coordinator one or 2 days in advance, indicating Date & time of meeting, Location and agenda of the meeting.
2. Quorum is (MS, Anaesthetist, Physician or Surgeon). The proceedings of the meeting are started once defined members are present.
3. First of all, minutes of last meeting are reviewed.
4. Minutes of every meeting are recorded by the coordinator and circulated among members.
   A copy is kept on record.
5. Corrective & preventive actions taken for any shortfall. Records for all CAPA (Corrective Actions & Preventive Actions) are to be maintained.
6. Format for taking and maintaining attendance of the meeting:

QUALITY INDICATORS:

Indicators that can be used for evaluating whether or not the code blue system is working efficiently and effectively, are given below

1. Average time to respond: that is time taken between announcements of code blue to reaching of code blue team to site.

2. Outcome percentage: that is percentage of patients survived by CPR.
3. Non- compliance rate: that is how many staff did not know the process of code blue.
4. Failure to activate: How many times the ABC Hospital failed to activate Code Blue.

****

CODE RED

Hospitals in India use code names to alert its staff to an emergency.

Announcement of an emergency by code names does not create panic among other patients and visitors. Simultaneously it allows trained hospital personnel to respond quickly and appropriately to various events.

These codes are communicated through a Public Address System which is available in almost all hospitals.

The announcement also tells the location of emergency. Hospital personnel are trained to respond to all codes used in the hospital.

Code Red is for **Fire, smoke, or smells of smoke & Internal Disaster**.

DEFINITION:

Code Red alerts hospital staff to a fire or probable fire. A Code Red may also be activated if someone smells or sees smoke. This code will often come with information about the fire's location and will typically require evacuation.

CODE ACTIVATION:

1. Code red shall be activated by any employee of the hospital who detects or is informed about unexpected fire flames, smoke, and smell of smoke, unusual heat or any other indication of fire.
2. The fire or fire like situation could be observed in any part of the hospital, including hospital's exteriors and terrace.
3. Code red should be activated even if it is uncertain, if the situation is caused because of fire or not.
4. For activating code red, the emergency intercom number should be called from the nearest intercom device and ***'Code Red'*** followed by the location details shall be spoken.
5. The announcement shall be repeated 3 times initially in clear voice and then shall be repeated intermittently after that.

PROCEDURE FOLLOWING CODE RED ALERT:

Remain calm and follow the acronym.

A. **Employee near to the area where fire is detected** – As soon as code red is announced, all employees who are near the location where fire is detected should immediately assess the severity of fire. Remain calm and follow the acronym.

   R.A.C.E.

   a. **Rescue/Remove** anyone from immediate danger to a safe area.
   b. **Alarm** others in the nearby area and call for help.
   c. **Confine** the fire by closing all doors/windows.

d. **Extinguish** the fire if the fire is small, by using fire extinguisher. Fire extinguisher should be used as per **P.A.S.S.** protocol, which is
   1. **Pull the pin** of fire extinguisher
   2. **Aim** the stream at the base of the fire
   3. **Squeeze** the lever slowly and gently
   4. **Sweep** from side to side

B. **Employees who are away from the fire location** - All other employee shall must note the location where fire has been announced and shall do following:
   1. Do not go towards the area where fire has been detected, unless and until specifically called upon or required.
   2. Listen for additional instructions and be ready to help in case required.
   3. Prevent and other outsiders in their vicinity from going towards the fire affected area.
   4. Keep all fire doors closed except while passing through them, to prevent spread of fire and smoke.
   5. Be ready to evacuate if directed and get assembled in assembly area of the hospital.
   6. Do not use elevators.

C. **Hospital administrator** – He will immediately reach the place and taking care of his own safety, assess the situation. He shall ensure that R.A.C.E protocol is initiated and shall also take decision on whether patients and others need to be evacuated and whether to call fire brigade immediately, without waiting for hospital's fire-fighting team to arrive. Any situational decisions shall be taken by him/her till the time of reaching of fire-fighting team after which the situation shall be handed over to them.

   In absence of hospital administrator, the in-charge of the area where fire is detected shall perform these functions.

D. **In-charge of Central oxygen supply -** He/she shall wait for instruction on whether Oxygen supply shall be closed to the area where fire is detected and do according to the instruction. He/she shall be available for any further instruction.

E. **Fire-fighting team** - The fire-fighting team is composed of 4 personnel from security and maintenance. The members of fire-fighting team are trained on fire-fighting measures. Three teams are constituted and it is ensured that one team is present in all shift. There is an in-charge of each team. The fire-fighting team must do following on listening **code red** alert
   a. Reach to the place where fire has occurred on an urgent basis
   b. Take charge of fire-fighting measures from the employees on sight
   c. Pass on necessary instructions to the people present over there for safety
   d. Start controlling the fire as per the training given to them.

F. **Fire-fighting team in-charge:** The in-charge should also reach the place along with other team members. The in-charge will lead the fire-fighting team and will also do following
   a. Assess the situation and determine, if the fire is severe enough to call for external help
   b. Decide whether evacuation plan needs to be initiated
   c. Decide whether Fire Brigade needs to be called
   d. Any other decision that needs to be taken

G. **Fire Brigade** – In case fire brigade is called, the fire-fighting team should continue their effort till the time it reaches. Focus should be on safety. As soon as the fire brigade arrives, the situation should be handed over to them and their direction should be followed.

EVACUATION:

In case evacuation needs to be done, hospital's evacuation plan for each area shall be followed. This should be supervised by the fire-fighting team.

CODE RED – ALL CLEAR

1. The fire-fighting team in-charge has the authority to declare if the situation has been tackled and is safe from fire. For this the in-charge calls back on emergency number and speaks
2. **'Code Red – All Clear'.** On getting this information, the operator then announces the same on public announcement system. Employee on listening 'Code Red – All Clear' can assume that the fire emergency has been taken care of and they can resume back to their normal work.
3. The employees, patient and visitors of the area where fire occurred shall be instructed, if the area can be used or not. Also, any patient or employee if injured during the incident shall immediately be taken to hospital's emergency for treatment.

DOCUMENTATION

1. Code red event whenever occurred (real or mock) must be documented to keep a record and for further improvement.
2. This shall be done by preparing a report within 3 days of occurrence of the incident.
3. The report shall be prepared by the in-charge of fire-fighting team in consultation with the employee of area where fire was detected.
4. The report must contain following points and shall be submitted to CEO
   a. Date and time of code red activation
   b. Severity of fire
   c. Measures taken for controlling fire (both by employee and team)
   d. Whether fire brigade was called?
   e. Whether evacuation was done?
   f. Losses – injuries, death, damage of property etc.
   g. Probable causes of fire
   h. Problems identified and corrective actions to be taken

SOP - Daily Checking of Fire Fighting System:

Firefighting system should be maintained so that it operates safely, smoothly and trouble free.

1. Inspect the firefighting system (Fire Pump Room) and check all the pumps as per SOP.
2. Check the Fire Panel in the Pump Room and ensure that all the pumps are in Auto Mode.
3. Ensure that the pressure gauges of the Hydrant and Sprinkler System are showing pressure between 5 to 7.5 kg/cm2.
4. Check the detectors and MCP's on all floors and ensure that they are working okay (Blinking properly). If not, then clean the detector and if required, call the supplier.
5. Take a round of all the fire staircases and ensure that there is no leakage from glands/pipe joints. Also inspect all the hose boxes.
6. Check all the Fire Extinguishers. Report to Facility Manager if the pressure shows low on any of the extinguishers.
7. Fill up the Daily Check Lists and report to Facility Manager.

SOP – Checking of Smoke Detectors:

It is to establish a procedure for testing of fire alarm system in the hospital.

1. Activate any detector on a pre designated floor using an Incense Stick.
2. Confirm that the correct address of the activated detector is displayed on the LCD of the fire panel.

3. Confirm the address (Zone, loop, detector no.) with the list (hard copy).
4. Confirm that the hooters of the concerned floor are activated instantly.
5. The person stationed near the Man Panel after confirming the correct address shall accept the alarm by pressing ACCEPT button on the fire Panel.
6. Silence the hooters by pressing SILENCE SOUNDERS on the fire panel.
7. Clean the detector and fit it back. Repeat this exercise for at least 3 locations on each floor.
8. Also include the detectors above the false ceiling and use random sampling method.
9. Break the glass of MCP on the designated floor and confirm the address is correct and matches with the indication on the fire panel.
10. Confirm that the hooters are activated on the concerned floor.
11. Accept the call and silence the hooters as stated above on the fire panel.
12. Replace the broken glass.
13. Repeat the above procedure on each floor as scheduled.

SOP – Fire Drill:

It is to establish a procedure for using of the Fire Extinguishers.

1. Create an artificial fire outside the main building near the Hydrant.
2. Open the hose door using the Key and roll out the hose reel hose and run towards the designated fire.
3. Aim at the Fire and open the valve of the hose reel hose to pour the water over the fire.
4. Repeat the same exercise using the hose pipe. Make sure that the hose is first fitted in the pipe and after laying the hose pipe, the nozzle is fitted. Then open the valve slowly after ensuring that the nozzle is held by the person firmly and aimed at the fire point.
5. The opening of the hose valve shall be done as per instructions and under personal supervision of the safety officer.
6. After the drill is over, remove the nozzle and roll back the pipe after ensuring that it has dried.
7. Repeat the above steps using a fire extinguisher as per SOP over the controlled fire.
8. Prepare the report and take signatures of all the attendees, and report to the Quality Cell of the hospital/Fire Safety Officer.

SOP – Fire Extinguisher Inspection:

All fire extinguishers in the hospital are to be inspected and maintained so that they are readily available and easily accessible whenever needed.

A. **MONTHLY INSPECTION:**

1. **CO2 Cylinders:**
    a. Weigh and check if extinguisher is full or not, with help of calibrated weighing scale. If weight is 10% less than standard weight, it should be sent for refilling.
    b. Check for access to the extinguisher. If any obstruction is observed, clear it.
    c. Inspect hose and horn. It must be in good condition and open (not choked)
    d. Check for lock pin for its positioning. If not ok, set it.
2. **Water CO2:**
    a. Weigh and check if extinguisher is full or not, with help of calibrated weighing scale. If weight is 10% less than standard weight, then fill up the extinguisher with fresh water.
    b. Check for access to the extinguisher. If any obstruction is observed, clear it.

c. Inspect hose or nozzle. It must be in good condition and open (not choked or damaged)
d. Check for neck guard of extinguisher. If it is not in position, do check the cartridge of extinguisher. If cartridge is punctured, replace it.

3. **Dry Chemical Powder:**
   a. Weigh and check if extinguisher is full or not, with help of calibrated weighing scale. If weight is 10% less than standard weight, send it for refilling.
   b. Check for access to the extinguisher. If any obstruction is observed, clear it.
   c. Inspect the hose. It must be in good condition and open (not choked or damaged)
   d. Check for neck guard of extinguisher. If it is not in position, do check the cartridge of extinguisher. If cartridge is punctured, replace it.

B. **YEARLY INSPECTION:**
1. **CO2 Cylinders:**
   a. Weigh and check if extinguisher is full or not, with help of calibrated weighing scale. If weight is 10% less than standard weight, it should be sent for refilling.
   b. Check for access to the extinguisher. If any obstruction is observed, clear it.
   c. Inspect hose and horn. It must be in good condition and open (not choked)
   d. Check for lock pin for its positioning. If not ok, set it.
2. **Water CO2:**
   a. Replace the water of the fire extinguisher.
   b. Check the cartridge of extinguisher. If cartridge is punctured or weight is not as per standard, replace it.
3. **Dry Chemical Powder:**
   a. Check the cartridge weight, if not as per standards, replace it.

C. **Inspection every five years: (external agency):**
1. Co2 cylinders:
   - Hydro test as per local standards
2. Water Co2:
   - Hydro test as per local standards
3. Dry chemical powder:
   - Hydro test as per local standards

SOP – Fire Hydrant Inspection - Checklist:

Hydrant and sprinkler system should be inspected and maintained so that it operates safely, smoothly and trouble free.

Monthly inspection:

1. Drain all hydrants for 2 minutes and check the flow of water (with hose)
2. Check the rubber gasket of each hydrant point. If not ok or missing, replace it.
3. Check hose box and panel key.
4. Check hose condition. If not good, replace it. And send old ones to repair.
5. Check for presence of rubber gaskets in hose. If missing, put new one.
6. Check the nozzle. If oxidation is formed, clean it. Also check nozzle for choking.
7. Check if hose fixes firmly on hydrant point and hose.
8. Check hydrant pipeline for rusting. Restore any deterioration immediately.

9. Check all hydrant section valves for water leakages. Adjust gland. If required, replace the gland packing.
10. Check free operation of hydrant valves. If not ok, grease it.

SOP – Pumps Inspection – Checklist:

1. Ensure voltage of 415 Volt in the volt meter of the panel.
2. Check all suction and discharge valves are in open position.
3. Hydrant pump should always in AUTO Mode & Jockey pump in to off mode.
4. Check the pump rotation it should rotate freely when rotated by hand.
5. Put the selector switch in to manual mode and Start the Jockey pump by pressing the start push button.
6. Check the flow discharge pressure at pressure gauge.
7. Stop the Jockey pump by pressing the stop push button.
8. Drain the water through any one of the hydrants point when pressure drop down to 4.5, Hydrant pump should start.
9. Check for any unusual sound and rectify the problem immediately.
10. Check the flow discharge pressure at pressure gauge.
11. Check for any unusual sound and rectify the problem immediately.
12. Check the Hydrant pump operation by draining the water through all the Hydrant Points.

For prevention or extinguishing a fire, it is most important that keeping fuel sources and ignition sources separate.

Fire to happen, there are three important elements. All three elements must be present for fire to ignite and spread. If any one element is taken away, the fire will be extinguished.

1. OXYGEN for combustion
2. HEAT to reach ignition temperature
3. FUEL or combustible material

TYPES OF FIRE EXTINGUISHER:

Type (Fire / Extinguisher)	CLASS A Combustible materials (e.g. paper & wood)	CLASS B Flammable liquids (e.g. paint & petrol)	CLASS C Flammable gases (e.g. butane and methane)	CLASS D Flammable metals (e.g. lithium & potassium)	Electrical Electrical equipment (e.g. computers & generators)	CLASS F Deep fat fryers (e.g. chip pans)	Comments
Water	✓	✗	✗	✗	✗	✗	Do not use on liquid or electric fires
Foam	✓	✓	✗	✗	✗	✗	Not suited to domestic use
Dry Powder	✓	✓	✓	✓	✓	✗	Can be used safely up to 1000 volts
CO2	✗	✓	✗	✗	✓	✗	Safe on both high and low voltage
Wet Chemical	✓	✗	✗	✗	✗	✓	Use on extremely high temperatures

There are different types of "Fire Extinguishers" available in the market for different types of fire.

Following are the commonly available:

1. Water (W/Co2): For 'A' Class of fire
2. Mechanical Foam: For 'A' & 'B' Class of fire
3. Carbon Dioxide (CO2): For 'B' & 'C' Class of fire
4. Dry Chemical (ABC): For 'A', 'B' & 'C' Class of fire
5. Dry Chemical (BC): For 'B' & 'C' Class of fire

1. **Water (W/Co2) Fire Extinguishers:**

   It is best suited for fire of ordinary carbonaceous materials like wood, paper, cloth, rubber etc.

   These work by taking away the "heat" element of the Fire.

   Water cannot be used on electrical fire. But if there is no option, make sure that the electrical equipment is un-plugged.

2. **Mechanical Foam Fire Extinguishers:**

   It works by forming a thick layer of foam over the fire there by cutting the supply of atmospheric oxygen. It also reduces the 'heat' element of the fire.

   These are designed for Class A & B fires: such as; Petrol, oil, naphtha, paints, alcohols & solvents.

3. **Carbon Dioxide Fire Extinguishers:**

   It again works by reducing the availability of oxygen required for fire to spread.

   These are used for Class B & C fire such as; Flammable Liquids and Electrical Sources fires.

4. **Dry Chemical (ABC) Fire Extinguishers:**

   They are the most common type of fire extinguishers and are commonly used in most type of fires.

   They cut of the oxygen supply and reduce heat.

   These are used to extinguish Class A, B and C fires.

5. **Dry Chemical (BC) Fire Extinguishers**

   It works on the same principal as ABC, but is not commonly used.

   These extinguishers are used for class B & C fires.

IMPORTANT POINTS:

1. Most important thing that the person trying to extinguish a fire must know "What is burning". It will help you in using correct type of extinguisher.
2. Though ABC type is commonly used but still to avoid any complication, one must understand about items that are burning are near the fire.
3. The nozzle of the extinguisher is to be directed at the beginning stages of the fire.
4. While fighting a fire, be sure that there is an exit point (escape route) on back side of you. It is essential to know – how to escape if fire spreads.

INSTALLATION OF FIRE ALARM & FIRE FIGHTING SYSTEM:

Following systems must be provided in the hospital building:

1. Hydrant System consisting of External Hydrant System and Internal Hydrant Risers.
2. Automatic Pumping System with Hydrant, Sprinkler and Jockey Pumps. Additionally, a standby engine operated pump is to be provided.
3. Sprinkler System covering all parts of the building other than the electrical areas.
4. Fire Alarm System for the entire Building, other than the parking areas of the Basement.
5. Emergency Public Address System for all areas.

6. Fire Extinguishers of required types.
7. Cable Fire Seals, Cable Tray protection on power cables.

Hydrant System: (Specifications)

1. The Hydrant System consists of number of risers of 150 mm diameter for the building. The Risers shall be located in the Fire Hose Cabinet (F H C).
2. On each floor with each riser there should be a Hydrant Station having a Hydrant, 2 numbers RRL Hose and a Short Branch Pipe. The reinforced rubber lined hose should be of 15 metres in length. They should be provided with gun metal quick jointing couplings. The Hydrant should be of gun metal and should be provided with a stainless-steel orifice plate to reduce water pressure to 3.5 bar so that the water pressure is manageable.
3. The Hydrant Station should also be provided with a First Aid Hose Reel consisting of a 36-metre length 20 mm diameter double braided rubber hose wound on a drum bracket with aluminium alloy bracket and piping. This set should be connected to the Hydrant Riser through a 25 mm diameter Ball Valve.
4. The Terrace should have an Air Vessel with drain and Pressure Gauge to absorb pressure surges and water hammer effect when any of the main pumps start.
5. Each Riser should also have a Fire Brigade Inlet (Four Way) outside the building. In case the Water Tank of the Building is exhausted, and additional water is required, then the Fire Brigade Inlet shall be used to pump water directly into the Riser through the Fire Brigade Riser.

Pumping System:

1. To cater for the Hydrant and Sprinkler Systems, a good pumping system should be provided:
2. Other than the Sprinkler Pump, all other Pumps should be able to feed the Hydrant System. All the Pumps should be able to feed the Sprinkler System.
3. There should be a common Suction Header of 250 mm diameter, which should be fed from the tank through Basket Strainers. Each Pump should have a Gate Valve on the Suction Side as well as Gate Valve and Non-Return Valve on the Delivery Side. The Delivery of each Pump shall be connected to the Common Delivery Header.
4. The Pumps should start automatically through use of Pressure Switches.
5. The Pumps should be single stage horizontal split casing coupled to motor at 1450 RPM. The engine driven pump should also be of 1450 RPM. The engine should be multi cylinder Heat Exchanger cooled type. All Pumps shall have mechanical seal.

Sprinkler System:

1. The Sprinkler System should have an independent Main Pump, with the engine driven pump being common for Hydrant System. The Sprinkler Pump shall be of 2850 LPM. There shall be a common tank for Hydrant and Sprinkler System.
2. The Sprinkler System should have an additional Over Head Tank of sufficient capacity that should feed directly to the Installation Control Valves.
3. The Installation Control Valve should be UL listed and have a turbine operated gong that should operate an audible alarm in case of a sprinkler discharge.
4. Sprinkler discharge should be based on an AMAO (assumed Maximum Area of Operation) of 360 M2 and a discharge density of 5 LPM/minute applicable for Ordinary Hazard areas. Approximate area coverage per sprinkler shall be 12 M2.

5. Sprinklers should be of quartzoid bulb type with an orifice of 15 mm diameter. Sprinklers should be either pendant or upright type. All areas with false ceiling should be provided with powder coated sprinklers with powder coated rosette plate. Certain special areas such as at the entry shall have powder coated concealed sprinklers.
6. All internal piping should be of Mild Steel Heavy Grade and should have welded jointing for pipes above 50 mm diameter. All pipes should be painted with a primer coat and two coats of post office red paint.
7. Each Floor should be provided with a Flow Switch (connected to the Fire Alarm System or the Sprinkler Annunciation Panel) so that in case of any sprinkler discharge on any floor, the alarm shall be indicated on the Panel.

Fire Alarm System:

1. It is advisable to have an Intelligent Addressable Fire Alarm System.
2. The building should be protected with Intelligent Smoke Detectors of Photo Electric type with Sensitivity level of about 0.8 % obscuration.
3. Each Detector should have coverage of 80 M2 per detector for flat surfaces. Wherever there is an obscuration of 450 mm or higher than additional detectors shall be installed.
4. Thermistor type rate of Rise Heat Detectors should be installed in areas that are susceptible to high dust intake such as open balconies and non-air-conditioned machine rooms.
5. Combination of Smoke and Heat Detectors should be installed in areas where it is felt that an additional heat sensor would be advisable.
6. Air conditioning units should have a Duct Detector to sample air from the area of conditioning. Probes should be fixed into the duct to sample air which is passed through a photo detector. The tubes should be used to lower the air velocity in the sampling chamber.
7. Relay signals should be used to trip AHUs in case of a fire in the floor, or to start extraction fans in the basement, or to actuate strobes and hooters.

Difference between Wireless & Wired Fire Alarm System:

SN	Category	Wireless Technology	Wired Technology
1	Disturbance in Frequency	1. Disturbance can be caused by the operating frequency as other facilities might have same frequency. 2. Weather can disturb the operation of the system, as they might disturb the RF Frequency, which results in malfunctioning of the system.	There's no problem regarding Frequency Licensing or Frequency Operating.
2	Mode of operation	We have to keep replacing their batteries from time to time.	There's no need to change batteries as they are connected through cables.
3	Third Party Integration	It's difficult to integrate with any other third party equipment	Wide ranges of equipment are available with it. Hence can be integrated with third party equipment like HVAC, Lift, Sprinklers etc
4	Scalability	Equipment that boosts signals are needed after certain distance. Hence due to this limitation they cannot be expanded at a farther distance.	This system can be expanded at any given time in the future according to user's needs.

The Hose Cabinet Shutters should also be monitored from the Fire Alarm System. In case the Hose Cabinet shutter is opened (unauthorised access to Hose Cabinet can result in theft of gun metal parts), the Magnetic Contact will give an alarm in the Panel with the exact location of the opening.

Main Points:

1. Sprinklers shall NOT be installed in the Electrical Panel Room, C. T. Scan, M.R.I., Cath lab and Operating Rooms.
2. One detector may or may not have coverage of 80 square meters so quantity maybe set as per building layout.
3. Main fire alarm panel should be located at 24 hrs manned area like security cabin, maintenance office or reception.

CODE PINK

Hospitals in India use code names to alert its staff to an emergency.

Announcement of an emergency by code names does not create panic among other patients and visitors. Simultaneously it allows trained hospital personnel to respond quickly and appropriately to various events.

These codes are communicated through a Public Address System which is available in almost all hospitals.

The announcement also tells the location of emergency. Hospital personnel are trained to respond to all codes used in the hospital.

What is code pink in hospital?

Code Pink is **when an infant less than 12 months of age is suspected or confirmed as missing**.

It is also used for any missing patient. In some hospitals Code Purple is called when a child greater than 12 months of age is suspected or confirmed as missing.

DEFINITION:

Code Pink is similar to Code Purple and denotes an infant abduction.

INTRODUCTION:

1. A missing child/baby from the place where he/she should have been should be taken as an emergency situation.
2. This policy is not only restricted to paediatric and neonatal areas, but is applicable across the **hospital** wherever incidence of missing child/baby happens.
3. Code Pink should be activated as soon as child/baby is considered to be missing.
4. The missing child could be admitted in hospital or a visitor.
5. Any staff of the hospital that first gets the information about the missing child must do a quick search in the nearby areas and take help of other staff/people around to find the missing child/baby.
6. If not found, **Code Pink** should be activated by the staff immediately. It is important that code pink should be activated as soon as there is a reasonable assurance that the child/baby is not around the place.
7. **Code pink** can be activated by any staff of the hospital by calling emergency number.
8. The basic description should be 'age', 'gender', 'name', 'type and colour of clothing' along with the location from where he/she is missing. This message should be repeated thrice to ensure that the receiver has understood.

PURPOSE:

- To facilitate speedy return of the child to a place of safety and to ensure awareness of staff of their roles and responsibilities

SOP – PROCEDURES:

A. **Area In-charge will:**
   1. The nurse will notify the Security/Manager - Admin and inform them that an infant/PERSON is missing.
   2. A description of the abductor shall be given if suspected.
   3. Will inform of the last known location and how long has been missing.
   4. Notify the patient's attending physician if the infant is an inpatient.
   5. Function as communication point and gather as much information as possible about the missing child. For example, when and wherever was the child/baby last seen, who all came to visit the area, any suspected event that took place, etc.
   6. Be available at the desk to maintain communication and coordination.
   7. Should also arrange for someone to look after the parents of the missing child/baby.
   8. Parents should be kept informed about the search process and its development. Parents should be encouraged to help as much as possible by providing all necessary information and maintaining their patience.

B. **In-charges of other wards**:
   - They should understand the description and start a search of the missing child/baby within and around their ward. She should seek help of other nurses and staff for the search, however critical patient care work should not be stopped for this.

C. **OPD and Emergency:**
   - As OPD and emergency has an entry/exit point, the in-charge must assign some staff from there department to monitor the gates and also the outside areas of the hospital.

D. **Security:**
   1. The security guard should close all the entry/exit points within the hospital building.
   2. The security in-charge must immediately position sufficient guards on all **entry/exit points** within the hospital building. Anyone exiting from the hospital must be frisked and inspected. In case of doubt the person should not be allowed to exit.
   3. Few security guards must be sent across the hospitals, including **exteriors, terrace, basements** to do a thorough search of the hospital for the missing baby. All security guards must listen to the announcement and understand the description. In case of doubt the In-charge of the area from where the child/baby is missing should be contacted.
   4. Any **suspicious person** within the hospital premise should be checked. Anyone carrying a large bag or wearing clothes in manner where baby/child could be hidden, or any one with unnatural behaviour must be suspected.
   5. All **employees on contract or outsourced manpower** must also be restricted from any movement outside the hospital. They shall be checked if suspected.
   6. The personnel manning the **CCTV camera** must closely examine all areas trough CCTV. An additional person should be deployed for careful scrutiny.
   7. Security In-charge/Safety officer must coordinate the work of security during Code Pink event.

E. **Other staff:**

- All other staff must look around their place of work and be vigilant about the missing baby/ child. If any staff finds a suspicious person, security in-charge should be contacted.

F. **Hospital Administrator:**

1. As soon as the hospital's administrator come to know about the incident, he should visit the area from where the child/baby is missing and take information about the situation.
2. He will quickly ascertain if code pink action plan is being implemented appropriately.
3. Hospital administrator should also meet the parents and assure them of all possible efforts on part of hospital.
4. Inform staff members in the area and designate staff to inform families on the unit that a police investigation will happen
5. Designate a counsellor to provide support for family members of the missing person.
6. Assign a staff member to stay with and support the family members of the missing infant that are present.
7. The family will be kept informed and updated on the search status through this staff member.

H. **Important Notes:**

1. The physical environment in the immediate vicinity of the incident will be left untouched and secured. All of the patient's belongings will be left in the patient's room.
2. The Nurse/manager will secure the medical records
3. All staff communication with news media related to the incident will be through or with the approval of the Chairman/Executive Director.
4. All staff on duty on the unit when abduction occurs (even if this occurs during change of shift) will remain on the unit until police personnel release the staff members.
5. If the person is recovered in a timely manner inside the hospital, he/she will be taken to the Emergency Room and examined by a physician.

CALLING CODE PINK OFF:

Code Pink shall remain activated till the time any one of the following out-come materialises.

1. The child/baby is found
2. If the child is not found up-to one hour after code pink activation, a decision to stop code pink can be taken by hospital administrator. The time could be extended or reduced as per the situational analysis.
3. In case child is not found, police should be informed before calling off the code pink. Instruction from police department must be adhered to.
4. For calling off code pink, the telephone operator should be informed and he/she will announce **'Code Pink – All Clear'**, three times. With this announcement all staff will resume back to their normal work and active search of the child/baby can be discontinued.

PROCEDURE AFTER "ALL OVER":

Hospital administrator, security in-charge and the in-charge of the department from where the child/baby was missing should complete following process after calling off code pink

1. If the child/baby is found alright a **quick physical examination** of the child/baby should be done to ensure that child/baby is in normal condition. He/she should then be handed over to the parent.
2. If the child/baby is found with minor injuries, first aid/treatment should be given.
3. If the child/baby is found with severe injuries or in dead condition, or in any condition which indicates a manhandling/abuse/crime, police shall immediately be informed and a medico-legal case must be documented.

4. If a suspect is found eloping with the child, the description of the suspect should be noted and police should be informed as soon as possible.
5. If child is not found within sufficient time, police should be informed.
6. The safety/security officer should prepare a detailed report on the code pink incident. The report must contain description of child, time of code pink activation, details of search operations, decisions taken and outcome of code pink.
7. Hospital administrator must analyse the code pink system and take corrective action to make it more robust.

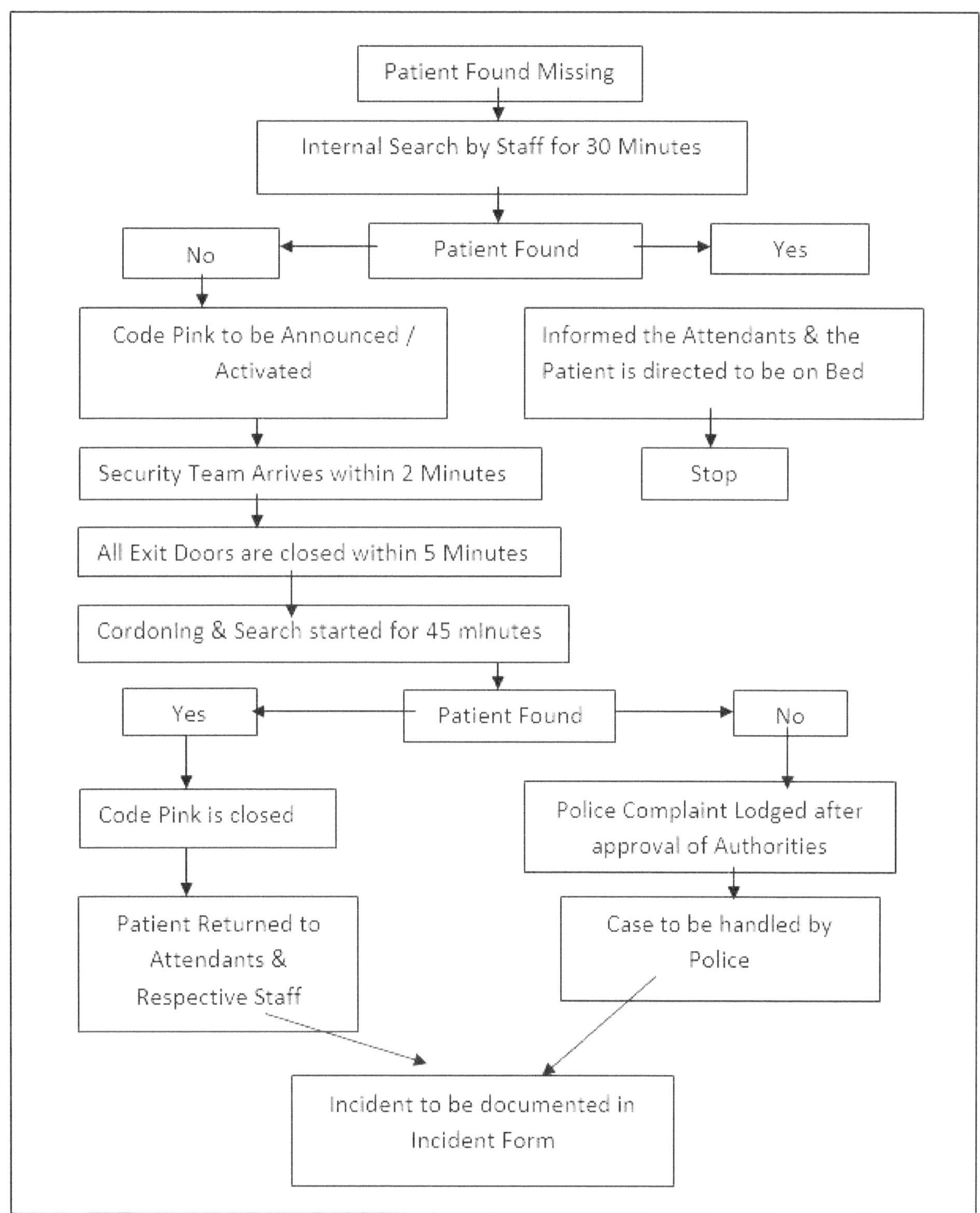

CODE ORANGE

Hospitals in India use code names to alert its staff to an emergency.

Announcement of an emergency by code names does not create panic among other patients and visitors. Simultaneously it allows trained hospital personnel to respond quickly and appropriately to various events.

These codes are communicated through a Public Address System which is available in almost all hospitals.

The announcement also tells the location of emergency. Hospital personnel are trained to respond to all codes used in the hospital.

INTRODUCTION:

It means a call for medical decontamination, typically due to a hazardous fluids spill, like chemicals or patient blood.

DEFINITION:

Code Orange is a call for medical decontamination, usually due to a hazardous fluids spill. For example, a **hospital** may call a **code orange** if toxic chemicals spill in an emergency room, or if a bag of patient blood spills on the floor.

Code Orange can vary; in some hospitals it also denotes a combative or aggressive person at some hospitals.

DEFINITION/TYPES:

1. A spill is defined as an uncontrolled release of a chemical.
2. Spills can be categorized into two types, depending on the volume, location and hazard of the substance spilt.
   a. Minor Spill
   b. Major Spill
      a. **Minor Spill:**
         1. Do not leave the site unattended.
         2. Notify fellow workers in vicinity of spill. Secure the area by restricting access and posting caution signage.
            DO NOT ATTEMPT TO CLEAN A MAJOR SPILL.
         3. Remove any potential ignition sources & unplug the nearby electrical equipment.
         4. Bring a spill kit.
         5. Wear personal protective equipment which includes impervious rubber gloves, safety glasses, protective apron.
      b. **Major Spill:**
         If any of the following apply, the spill is considered major.
         1. Quantity – As a guide, if more than 100 ml/10 grams of highly hazardous chemical.
         2. Hazard - If the chemical presents an immediate threat to human health or safety or the environment; is unknown, or is an immediate hazard.
         3. Location – If the chemical is outside of the laboratory or outside of the area where the material is normally used, and/or there is no trained person available to clean up the spill.

SPILL KIT/HAZMAT KIT:

1. **HAZMAT** is a term used to describe incidents involving **Hazardous Materials**
2. **Hazardous Materials** are defined as substances that have the potential to harm a person or the environment upon contact.
3. These can be gases, liquids, or solids and include radioactive and chemical materials.
4. Biological organisms, such as viruses and bacteria, are not included as Hazardous.

Contents of the Kit:

1. Rubber Gloves
2. Safety Glasses
3. 1 Kg of Sand
4. One large bag marked "Hazardous Material"
5. Gum Boots
6. Protective Clothing (Apron)
7. Dust Pan
8. Scoop & Brush

PROCEDURE:

a. **General Precautions:**
   1. Do not touch spilled material
   2. If spilled on cloth – take off contaminated clothing – Rinse skin immediately with plenty of water for 15- 20 minutes
   3. If contact in eyes – Flush with plenty of water for 15 minutes
   4. If ingestion – Rinse mouth with water do not induce vomiting

b. **Small Spill (10 cm diameter or 100 ml):**
   1. Select appropriate PPE.
   2. Mark the site.
   3. Place absorbent paper and pour 1% hypochlorite over it.
   4. Wait for 15 minutes.
   5. Collect the contaminated absorbent paper and discard it into yellow plastic bag.
   6. Wipe the area with regular disinfectant.
   7. After all the visible traces have been removed, thoroughly clean the area (Water wet mop) and regular disinfectants.
   8. Carefully remove PPE, Place non-reusable items in disposal container.
   9. Perform Hand Hygiene.
   10. Replenish spill kit.

c. **Large Spill (Greater than 10 cm or more than 100 ml):**
   1. Activate Code orange.
   2. Do not leave the site unattended. Notify fellow workers in vicinity of spill. Secure the area by restricting access and posting caution signage.
      DO NOT ATTEMPT TO CLEAN A MAJOR SPILL.
   3. Remove any potential ignition sources & unplug the nearby electrical equipment.
   4. Wear personal protective equipment which includes impervious rubber gloves, safety glasses, protective apron.
   5. Put sand on the material.

6. Dispose the sand in a container/bag marked as Hazardous Material.
7. After all the visible traces have been removed, thoroughly clean the area (Water wet mop).
8. Carefully remove PPE, Place non-reusable items in disposal container & thoroughly wash Hands.
9. Replenish spill kit.

d. **Blood Spillage:**

1. Whenever there is a spill of blood or body fluid, consider it INFECTIOUS.
2. Block the area from others.
3. Cover the spill with cotton or paper towels.
4. Put on disposable latex gloves to prevent contamination of hands.
5. Gently pour 1% bleach solution onto the blood/cotton.
6. Wait for 20 minutes
7. Pick the cotton and throw in yellow bag
8. Clean the area with wet cotton and throw it in yellow bag. If spill is large, then clean the area with wet mop. After cleaning, dip the mop in sodium hypochlorite/bleach solution for 20 minutes
9. discard the used gloves in yellow bag
10. Thoroughly wash hands with soap and water

e. **Chemical Spill Protocol**:

i. **Minor Chemical Spill: -**

A minor chemical spill is one that:

1. The staffs are capable of handling safely without assistance.
2. Staffs have knowledge of the chemical.
3. A small quantity has been spilled.
4. Staffs know how to properly clean-up the spilled material.
5. No immediate toxicity to staff exposed.

Procedure: Alert people in immediate area of spill, wear appropriate protective equipment, including safety goggles, gloves, and long-sleeve lab coat.

1. Avoid breathing vapours from spills.
2. Use appropriate spill kit or absorb the spill with tissue paper & Collect residue, place in a waste disposal bag.
3. Record: staff involved in the clean-up, department, and chemical contaminant.
4. Clean spill area with water.

ii. **Major Chemical Spill (all other spills)**: -

Procedures: Alert people in the immediate area to evacuate.

1. If spilled material is flammable, turn off ignition and heat sources.
2. Close doors to affected area.

ETO GAS SPILL MANAGEMENT:

Ethylene oxide (also known as **EO or ETO**) is a low temperature gaseous process widely used to sterilize a variety of healthcare products.

- Since ETO is a gas at room temperature, you are dealing with the gaseous form of ETO predominantly in your work air that will not produce a spill.
- For example, when ETO leaks from a high-pressure vessel, the ETO would be in a liquid form for only a short period of time as it leaks into the air.

- It then quickly equilibrates with the room air to form a gas. Both the gaseous and, when necessary, the liquid phase of ETO exposure must be taken into consideration.

PROCEDURE:

1. There should be an automatic exhaust system in the ETO Room which should start as soon as the gas is released.
2. The autoclave personnel have to enter the room wearing all the PPE's.
3. He/she should switch off the ETO machine immediately.
4. The person should convey the incident ASAP. So that the preventive action can be taken.

MERCURY SPILL MANAGEMENT:

- **MERCURY** is a known **neurotoxin** that is extremely toxic even in small amounts.
- It directly affects the central nervous and renal systems, causing developmental delays and motor and brain problems like those associated with autism.
- Mercury's hidden danger also lies in, when at room temperature, when exposed it vaporizes readily.
- Once it has become an aerosol, it is absorbed into the lungs and spreads throughout the body.
- Chronic mercury poisoning is more common due to long-term exposure by inhalation of dust or vapours, and knowledge to prevent such incidents is vital in mercury collection and clean-up.

Clean-up Procedures:

1. The most common form of a mercury spill is in liquid form.
2. When liquefied, the small beads that form are difficult to pick up and contain, and measures should be taken accordingly to ensure workers are protected and do not come in contact with the contaminated area without wearing proper protection.
3. A broken light fixture, while not spread out, is just as much of risk to the employees because the dust very readily spreads and can be inhaled.

Mercury Spill Kit:

1. PPE (Personal Protective Equipment)
2. X-Ray Films
3. Container With Water
4. Absorbent Tape
5. Syringe
6. Bag
7. Incident Form

How to handle Mercury?

1. Ventilation is the primary concern at the contaminated area because the free mercury readily vaporizes and will continue to do so until collected.
2. It is recommended to shut down the air conditioning or heating, if applicable.
3. Open the windows to get the maximum amount of air in the room and allow the vapours to flow outside.
4. Do not touch mercury
5. Remove any jewellery or watch
6. Wear appropriate PPE

7. Locate spilled mercury with flashlight as it is difficult to locate the same with open eyes
8. Use cardboard sheets/X-Ray film to push beards in 1 place
9. One can also use syringe to push mercury beads in 1 place
10. After collecting the mercury place it in a container with water
11. Use absorbent on mercury spillage area. (zinc-ferrous based magnetic mercury amalgamation powder)
12. If spillage is still there – use stick tape
13. Place contaminated items in a bag with used syringe, cardboard and gloves
14. Label the bag as mercury waste
15. Handover the mercury waste to BME
16. Document the incident and report it to the in-charge.

NOTIFY:

1. Designated Safety Officer
2. Keep people away
3. Obtain MSDS on chemical

LIST OF HAZARDOUS MATERIALS:

1. Bacillocid Extra
2. Formalin (Liquid & Tablets)
3. Handrub – 3M
4. Korsolex
5. Medispirit
6. Hydrogen peroxide
7. Microgen – D- 125
8. Sodium hypochlorite
9. Wonder Pine Phenyl
10. Wonder shine Glass
11. X – Ray Chemicals
12. Biomedical Waste
13. Diesel
14. LPG
15. Paints

CODE VIOLET

Hospitals in India use code names to alert its staff to an emergency.

Announcement of an emergency by code names does not create panic among other patients and visitors. Simultaneously it allows trained hospital personnel to respond quickly and appropriately to various events.

These codes are communicated through a Public Address System which is available in almost all hospitals.

The announcement also tells the location of emergency. Hospital personnel are trained to respond to all codes used in the hospital.

DEFINITION:

Code Violet stands for violence.

Code Violet alludes the hospital's response to violent and/or combative persons when they pose a threat to self and/or others.

Code Violet is used for such circumstances in the hospital.

PURPOSE:

- To identify measures which prevent and mitigate potentially violent situations and ensure the safety of staff, patient or visitors at this hospital.

CODE VIOLET SITUATIONS:

1. Behaviour involving physical force intended to hurt, damage, or kill someone or something.
2. Strength of emotion or an unpleasant or destructive natural force.

OVERALL RESPONSIBILITY:

- Security Officer

PROCEDURE (SOP):

At the onset of any visible disturbance or impending violence, a message of Code Violet mentioning the exact location of the incident shall be announced over the hospital's public address system. This will disseminate information indicating an imminent attack by relatives of patient expecting a prompt action by the staff.

1. The operator will make an "all call" announcement over the internal public address system and state 3 times **"Code Violet"** with location.
2. Security will respond immediately and provide assistance as needed.
3. The personnel involved have to be extremely quiet, and avoid any altercation/discussion which can escalate the situation.
4. A senior member of staff (can be designated before) who himself is not directly involved in treatment in that particular case shall politely communicate with relatives of patients and try to verbally De-escalate a threatening situation.
5. In this situation, there should not be argument on part of the hospital staff and the designated member should give enough opportunity to the disgruntled patient/attendant to explain their grievances.
6. All the members of staff shall exercise restraint and shall not lose their cool under any circumstance.
7. Once the situation is under control, the operator will make an announcement over the internal public address system and state 3 times **"Code Violet- All Clear."**
8. If the situation is not under control and law and order situation arises in the form of assault, external help shall be sought from nearby hospitals and Police.

PREVENTION OF SUCH INCIDENCES:

1. Create a safety culture.
2. Train workers for Early Recognition and Reporting.
3. The security of hospital should be strengthened and the security personnel should be directed not to allow entry of any unauthorized person inside Hospital. There should be absolute weapons prohibition inside premises of hospital.

4. CCTV cameras should be installed at all important places especially near reception, accounts department, Operation Theatre and ICU to identify and catch the miscreants. It should be displayed in bold letters that "**This Hospital is under surveillance of CCTV Cameras "so** that it acts as a deterrent.
5. The Visitor time should be specified and restricted and only limited and valid visitors should be allowed by turn during visiting time.
6. Hospitals should be declared safe zones and gathering of people should not be allowed outside the critical areas.
7. Relatives sitting area should be far away from the critical area and the dead body whenever shifted should never be shifted from the area where the relatives of the patient are sitting.

CODE YELLOW

Hospitals in India use code names to alert its staff to an emergency.

Announcement of an emergency by code names does not create panic among other patients and visitors. Simultaneously it allows trained hospital personnel to respond quickly and appropriately to various events.

These codes are communicated through a Public Address System which is available in almost all hospitals.

The announcement also tells the location of emergency. Hospital personnel are trained to respond to all codes used in the hospital.

DEFINITION:

Code yellow in typically "An External Disaster"

Disaster is a sudden, calamitous event bringing great damage, loss, and destruction and devastation to life and property.

A disaster that has occurred outside the hospital, such as bus/train accident, wide-spread food poisoning, epidemic, fire in a building, bomb blast etc.

The hospital is the place where the victims of external disaster will be brought for medical care.

Hence the objective of the hospital in external disaster is to handle mass casualty situation.

TYPES OF DISASTER:

A. **It may be;**
   1. Minor external disasters: incidents involving ≤10 casualties.
   2. Major external disasters: incidents involving: >10 casualties.

B. **It may be;**
   1. Natural
   2. Manmade
   3. Internal Disasters

Following are Natural Disasters:

1. Flood
2. Cyclone
3. Drought

4. Earthquake
5. Tsunami

Man – Made Disasters:

1. Wars
2. Road/train accidents
3. Riots
4. Chemical Explosion
5. Industrial Accident
6. Building collapse

Internal Disaster:

1. Fire
2. Hazardous materials
3. Loss of environmental supplies
4. Loss of medical gases
5. Explosions
6. Violence
7. Police Action
8. Enemy attack inside the premises

STEPS:

1. There should be an identified person or team who will take charge in case of declaration of mass casualty.
2. The hospital should have a list of people (doctors, nurses and support staff) who will be called in case of mass casualty should.
3. There should be a document "Disaster Management" with defined role and responsibility of each staff during mass casualty handling.
4. The hospital should have an earmarked place for accommodating such victims.
5. The hospital already has defined process of **triaging** and place for each category of triage.
6. The hospital should be prepared to identify on-site morgue for temporarily keeping dead bodies.
7. Dedicated store of medicine, consumable and other materials to be used only during mass casualty situations.
8. Availability of ambulances for shifting of patients.
9. Identified places (internally and externally) where patients will be shifted/referred after managing emergency care.

PROCEDURE:

The hospital has got experience in handling casualties for the last so many years. The only difference in this situation is that the casualties are in mass.

During any external medical emergency, casualties are treated as per hospital protocol.

Triage

Triage refers to the evaluation and categorization of the sick or wounded when there are insufficient resources for medical care of everyone at once.

Historically, triage is believed to have arisen from systems developed for categorization and transport of wounded soldiers on the battlefield in World War I.

a. In a disaster or mass casualty situation, different systems for triage have been developed. One system is known as START (Simple Triage and Rapid Treatment).
   - In START, victims are grouped into four categories, depending on the urgency of their need for evacuation.
   - If necessary, START can be implemented by persons without a high level of training.

   The categories in START are:
   1. The deceased, who are beyond help
   2. The injured who could be helped by immediate transportation
   3. The injured with less severe injuries whose transport can be delayed
   4. Those with minor injuries not requiring urgent care.

b. Another system that has been used in mass casualty situations is an example of advanced triage implemented by nurses or other skilled personnel.

   This advanced triage system involves a colour-coding scheme using red, yellow, green, and black tags:

Category	Priority	Colour	Conditions
Immediate	1	Red	Victims whose injuries demand urgent medical attention
Delayed Treatment within 10 minutes	2	Yellow	Victims whose injuries require medical care but can be somewhat delayed
Minimal treatment within 30 minutes	3	Green	Victims whose injuries are so minor that they can be managed by self-help or volunteer assistance.
Deceased	4	Black	Dead Victims

DISASTER MANAGEMENT:

Introduction:

Hospitals play an important role during any disaster by providing medical care to the community and helping in reducing mortality & morbidity.

A well written document should achieve; (1) Continuity of essential services; (2) well-coordinated implementation of hospital operations at every level; (3) clear and accurate internal and external communication; (4) swift adaptation to increased demands; (5) the effective use of scarce resources; and (6) a safe environment for health-care workers.

Scope:

Entire Hospital including all Doctors, Staff, Patients and Attendants including contractual Workers

Definitions:

1. **A disaster** is a serious disruption occurring over a relatively short period of time that causes widespread human, material, economic or environmental loss which exceeds the ability of the affected community or society to cope on a timely basis using its own resources.

   (Disaster: https://en.wikipedia.org/wiki/Disaster)

2. **All Clear**: This announcement is made when the disaster has been taken care and now there is no need to be on high alert and now normal work can resume in the hospital.
3. **Critical**: The patient has unstable vital signs and parameters are not within normal limits. Patient may be acutely ill or unconscious.
4. **Non-Critical:** The patient is stable and vitals are within normal limits. Patient is conscious and can be uncomfortable but all indicators are favourable.
5. **Command Centre:** The central station from where all commands originates. A central commanding centre is very much essential for proper handling of the situation and to avoid confusions.

Purpose:

a. To provide a standard procedure for hospital response in case of any emergency situation because of factors which are natural or manmade and which may affect the hospital, its staff, patients and visitors.
b. To lay down duties and responsibilities of various key personnel/departments of the hospital during such situation.
c. A Mock Drill shall be conducted every year to test this plan.
d. External disasters are announced in the hospital as "Code Yellow".

Types of Disasters:

1. Natural Disasters: such as
   a. Earthquake
   b. Tsunami
   c. Volcanic Eruptions
   d. Landslides
   e. Wild fires & floods
   f. etc
2. Man-made Disasters:
   a. War
   b. Act of Terrorism/Violence
   c. Fire
   d. Stampede
   e. Major Accidents, industrial as well as elsewhere.

Key Components of a Well Organised Plan are: (As per WHO Guidelines)

1. Command and control: A well-functioning command-and-control system is essential for effective hospital emergency management operations.
2. Communication: Clear, accurate and timely communication is necessary to ensure informed decision-making, effective collaboration and cooperation, and public awareness and trust.
3. Safety and security: Well-developed safety and security procedures are essential for the maintenance of hospital functions and for incident response operations during a disaster.
4. Triage: Maintaining patient triage operations, on the basis of a well-functioning mass-casualty triage protocol, is essential for the appropriate organization of patient care.
5. Surge capacity: Surge capacity – defined as the ability of a health service to expand beyond normal capacity to meet increased demand for clinical care – is an important factor of hospital disaster response and should be addressed early in the planning process.

6. Continuity of essential services: A disaster does not remove the day-to-day requirement for essential medical and surgical services (e.g., emergency care, urgent operations, maternal and child care) that exists under normal circumstances. Rather, the availability of essential services needs to continue in parallel with the activation of a hospital emergency response plan.
7. Human resources: Effective human resource management is essential to ensure adequate staff capacity and the continuity of operations during any incident that increases the demand for human resources.
8. Logistics and supply management: Continuity of the hospital supply and delivery chain is often an underestimated challenge during a disaster, requiring attentive contingency planning and response.
9. Post-disaster recovery: post-disaster recovery planning should be performed at the onset of response activities. Prompt implementation of recovery efforts can help mitigate a disaster's long-term impact on hospital operations.

Planning in Various Phases of a Disaster:

A. **Pre-Disaster Planning:**

   The hospital should start planning for worst from the day one, if it is providing emergency services to the community. Following actions should be put in place;

B. **Disaster Management Committee:**

   Following should be the members of this committee.

   1. Head of the Hospital
   2. Heads of Casualty, Orthopaedics, Neurosurgery
   3. Nursing Superintendent
   4. Store In-charge
   5. ....

C. **Central Command:**

   To ensure effectiveness and avoid duplication, *ABC Hospital* has set up a Command Centre for emergency purposes. The Command Centre only comes in function on announcement of a disaster.

   Members of command centre are;

   1. Managing Director .... (Cell No.)
   2. Medical Superintendent .... (Cell No.)
   3. PRO/Liaison Officer
   4. ....

   All members will immediately assemble in MD's room/office on announcement of a disaster.

D. **Job Description:**

   Each and every person in the Disaster Management should have a clear-cut defined job description in such situations. Everybody will be in contact with command centre for any requirement. All leaves are automatically cancelled. Every staff member shall report to hospital as soon as he/she come to know about a disaster. Nobody shall refuse to work for extra hours and more than what is defined in his job description.

   1. Medical Superintendent/Medical Director:
      a. Shall check with local authorities to verify the disaster, nature and type of disaster and shall obtain additional information.
      b. Shall ask front-office to make announcement for all hospital staff.

   c. Shall ask for external help for men and material as deemed necessary.
   d. Shall be available in the hospital to assist various functions.
2. Nursing Supervisor:
   a. Shall function as head of committee, if seniors are not available.
   b. Shall establish the command centre and will work as its head. All departmental heads shall report to her before proceeding to their departments.
   c. Shall arrange adequate number of staff for all departments; clinical and non-clinical both.
   d. Shall be authorised to cancel leave of a staff member and to call anybody on duty. No staff shall refuse duty at any time during day or night. (Re-deploying existing employees and recalling other staff)
   e. Shall arrange extra beds as much as possible.
3. Maintenance:
   a. The HOD maintenance shall ensure that all support services are available round the clock without any interruption.
   b. All entry exit doors shall be locked and manned by security.
   c. Maintenance staff shall not hesitate to help in transporting patients and bringing supplies to them.
4. Front Desk:
   a. Shall ensure that telephone services are manned round the clock.
   b. Shall be vigilant in making all announcements.
5. Blood bank & Laboratory:
   a. Shall arrange for extra blood. May arrange donations from staff and other volunteers.
   b. Keep extra manpower by cancelling leaves and increasing duty hours.
6. Security:
   a. To cordon off the affected area.
   b. To safeguard belongings of victims.
   c. To make parking arrangements.
   d. To regulate entry of extra persons.
7. Food Services:
   a. To arrange safe drinking water for all.
   b. To maintain adequate supplies for patients.
8. Bio-Medical Engineer:
   a. To arrange for extra critical equipment.
   b. To oversee functioning of critical equipment and to troubleshoot ASAP.
9. Housekeeping & Laundry:
   a. To arrange for extra linen as per need.
   b. To keep area clean and to carry on cleaning continuously.
10. OT, Recovery & ICU:
   a. To keep theatre ready on 24 x 7 basis.
   b. To keep backup for men and material.
   c. ICU staff will try to discharge or shift patients who are already admitted there based on their clinical condition. Will try to free beds for disaster patients)
11. Diagnostic Services:
   a. Shall call any or all personnel of this department to report on duty.
   b. Shall arrange for extra supplies from the market and nearby healthcare organisations.

c. Shall give priority to more critical patients. May not follow usual system of calling persons on their turn.

12. Pharmacy:

a. The pharmacy shall play very crucial role. Supervisor shall make sure that it does not run out of supplies.
b. Shall make extra arrangements to deliver medicines at patients' bedside.
c. Shall ensure backup supply of life saving medicines.

E. **Activation of Contingency Plan:**

1. Information for any External Disasters may be received at the EPABX through Hospital external phone no 0000000000/0000000000
2. On receiving information of an emergency from any source like police, fire service or individuals from the accident site, the operator on duty shall identify the person giving the information and then inquire about the nature and magnitude of the emergency, the location, and time, possible number of victims and approximate time of arrival.
3. The Operator on Duty will then immediately inform the members of Command Centre on their Internal No's or Mobile No's
4. The Managing Director/Head Operation shall assess the situation and activate the External Disaster Plan by declaring CODE YELLOW. Only MANAGING DIRECTOR/MS can authorise announcement of CODE YELLOW.
5. The Telephone Operator on Duty in shall be intimated immediately by the Director/DMS to announce CODE YELLOW on the Hospital Public Address (PA) system and to inform all the concerned Heads of the Departments as per laid down protocols, herein.

Communication of Code Yellow:

The front office will be the HUB for all communications at *ABC Hospital*. The front office has the following contact numbers:

External Contact Number: ....

Internal Contact Number for CODE YELLOW: ....

6. On activation of CODE YELLOW all concerned people shall be informed regarding the External Disaster by the Operator on Duty as per the following sequence:
   a. Operator on Duty (OOD) on declaration of CODE YELLOW by Managing Director/Head Operation/MS shall announce CODE YELLOW over the Public Address System (PA) of the hospital.
   b. The announcement shall be made 3 times at a time after every 30 seconds, at least thrice.
   c. The front office will make the following announcement based on the orders from command centre;
      - "Code YELLOW" and Details of Location
      - The announcement should be made thrice.
      - In case of a minor mock drill announcement will be made accordingly.
      - The announcement would be made based on the orders from command centre.
7. The following Department Heads shall then be informed so that they can perform the assigned duties in case of External Disasters.

SN	Department	Person	Contact No.
1	MD	Dr.	....
2	MS	Dr.	....
3			

8. The Operator on Duty shall remain alert after that for communication of any information as and when required. When there is a change in shift, the Operator on Duty shall pass on all the information in details to the next person on duty.

F. **Public Information Centre**

The Hospital shall set up a Centre headed by HOD marketing to deal with communications. It shall be activated in case of any External Disaster. It will operate from the Front Desk of the hospital.

G. **Action Plan:**

Administrative:

1. Once CODE YELLOW has been announced and the Disaster Management Plan activated, the Members of the Command Centre shall meet in Director Office to assess the situation to ensure that the Disaster is managed efficiently and proper communications are established.
2. Casualty Triage shall be immediately established in the Emergency and area and all the designated trolleys and supplies shall be moved to the area.
3. All departments shall activate their established procedures to provide immediate and necessary support. The HODs shall be assigned key areas where additional staff is to be provided as needed. Expansion of the existing hospital beds shall be managed by Hospital Managing Director/Head Operation in coordination with House Keeping Manager/ Supervisor.

Clinical:

G.1 Triage Criteria: These are same as described in the 'Emergency Manual'.

Patients shall be received in the Emergency and Triage will be carried out as per established norms.

MOST URGENT PRIORITY 1 (RED COLOUR)

1. Any injury with respiratory or circulatory compromise
2. Injuries to the face, trachea, neck (which will lead to respiratory compromise)
3. Patient is critical but can survive.
4. …………

URGENT PRIORITY 2 (YELLOW COLOUR)

1. Compound fracture without vascular compromise.
2. Other fractures without vascular compromise.
3. ……………

NON-URGENT PRIORITY 3 (GREEN COLOUR)

1. Minor cuts, bruises, abrasions
2. ………

DEAD (BLACK COLOUR)

1. In Cardiac arrest on arrival to hospital.
2. Massive injuries incompatible with life.

Detailed management has already been described in Policies for Emergency Department.

H. **Once the emergency is over**, Head of the Command Centre will announce "All Clear" in the same way as other codes is announced.

I. **Dealing with Fatalities:**

1. Though the local police are primarily responsible for dealing with deaths in case of a disaster, the hospital is also an affected party so equally interested in transporting dead patients from ward, ICU, emergency etc.

2. All dead bodies are to be tagged and wrapped after police nod.
3. Any hospital staff shall not remove a dead body to mortuary or hand it over to family members without police permission.
4. The police, in consultation with the local authority, are responsible for identifying body holding areas and temporary mortuaries.

FACTORS:

The factors to be considered are given below: -

a. A warning rarely precedes disasters of the type envisaged above. Such accidents can occur at any time of day or night and anywhere.
b. The number of casualties is unpredictable. For the purpose of this plan, it has been assumed that there will be about 50 casualties, mainly surgical (including burns.)
c. Many casualties are likely to succumb to serious haemorrhage at the scene of accident, if not given prompt first aid.
d. Distances of the scene of accident from the hospital can create problems for rushing assistance to the spot and evacuating casualties to the hospital.
e. The sudden arrival of a large number of casualties will throw a heavy strain on the resources of the hospital. There may not be adequate number of vacant beds to receive the casualties. There will be a sudden demand for large quantities of sterile dressings, syringes, drugs (Morphine, Pethidine, and Antibiotics). Available staff will have to work methodically and over time. Large quantities of fresh blood and plasma expanders may be required. General stores like beds, mattresses, blankets etc may fall short. Refreshments will be required. Inter-communication may become difficult due to over load on available telephones. Available transport may not be enough for speedy evacuation.
f. Besides the above problems, the arrival of mass casualties along with anxious relatives and curious spectators may create problems of security of cash and valuables on the disabled patients.

Procedure Summarised:

1. Immediately on receipt of information regarding the accident, the appropriate alarm will be sounded. All members of staff will report to their respective places of duty in the hospital except those who are detailed to reinforce the reception arrangements in the casualty. One medical officer accompanied by two staff nurses, two nursing assistants and two ward assistants will take the emergency medical equipment in an ambulance and rush to the scene of accident. The ambulance car should be equipped with a walkie-talkie set to facilitate easy intercommunication. On arrival at the scene of accident the Medical Officer will access the seriousness of the situation, and inform the hospital about nature and number of casualties. And ask for additional help if required. Immediately after rendering lifesaving first aid, the Medical Officer will start evacuating casualties to the hospital by ambulance and any other available vehicles.
2. Presuming that only one medical Officer has gone to the scene of accident, there will be 4 lefts in the Casualty & Emergency Department. They will ensure arrangements for reception of the casualties, adequate supplies of sterile dressings and drugs and if necessary, seek the assistance of the required specialist in sorting out casualties.
3. Stretchers, trolleys and wheel chairs together with adequate manpower to handle these will be stationed in front of the casualty department. As soon as the casualties arrive, they will

be shifted quickly to the assembly area of the main reception hall. Entry into this area will be strictly controlled to ensure that the medical staff can attend to the casualties unhampered by spectators.

4. A senior doctor, preferably a surgical registrar, will quickly examine the casualties and classify them into 3 groups as follows.

   a. FIRST PRIORITY: Cases requiring resuscitation and urgent surgery: Asphyxia due to respiratory obstruction, sucking chest wounds and tension pneumo-thorax, shock due to major haemorrhage, visceral injuries, cardio-pericardial injuries, massive muscle damage, extensive burns, severe multiple wounds and major fractures.

      These conditions will be dealt with, if possible, before shock develops.

   b. SECOND PRIORITY: Cases requiring early surgery and possible resuscitation, perforations of gastrointestinal tract, genitourinary tract, biliary system and pancreatic system not bleeding severely.

   c. THIRD PRIORITY: Spinal injuries requiring decompression, soft tissue injuries of less than major degree requiring wound toilet, lesser fractures and dislocations, eye injuries and maxillo-facial injuries.

5. The clerks detailed for the purpose will start preparing medical documents for the casualties in the order of their priorities. The doctor will enter brief details of injury and assessment in the documents. Priority I casualties will then be sent to the ward prepared for them, where the surgical team will take charge,
6. Priority II and III casualties will be retained in the casualty and Emergency service Department, given treatment and made as comfortable as possible until the surgical team is ready to take them over or the casualty is fit to be discharged.
7. This hospital will hold a complete set of equipment for 50 beds known as crisis Expansion beds for use in emergencies of the type envisaged in this plan. List of equipment is already explained elsewhere. This store and equipment will be periodically checked and turned over.
8. On receipt of first information about a major accident, the Resident Surgeon will arrange to place two additional beds in each of the 4 bedded cubicles in the general wards, irrespective of whether these are surgical or medical.
9. As many of the patients in general wards close to the OT as possible will be moved towards away from the OT to take the first rush of priority I casualties.
10. The blood bank will call up donors and keep a minimum amount of blood ready to meet immediate requirements. Thereafter recipients and donor's blood will be a cross-matched and appropriate donor bled as necessary.
11. The Resident Anaesthetist will supervise arrangements for resuscitation of priority I casualties. Other anaesthetists will work in the casualty and the OTs. The sister in-charge will get the OT ready for surgery on priority I case.
12. The CSSD will send adequate supplies of dressings, syringes etc to the Casualty and OT.
13. The laboratory and X-ray department, medical stores and dispensary will be ready to meet urgent demands.
14. The mortuary will be kept ready to receive the dead bodies.
15. The AO will supervise all administrative support to the above plan.
16. The MS will arrange to collect all information about the casualties, feed the same to the Central Inquiry Office, meet members of the police inquiring into the accident, and arrange for post-mortems and disposal of dead bodies.

17. The telephone exchange will be fully manned to attend to the anticipated rush of calls and central broadcasting system.
18. All lifts will be operative.
19. Kitchen staff will be ready to prepare and supply refreshments according to requirements.
20. The Public Relation Officer/Social Worker and Reception staff will ensure that relatives of victims are looked after and reassured.
21. The Security Officer will control traffic and remain alert to prevent pilferage.
22. The electrician will be at his post to attend to break downs in power supply.
23. The MS and Matron will visit all departments periodically to ensure that the plan is being implemented efficiently and to render any additional assistance that may be required.
24. As different departments will be committed to varying extents, it is not proposed to sound a 'Stand Down' alarm. Each departmental head will assess the situation after all casualties have been attended to, detail the minimum staff that may be required and permit remainder to break off.

CONCLUSION:

a. It is obvious that the hospital should prepare a plan to mobilise the resources of the hospital at a short notice and practice the plan periodically to ensure that every member of the staff knows what is expected from him. Such practices will not only reveal the lacunae, which have to be plugged but also give confidence to the participants.
b. There should be an efficient warning system to alert all members of staff whether on duty or not, so that they can report immediately to the allotted stations.
c. Certain reserve capacities of the hospital services and equipment have to be established. As regard transport, an understanding has to be arrived at with nearby factories and institutions to provide the extra transport required for collection and evacuation of casualties.
d. While a few beds can be released by discharging patients who can afford to take treatment as outpatient, additional beds will have to be placed in available space.
e. The blood bank of the hospital should have an adequate number of donors on its donor panel and ensure the promptness of response from such donors when called up in emergency.
f. The reception arrangements should be such that the hospital staff can function quickly and effectively, unhampered by outsiders.
g. The security staff has to be on the alert to prevent breaches of security.

LIST OF CONTACT NUMBERS TO BE DISPLAYED IN THE CONTROL ROOM:

1. Staff which is mentioned in the incident command.
2. Other Hospitals in Network
3. District Medical Authorities
4. District Administration
5. Police
6. Ambulance Services
7. Hearse Van
8. Fire Services
9. Private Physicians
10. Blood Banks
11. NGOs and other organizations which can be contacted if external help is needed.

CODE BLACK

Hospitals in India use code names to alert its staff to an emergency.

Announcement of an emergency by code names does not create panic among other patients and visitors. Simultaneously it allows trained hospital personnel to respond quickly and appropriately to various events.

These codes are communicated through a Public Address System which is available in almost all hospitals.

The announcement also tells the location of emergency. Hospital personnel are trained to respond to all codes used in the hospital.

DEFINITION:

Code black most often indicates a bomb threat. Code black may be activated if there has been a threat made to the facility from an internal or external source, or if staff or law enforcement officials have identified a possible bomb in or near the facility.

Bomb Threats generally emanate from terrorists, anti-social elements, pranksters etc. These are designed to create panic as well as to cause damage to life and property.

Threats may assume in both **overt and covert forms**. While generally these calls are hoax, yet will be treated and dealt as true.

TYPES:

A. **Overt Bomb Threat:**

These bomb threat calls may come through telephone from an anonymous/assumed name/ designation person to convey a message about an impending placement/blowing off of a bomb in the hospital or particular location in the hospital.

On receipt of such a call, the following action is taken:

1. The recipient of the call should try to prolong the conversation with the caller & seek information of the area/location of the bomb, nature of the bomb and other relevant information.
2. The recipient of the call should record the time & exact conversation, soon after the call is over. Effort should be made to gather as much information as possible. Details to be noted down as per Bomb Threat action card given as Appendix's"
3. The recipient of the call should not disconnect the call, but try to have it traced through the telephone exchange.
4. The recipient of the call should immediately pass this information to Security. The security will inform the Chairman Emergency who would give instructions in regard to further course of action.
5. Departmental Teams should be briefed to search their areas and identify doubtful objects. They should not touch/remove any such object found/located. They should also cordon off the area.

B. **Covert Bomb Threat:**

This will generally take the form of placement of Bombs/similar exploding devices in a concealed form in a particular place or places.

On receipt of such information all likely places where such devices could be possibly placed, would be searched with a view to identification and location of such devices. Same is discussed in Appendix" A"

Important:

- Staff member shall be briefed not to make any communication about the bomb threat to any Patient/Visitor, at any stage.
- All Queries in this regard would be referred to the Director Operations.

PROCEDURE:

1. Once the code is announced, a "Emergency Response Team" (ERT) of the hospital reaches the spot.
2. Police is informed.
3. Once police reach the spot, they take action as per their protocol. But till that time, the hospital ERT takes charge.
4. The team is divided into four parts;
   a. Scanning Party
   b. Cordon Party
   c. Salvage Party
   d. Rescue Party

Scanning Party:

Scanning will be carried out to look for any suspicious object. All members will ensure that throughout the scanning operations no object will be touched. After the scanning is completed the room/area will be marked to remove the possibility of rechecks of same area my mistake.

1. Area for scanning will be defined for all ERT members.
2. Area will first be scanned from ground to belt level.
3. Area will then be scanned from belt to head level.
4. Finally, it will be scanned above head level.

Cordon Party:

1. Will cordon the area require to be scanned?
2. Will ensure that only required in and out movement to the area.

Salvage Party:

- Will take out material around the area require to be scanned on the instructions from authorities.

Rescue Party

- Will ensure that the Patients/Visitors, employees and all others are evacuated from the area of scanning.

On identification the device would be isolated, without being physically handled in any way. The police would be contacted and appraised of the situation with a view for getting help to neutralize the bomb. Emergency Chairman will take all the decision on calling police, bomb squad, fire tenders and evacuation.

ACTIONS - ON DETECTION OF A BOMB/SUSPICIOUS OBJECT:

Action by the Individual on Detection

1. Inform Security Officer.
2. Do not raise an alarm, under any circumstances.

3. Keep distance from the object and under no circumstance touch the object.
4. Do not let the object to be out of your sight.
5. Do not let anyone go near the object by purpose or by default.
6. Do not give away the feeling to the Patients/visitors that something is wrong.
7. Do not open doors/windows with force as the trigger mechanism of the explosive may go off.
8. If you hear symptomatic behaviour of the object like the ticking sound or protruding wires or batteries or gunpowder smell the spare no time to inform the security immediately.

Action by Security Officer

1. Security Officer will ensure that the object is covered with Bomb suppression Blanket & Security personnel is posted.
2. Area to be cordoned off up to the arrival Bomb squad team
3. Surrounding area to be vacated.
4. Inform Police Control (Tel. 100) for Bomb Disposal Team.
5. Provide all assistance to Police/Bomb Disposal Team on arrival.
6. Render detailed report to Executive Director

BIBLIOGRAPHY, REFERENCES & ACKNOWLEDGMENTS:

1. NABH 5th Edition
2. BBC Heart care & Purthi Hospital, Jalandhar City, Punjab
3. Amcare Hospital, Zirakpur, Punjab
4. Campus Safety Magazine, Emerald Expositions, Framingham, MA 01702, USA
5. Singh S, Sharma DK, Bhoi S, Sardana SR, Chauhan S. Code Blue Policy for a Tertiary Care Trauma Hospital in India. Int J Res Foundation Hosp Health & Adm 2015;3(2):114-122.
6. The Healthcare Manager Blogspot, 29 March 2018 (https://expresshealthcaremanagement.blogspot.com/2018/03/code-blue-system-in-hospitals.html)
7. Rockland Hospitals
8. https://www.youtube.com/watch?v=18xjzoOoCNY
9. Hospital emergency response checklist, World Health Organization, Regional Office for Europe, Scherfigsvej 8, DK-2100 Copenhagen Ø, Denmark

Chapter – 11

DEPARTMENT OF ENDOCRINOLOGY

INDEX

INTRODUCTION:

Endocrinology is the study of the medical aspects of hormones, including diseases and conditions associated with hormonal imbalance, damage to the glands that make hormones, or the use of synthetic or natural hormonal drugs.

The department interacts very closely with the other departments of Gynaecology & Obstetrics, Orthopaedics, Neurology, Ophthalmology, Cardiology, Nephrology etc. in order to provide comprehensive management.

Endocrinology involves a wide range of systems in the human body. The endocrinal glands in the body include:

1. Adrenal gland,
2. Hypothalamus,
3. Pituitary,
4. Thyroid & Parathyroid,
5. Ovaries,
6. And Testis.

The department provided comprehensive management of all such disorders.

AIM, VISION & MISSION:

1. To provide best endocrine care to patients
2. To improve research into new technologies to bring these improvements to our patients.
3. To provide the highest quality of compassionate, comprehensive, coordinated, and value-based health care.
4. To ensure that optimum care is given to all endocrine patients using available resources and appropriate facilities.

INFRASTRUCTURE & EQUIPMENT:

1. OPDs is located on ground floor of the hospital.
2. Wards are on Second floor
3. Operation theatres are located on fourth floor of the hospital

Equipment:

1. Insulin Pump
2. Thyroid Scan
3. Ambulatory Glucose Monitoring (CGMS)
4. Bone Densitometer

Facilities Available:

1. Daily OPD
2. Admission facility for Indoor treatment
3. Diagnostic Facilities
4. Ultrasound
5. Biopsy

SERVICES OFFERED:

The department deals with disorders of;

1. The department deals with disorders of; Diabetes, Thyroid, Growth, Bone, abnormal hair growth in female, pubertal abnormalities in children, infertility in male and female, osteoporosis, pituitary and adrenal disorder, obesity management, hormone replacement therapy and various other hormone disorders.
2. Paediatric Endocrinology

DISEASES TREATED:

1. Diabetes in adults and children
2. Obesity
3. Thyroid Diseases (thyroid swelling, thyroid cancer, hyperthyroidism, hypothyroidism)
4. Hirsutism & Gynaecomastia
5. Precocious Puberty
6. Menstrual Problems (Oligomenorrhoea & Amenorrhoea, Menopausal Syndrome))
7. Metabolic Bone Disease
8. Diseases of Adrenal & Pituitary Glands
9. Sexual Problems and Infertility
10. Lack or delayed sexual development
11. Growth Retardation (Being too short or too long
12. Ambiguous Genitalia
13. Osteoporosis

14. Recurrent Kidney Stones
15. Young hypertension (age less than 30 years)
16. Excessive hair growth in females

FACILITIES:

Diagnostic Facilities:

1. Hormone Assay Facility in the department of Pathology
2. Molecular Endocrine Laboratory
3. DEXA Scan
4. Peripheral Vascular Studies
5. Radiological Investigations

Surgical Facilities:

1. Day care thyroid surgeries
2. Thyroid & Parathyroid surgeries
3. Endoscopic Thymectomy
4. Laparoscopic Adrenalectomy
5. Minimally Invasive breast surgeries

Inpatients Dynamic Testing:

1. ACTH Stimulation testing
2. Growth Hormone Stimulation testing (Clonidine/glucagon)
3. GnRH analogue stimulation testing
4. Dexamethasone suppression test
5. HCG stimulation test
6. Growth Hormone Suppression testing
7. Saline suppression testing
8. Water deprivation test

Facilities for Treating following Disorders:

Thyroid:

Diagnostic Facilities:

FNAC Thyroid, FT3, FT4, TSH

Thyroid Antibodies, Thyroid Scan

RAIU 24 hrs

Therapeutic Facilities:

Medical Treatment of Thyroid disorders

Thyroid Surgery I-131, Ablation

Parathyroid:

Diagnostic Facilities:

Sestambi Scan, Sc Ca/PO4/Alkaline Phophotase

Se PTH, Vit D assays

Therapeutic Facilities:

Medical Treatment of Parathyroid Disorders

Parathyroid Surgery

Adrenals:

Diagnostic Facilities:

CT + MRI, Serum Catecholamines

Se Cortisol/Plasma ACTH, Se DHEA's

Se 17 Alpha OH Progesterone

Therapeutic Facilities:

Medical and Surgical treatment of Adrenal Disorders

Testis:

Diagnostic Facilities:

Se Testosterone, LH, FSH, Ultrasound

Colour Doppler for Penile Blood Flow

Therapeutic Facilities:

Medical & Surgical Treatment of Infertility, Impotence, Hypogonadism

Ovaries:

Diagnostic Facilities:

Se LH, FSH, Estradiol, Ultrasound Pelvis, Ultrasound Ovarian Biopsy

Therapeutic Facilities:

Medical & Surgical Treatment of Ovarian Disorders

Pituitary:

Diagnostic Facilities:

MRI of Pituitary & Hormone Assays, CT

Therapeutic Facilities:

Medical & Surgical Treatment of Pituitary disorders

Diabetes:

Diagnostic Facilities:

HbA1c & Se Fructosamine, Glucometer in every ward, Micro Albumin Assessment

Fluorescein & Angiography Eyes, Colour Doppler lower limbs

Therapeutic Facilities:

Insulin Pumps

All kinds of diabetic emergencies can be managed

Medicines Available/Required for this Department:

1. Human Chorionic Gonadotropin Injection 1000 & 5000 IU
2. Tablets of Methylprednisolone 8 mg, 32 mg
3. Injections of Methylprednisolone 40/500 mg/ml
4. Tablets: Ethinylestradiol + Levonorgestrel 0.03 mg + 0.15 mg
5. Tablets: Ormeloxifene 30 mg & Ethinylestradiol 0.010.05 mg
6. Tablets: Ethinylestradiol 0.05 mg & Levonorgestrel 1.5/0.75 mg
7. Tablet: Glimepiride 1/2 mg
8. Tablet: Gliclazide 40 mg
9. Injection Insulin (Soluble) 40 IU/ml
10. Injection Insulin Rapid & Mixtard
11. Tablets of Metformin
12. Etc.

SPECIALTY CLINICS:

1. Diabetes Clinic
2. Obesity Clinic
3. Thyroid Clinic
4. Infertility Clinic
5. Growth Clinic
6. Dietetic Clinic (Diet Counselling)
7. Diabetic Foot Clinic

OBESITY:

Obesity is a state in which there is generalised accumulation of excess fat in the body leading to a body weight of more than 20% of the ideal body weight.

The BMI defines an individual as being overweight if he/she has a BMI of 25-30kg/m^2 and obese if he/she has a BMI of >30 kg/m^2

$$BMI = Weight (kg)/Height (m^2).$$

Height – Weight calculator

The chart given below summarizes the ideal height-weight ratio among Indians.

Height – Weight Chart

Men

Height (centimetres)	Small frame (Weight in kgs)	Medium frame (Weight in kgs)	Large frame (Weight in kgs)
157.5	58.1 - 60.8	59.4 - 64.0	62.6 - 68.0
160.0	59.0 - 61.7	60.3 - 64.9	63.5 - 69.4
162.6	59.9 - 62.6	61.2 - 65.8	64.4 – 70.7
165.1	60.8 - 63.5	62.1 - 67.1	65.3 - 72.6
167.6	61.7 - 64.4	63.0 - 68.5	66.2 - 74.4

Height (centimetres)	Small frame (Weight in kgs)	Medium frame (Weight in kgs)	Large frame (Weight in kgs)
170.2	62.6 - 65.8	64.4 - 69.8	67.6 - 76.2
172.7	63.5 - 67.1	65.8 - 71.2	68.9 - 78.0
175.3	64.4 - 68.5	67.1 - 72.6	70.3 - 79.8
177.8	65.3 - 69.8	68.5 - 73.9	71.7 - 81.6
180.3	66.2 - 71.2	69.8 - 75.3	73.0 - 83.5
182.9	67.6 - 72.6	71.2 - 77.1	74.4 - 85.3
185.4	68.9 - 74.4	72.6 - 78.9	76.2 - 87.1
188.0	70.3 - 76.2	74.4 - 80.7	78.0 - 89.4
190.5	71.7 - 78.0	75.7 - 82.6	79.8 - 91.6
193.0	73.5 - 79.8	77.6 - 84.8	82.1 - 93.9

Women

Height (centimetres)	Small frame (Weight in kgs)	Medium frame (Weight in kgs)	Large frame (Weight in kgs)
147.3	45.9 - 49.9	49.0 - 54.0	53.1 - 58.9
149.9	46.3 - 50.8	49.9 - 55.3	54.0 - 60.3
152.4	46.8 - 51.7	50.8 - 56.7	54.9 - 61.6
154.9	47.7 - 53.1	51.7 - 58.0	56.2 - 63.0
157.5	48.6 - 54.4	53.1 - 59.4	57.6 - 64.3
160.0	49.9 - 55.8	54.4 - 60.7	58.9 - 66.1
162.6	51.3 - 57.1	55.8 - 62.1	66.3 - 67.9
165.1	52.6 - 58.5	57.1 - 63.4	61.6 - 69.7
167.6	54.0 - 59.8	58.5 - 64.8	63.0 - 71.5
170.2	55.3 - 61.2	59.3 - 66.1	64.3 - 73.3
172.7	56.7 - 62.5	61.2 - 67.5	65.7 - 75.4
175.3	58.5 - 63.9	62.5 - 68.8	67.5 - 76.5
177.8	59.4 - 65.2	63.9 - 70.2	68.4 - 77.8
180.3	60.7 - 66.6	65.2 - 71.5	69.7 - 79.2
182.9	62.1 - 67.9	66.6 - 72.9	71.1 - 80.5

Sliding Scale:

Blood glucose level (mg/dL)	Breakfast	Lunch	Dinner
151-200	4U	4U	5U
201-250	5U	5U	7U
>250	6U	5U	8U

Diagnostic Points:

1. A random plasma glucose value (taken any time of day) of 200 mg/dl or more along with the presence of diabetes symptoms.

2. A plasma glucose value of 126 mg/dl or more after a person has fasted for 8 hours.
3. An oral GTT plasma glucose value of 200 mg/dl or more in the blood samples, taken after 2 hours after a person has consumed a drink containing 75 grams of glucose dissolved in water.
4. Glycated Haemoglobin (HbA1c) indicates blood glucose control over a period of approximately 3 months. Normal range is usually 4-7% correlating the average blood glucose of 60-150 mg/dl (3.3-8.3 mmol/l). Patient does not need to be fasting for this test.

Complications of Obesity:

1. Obesity: may cause
   a. Disturbed/Excessive sleep
   b. Stroke
   c. Breathlessness
   d. High Cholesterol/Blood Pressure
   e. Heart Attack
   f. Diabetes
   g. Impotence/Infertility
   h. Arthritis

Factors contributing to Obesity:

A sedentary lifestyle, dependence on television and computers for leisure and a less physically active lifestyle and stress have been significant contributors to obesity and related health complications. However, the major contribution has come from the wrong kind of nutrition – increased consumption of processed, complex carbohydrate-rich food is the main culprit in contributing to this fast-growing 'epidemic'.

Advice for Patients on Obesity:

Do's of diabetic diets:

1. Be consistent in diet and meal timings according to medicines.
2. Take multivitamin containing an antioxidant such as vitamin A, beta-carotene, vitamins C and E.
3. The diet should have minimum of 1,200 kcal/day for women and 1,500 kcal/day for men.
4. Salt intake should be maintained between 2.4 and 3.0 gm/day for people without hypertension and ≥ 2.4 gm/day for people with mild to moderate hypertension.
5. Consume fibre of approximately 20-35 gm/day from a variety of food sources should be consumed.

Don'ts of diabetic diet:

1. Avoid alcohol especially if diabetes is not in control.
2. Avoid in-between meals. Adhere to the time and size of the meal decided.
3. Avoid fasts as fasting alters body metabolism, adversely affecting the diabetic state.

You're Diet?

1. Pulses with husk
2. All green seasonal vegetables either as salad or cooked.
3. Skimmed or toned milk/curd
4. Fresh lime/clear soups/butter milk/tea/coffee.
5. Egg or paneer or chicken or fish.

6. Fruits – papaya/apple/mausami/orange/guava/pears.
7. Marie biscuits or rusk.
8. Dalia/wheat flakes/sooji.
9. Refined oil/mustard oil up to 10 - 15 Gm per day
10. Diabetes with heart diseases to take:
    Corn oil/saffola oil – 10- 15 gm day/2-3 TSP per day.

Please Avoid:

1. Vegetables – Potato, Sweet Potato, Shaljam, Zimikand, Beetroot, Arbi.
2. Fruits – Banana, Lichi, Mango, Grapes, Tinned fruits and fruit juices.
3. All sweets – Cakes/Ice Cream/Honey/Jaggery/Glucose/Jam.
4. Bournvita – Horlicks etc.
5. Alcoholic Drinks.
6. Red Meat/Cheese.
7. Fried Food – e.g., Puri, Parantha, Samosa, Patty, Pakora.
8. Dry fruits and nuts.
9. Butter, Pure Ghee, Cream, vanaspati.

PAEDIATRIC ENDOCRINOLOGY:

Hormones are chemicals produced in the body that affect the physiology of the body.

They are essential for the growth and development (both physical and mental) of a child. A child grows to his/her genetic potential and matures into an adult on appropriate time, only if his/her hormone system works well. Hormones like Thyroxine and Growth hormone are vital in this process.

Paediatric endocrinologists work closely with primary care paediatricians to provide coordinated and comprehensive care.

Following problems are dealt by this department:

1. Growth problems, such as short stature
2. Early or delayed puberty
3. Enlarged thyroid gland (goitre)
4. Underactive or overactive thyroid gland
5. Pituitary gland hypo/hyper function
6. Adrenal gland hypo/hyper function
7. Ambiguous genitals/intersex
8. Ovarian and testicular dysfunction
9. Paediatric age Diabetes
10. Low blood sugar (hypoglycaemia)
11. Obesity
12. Problems with Vitamin D (rickets, hypocalcaemia)

STAFFING:

The department has experienced doctors, a team of stroke coordinators, surgeons and trained nurses for the best treatment.

DUTIES & RESPONSIBILITIES:

A. Duties of an Endocrinologist:

Endocrinologist is a physician who specializes in the management of hormone conditions. Duties are similar to that of a specialist.

1. In short: history taking, physical examination, ordering investigations, prescribing treatment.
2. To explain treatment options and advises them on dietary changes, medications and lifestyle and other preventive measures.
3. Advising, ordering, and interpreting the results.
4. To follow-up appointments, monitor patient progress, adjust treatment plans and medications.
5. To maintain patients' medical records systemically and updating patient records.
6. To remain up-to-date on current discoveries, developments, trends, research, and technology.
7. To carry out basic administrative work such as supervising their subordinate staff for their turn out.
8. To take informed consent whenever it is required.
9. To advise surgery whenever necessary.
10. To carry out procedures.
11. To attend meetings whenever asked for.
12. To ensure smooth functioning of the department.
13. To advice other departments whenever asked for.
14. To strive to achieve the best patient and family centred care.
15. To conduct CMEs and lectures.
16. To follow hospital rules and regulations

B. Duties of a Nurse of This Department:

Similar to any nurse.

1. To explain the advised treatment to patients and relatives.
2. To monitor patients on specialised therapies.

C. Duties of a Dietician:

1. To calculate calorie intake required by the patient.
2. To explain patient about dietary regime.
3. To modify diets during treatment, if needed.

D. Technicians:

Duties are same as that of any other technician.

1. Taking samples of specimen.
2. Installing special devices such as Insulin Pump, CGMS

PROCEDURES (SOP):

A. For OPD

Same as that of any super-specialty OPD

B. For IPD

Similar to any other admission process

C. For Endocrinology Lab:

The hospital has a separate lab/common lab for carrying out investigations on patients of this department.

Following precautions are to be taken before collection of blood samples:

1. Wash hands before and after the collection of Samples.
2. Collection of the specimen before the administration of agents.
3. Prevention of contamination of the specimen.
4. Collect the specimen at the appropriate phase of disease.
5. Collect or place the specimen aseptically in a sterile and/or appropriate container.
6. Close the container tightly so that its contents do not leak during transportation.
7. Makes records in separate registers for each investigation.
8. Label and date the container appropriately.
9. Arrange for immediate transfer of the specimen to the specific laboratory.

TOPICS FOR CME:

1. Endocrinology simplified for Physicians/GPs
2. Endocrinology for Paediatricians
3. Etc.

ADVICE FOR PATIENTS:

Go for Diabetes screening if you are having;

1. Family history of diabetes
2. Any Cardiovascular disease, Hypertension
3. You are overweight or obese
4. If you are on steroids
5. If you were born with a Low Birth Weight (LBW)
6. Polycystic ovary syndrome

VARIOUS CHECKLISTS FOR THIS DEPARTMENT:

Checklist for Patients on Discharge:

1. Do you clearly understand name and doses of your post discharge medications?
2. Do you have a portable Glucometer (Blood Glucose Meter) at home and you are aware of its use?
3. Keep a record of all your Blood Sugar Tests results.
4. You know how often blood is to be tested for Glucose?
5. You know about your diet details after discharge?
6. You know symptoms and signs of High and Low sugar level?
7. You have contact numbers of the hospital and your doctor?

KEY PERFORMANCE INDICATORS (KPI):

KPI can be broadly grouped as follows:

A. Omission Errors

Omission errors include errors related to the patient's biodata, such as name, address, age, and gender.

B. Commission Errors

The errors are related to the prescriber biodata such as name, address, and also errors in dose, duration, dosage form, frequency, and strength.

C. Drug Interactions

Normal KPIs are;

1. % of error in patients bio data in the prescription:
2. % of drug prescribed in generic name:
3. % of adverse drug reaction and/or drug-drug interaction:
4. Waiting list in the out-patient clinic:
   Benchmark should be Zero but less than 20 minutes
   Frequency: Monthly

KPIs dedicated to Endocrinology:

1. Percentage of cases with diabetes attending Medicine and Endocrinology Clinics
2. Percentage of cases with thyroid attending Medicine and Endocrinology Clinics
3. Percentage of cases with Puberty and Growth disorders attending Medicine and Endocrinology Clinics
4. Patient readmission within 30 days of the initial admission:
   Benchmark should be less than 5 percent
5. Percentage of hypothyroid patients achieved euthyroid status after 6 months of first consultation by Endocrinologist
   Benchmark: More than 80 %
   Frequency: Six monthly
6. Percentage of insulin-treated in-patients experiencing severe hypoglycaemia
   Benchmark: Should be less than 5 percent
   Frequency: Monthly
7. Morbidity following thyroid and parathyroid surgery
8. Other QI are as for any IPD/OPD case.

KPI Data Collection Formats:

These are already available elsewhere.

QUALITY ASSURANCE:

1. Quality assurance in laboratory services, aimed at improving reliability, efficiency and facilitating inter-laboratory comparability in testing.
2. Quality controls of investigation kits once in a week or every time before a new batch of investigation kit.

3. These quality control strains are tested using exactly the same procedure as for the test organisms.
4. When the results regularly fall outside this range, they should be regarded as evidence that a technical error has been introduced into the test.

General laboratory directions for safety:

1. Long hair should be bound back neatly away from shoulders.
2. Do not wear any jewellery to laboratory sessions.
3. Keep fingers, pencils, bacteriological loops etc. out of your mouth.
4. Do not smoke in the laboratory.
5. Do not lick labels with tongue (use tap water).
6. Do not drink from laboratory glassware.

FUTURE PLANS:

1. To provide facility for ambulatory Insulin Infusion.

BIBLIOGRAPHY, REFERENCES & ACKNOWLEDGMENTS:

1. Indian Public Health Standards (IPHS)
   Guidelines for District Hospitals (101 to 500 Bedded) Revised 2012 Directorate General of Health Services Ministry of Health & Family Welfare, Government of India
2. "Standard Operating Procedures SOP For Hospitals 2nd Edition" by Dr. Arun K. Agarwal
3. "Duties & Responsibilities of Hospital Staff" by Dr. Arun Kumar
4. "Checklists for Hospitals" by Dr. Arun K. Agarwal
5. Aligarh Muslim University, Aligarh, India
6. "Technical Dossier" from Ochoa Laboratories Ltd. E-406, Greater Kailash-II, New Delhi-110 048, (Year 2005)
7. A Comprehensive Guide to Diabetes", Published from 'Novo Nordisk' Private Limited, Bangalore, India Year 2003-2004
8. Six Sigma Multispeciality Hospital, Nasik, India
9. Khan M, Ullah R, Khan A, Ur-Rahman N, Khan S, Riaz M. Assessment of Prescriptions in the Endocrinology Department of a Tertiary Care Hospital in Pakistan Using World Health Organization Guidelines. Adv Prev Med. 2020 May 30;2020:3705704. doi: 10.1155/2020/3705704. PMID: 32551141; PMCID: PMC7277054.

Chapter – 12

DEPARTMENT OF ENT

INDEX

1. Introduction
2. Aim, Vision, Mission
3. Objectives
4. Best Practices
5. Infrastructure
6. Facilities
7. Equipment
8. Medicines Required
9. Diseases Treated
10. Services Provided/Facilities
    a. OPD Procedures
    b. Minor Procedures
    c. Nose Surgery
    d. Ear Surgery
    e. Throat Surgery
    f. Endoscopic ENT Procedures
    g. General ENT Surgeries
    h. Rehabilitation Services
11. Specialty Clinics
12. Staffing
13. Duties & Responsibilities
    a. Otolaryngologist
    b. Audiologist
    c. ENT Technician
    d. Speech Therapist
14. Standard Operating Procedures (SOP)
    a. OPD Services Procedure
    b. IPD Procedure
15. Check Lists
    a. Checklist ENT Instruments
    b. Checklist ENT Surgical Sets
        i. ENT Instruments Sets Details
            1. Instruments for Tympanoplasty/Mastoidectomy
            2. FESS/Septoplasty

3. Tonsillectomy/Adenoidectomy
4. Direct Laryngoscopy & Biopsy
5. Tracheostomy Set

c. Checklist ENT Surgery
d. Checklist ENT Surgery Patients

16. Key Performance Indicators
17. Topics For CME/Lectures/Conferences
18. Future Plans
19. Stationary Formats
    a. Audiogram
    b. ENT Case Sheet
20. Bibliography, References & Acknowledgments

INTRODUCTION:

Otorhinolaryngology (also called otolaryngology) is the area of medicine that deals with conditions of the ear, nose, and throat (ENT) region. The specialty is often treated as a unit with surgery of the head and neck (otolaryngology–head and neck surgery, or OHNS). Doctors who specialize in this area are called otorhinolaryngologists, otolaryngologists, ENT doctors, ENT surgeons, or head and neck surgeons. Patients seek treatment from an otorhinolaryngologist for diseases of the ear, nose, throat, or base of the skull, and for the surgical management of cancers and benign tumours of the head and neck. [Otorhinolaryngology; From Wikipedia, the free encyclopedia. *https://en.wikipedia.org/wiki/Otorhinolaryngology*]

This department in this hospital provides comprehensive medical and surgical care to both adult and paediatric patients. The department takes care of diagnosis and treatment of various conditions of Ear, Nose and Throat. The department also oversees problems of other areas in Head & Neck region.

The Department of ENT in this hospital provides diagnosis and treatment for problems of the ear, nose and throat, and other problems of the head and the neck area. Facilities include all kind of diagnostic and therapeutic ENT Endoscopies, Routine ENT surgeries like Endoscopic Sinus Surgeries, Microscopic ENT Ear surgeries, etc.

The department is equipped with all kinds of advanced investigations like BERA, CT-scan, MRI and Polysomnography. Department is efficient enough to handle advanced procedures.

AIMS, VISION & MISSION:

Vision:

1. To create a dedicated, competent & compassionate doctor whose ultimate goal is to serve humanity & uphold the ideals of our noble profession.
2. To provide medical facilities of the highest standard at an affordable cost to all segments of society.
3. To be at the fore front of patient care in the field of Ear, Nose, Throat and Head & Neck Surgery.

Mission:

1. The mission of the Department of Otolaryngology and Head – Neck Surgery is to improve health care by enhancing the field of otolaryngology and head - neck surgery by advancing its clinical application. We are committed to the delivery of comprehensive, compassionate and cost-effective health care.
2. To provide therapeutic services to patients at single point.
3. To strengthen IEC activities for curative and preventive services.

4. The department, working as a team is dedicated to fulfilling this mission.
5. Curative medical services to community at single point.
6. Promoting outreach activities and public awareness through innovative activities for preventive services to patient and their relatives in community.
7. Strengthening IEC activities for curative and preventive services.
8. To offer cutting edge facilities in the field of ENT and Head & Neck surgeries at reasonable costs.
9. To improve the quality of life of people with hearing loss and related disorders through scientific research, patient care, and the sharing of knowledge.
10. To be at the forefront of medical research in the field of Ear, Nose, Throat and Head & Neck Surgery.

OBJECTIVES

1. Creating awareness among general population of conditions and ailments prone to the area in a tertiary care centre providing sufficient management modalities to diagnose and/or treat disability, disorder of disease, and also highlighting preventive Measure.
2. Attend to medical or surgical emergencies to those seeking immediate care in the hospital around the clock.
3. Orienting the patient and family to the disease condition, its prognosis, and different treatment modalities available based on their affordability.

BEST PRACTICES:

1. Implementing national programme for prevention and control of deafness.
2. Word class endoscopic services.
3. Sound proof room for correct diagnosis of hearing impairment.
4. Collection of reference books in hospital's central library.

INFRASTRUCTURE:

ENT – OPD is well equipped with basic examination tools.

A good sound proof room has been provided for hearing tests.

FACILITIES:

A. **Diagnostic Facilities:**
   1. Audiometry
   2. Tympanogram
   3. Impedance Audiometery
   4. Free Field Audiogram
   5. Hearing Aid Analysis
   6. BERA
   7. Nasal Endoscopy
   8. Direct Laryngoscopy
   9. Bronchoscopy

B. **Therapeutic Facilities:**
   1. Endoscopic Sinus Surgery
   2. Tympanoplasty

3. Stapedectomy
4. Septo-Rhinoplasty
5. Cochlear Implant Surgery
6. Surgery for Angiofibroma
7. Micro laryngeal Surgery
8. Facial Nerve Decompression
9. Trans Nasal Pituitary Surgery
10. Surgery for CSF Rhinorrhoea
11. Endoscopy for Foreign Body of Oesophagus & Bronchus

EQUIPMENT:

1. ENT Work Station
2. Audiometer
3. BERA (Brainstem Evoked Response Audiometer) & OAE Screening
4. Electronystagmography
5. Sinuscope
6. Fibre-optic Endoscopes
7. Operation Microscope
8. CO2 Laser for Surgery
9. Pure tone and impedance audiometer
10. Micro motor Drill System
11. Laryngoscope Set

Equipment & Instruments in OPD:

1. General examination instruments,
2. Ear & nasal Suction machine,
3. Otoscope,
4. Jobson Horne probe,
5. Head lamp
6. Nasal Speculum,
7. Laryngeal mirror,
8. Nasopharyngeal mirrors
9. Aural speculum
10. Siegles speculum,
11. Tuning fork (512 Hz),
12. Bayonet forces,

MEDICINES REQUIRED (for this Department):

Ciprofloxacin Drops 0.3%	Clotrimazole Drops 1%
Xylometazoline Nasal Drops 0.05 %, 0.1%	Ciprofloxacin Drops 0.3%
Wax Solvent Ear Drops: Benzocaine, Paradichlorobenzene, Turpentine oil	Normal Saline Nasal Drops: Sodium Chloride Drops 0.05% w/v

Boro-spirit Ear Drop S-0.183 gm Boric Acid in 2.08 ml of Alcohol	Combo Ear Drops-Chloramphenicol 5% w/v + Clotrimazole 1% + Lignocaine Hydrochloride 2%
Ofloxacin Tablet 200/400 mg	Clotrimazole Drops 1%
Other General Medicines	

Emergency Kit:

1. Medicine saline and xylometazolidine nasal drops,
2. Antibiotic and anti -fungal ear drops,
3. Betadine gargle,
4. Antihistamine,
5. 10% xylocaine spray,
6. Betadine Solution,
7. For Epistaxis-Killian's nasal Speculum, Tilley's Forceps, Tongue depressor, Bowl,
8. Nasal packs-anterior/posterior

DISEASES TREATED:

A. Ear conditions include:
   1. Otosclerosis (a condition of the middle ear that causes hearing loss) and other problems with hearing and deafness
   2. Otitis media with effusion – a common condition of childhood (also known as glue ear) in which the middle ear becomes blocked with fluid
   3. Age related hearing loss
   4. Tinnitus (ringing in the ears) and eustachian tube dysfunction
   5. Dizziness and vertigo

B. Nose conditions include:
   1. Sinus infection and rhino-sinusitis, including in children
   2. Nasal injuries
   3. Nasal polyps
   4. Tumours of the nose

C. Throat conditions include:
   1. Adenoid problems – surgical removal of these small glands in the throat at the back of the nose is sometimes needed and is usually performed in childhood
   2. Tonsillitis, sometimes requiring surgical removal of the tonsils, usually in childhood
   3. Hoarseness and laryngitis

SERVICES PROVIDED: (in short)

1. OPD ENT diagnostics including endoscopy,
2. Syringing, Wax Removal
3. Emergency ENT procedures,
4. Epistaxis Management
5. Tracheostomy,
6. Foreign Body removal (nasal and aural),

7. Nasal packing,
8. Incision and drainage of head & neck abscess,
9. Bronchoscopy,
10. Naso-endoscopic Surgeries,
11. Microscopic, endoscopic and open ENT surgeries,
12. Skull base surgery

SERVICES:

In short, the department takes care of:

1. General diseases of ear, nose & throat.
2. Speech problems (Speech Therapy).
3. Cancers of head & neck.
4. Hearing & body balancing problems.
5. Problems of 'tear duct'.
6. Problems of salivary glands.
7. Problems of 'Thyroid Gland'.
8. Problems of 'facial Nerve'.
9. Cosmetic surgery.
10. Swallowing disorders.

A. OPD Procedures:

1. Foreign Body Removal (Ear and Nose)
2. Stitching of CLW's
3. Dressings
4. Syringing of Ear
5. Chemical Cauterization (Nose & Ear)
6. Eustachian Tube Function Test
7. Vestibular Function Test/Caloric Test
8. Audiogram

B. Minor Procedures:

1. Therapeutic Removal of Granulations (Nasal, Aural, Oropharynx)
2. Punch Biopsy (Oral Cavity & Oropharynx)
3. Cauterization (Oral, Oropharynx, Aural & nasal)

C. Nose Surgery:

1. Nasal Endoscopy & Endoscopic Sinus Surgery
2. Packing (Anterior & Posterior Nasal)
3. Antral Puncture (Unilateral & Bilateral)
4. Inter Nasal Antrostomy (Unilateral & Bilateral)
5. I & D Septal Abscess (Unilateral & Bilateral)
6. SMR

7. Septoplasty
8. Fracture Reduction Nose
9. Fracture Reduction Nose with Septal Correction
10. Transantral Procedures (Biopsy, Excision of cyst and Angiofibroma Excision)
11. Transantral Biopsy
12. Rhinoplasty
13. Septoplasty with reduction of turbinate (SMD)

D. Ear Surgery:

1. Mastoid Abscess I & D
2. Mastoidectomy
3. Stapedotomy
4. Examination under Microscope
5. Myringotomy & Myringoplasty
6. Tympanoplasty
7. Ear Piercing
8. Hearing Aid Analysis and Selection

E. Throat Surgery:

1. Adenoidectomy
2. Tonsillectomy
3. Adenoidectomy + Tonsillectomy
4. Tongue Tie excision

F. Endoscopic ENT Procedures:

1. Direct Laryngoscopy
2. Hypopharyngoscopy
3. Direct Laryngoscopy & Biopsy
4. Broncoscopic Diagnostic
5. Broncoscopic & F B Removal

G. General ENT Surgery:

1. Stitching of LCW (Nose & Ear)
2. Preauricular Sinus Excision
3. Tracheostomy

H. Rehabilitation Services:

1. Hearing Aid Fitting
2. Speech Therapy

SPECIALITY CLINICS:

1. Voice Clinic
2. Audio-vestibular clinic

3. Vertigo Clinic
4. Headache Clinic
5. Head & Neck cancer Screening
6. Sleep Clinic

STAFFING:

1. Otolaryngologist (ENT Consultant)
2. Audiologists
3. ENT Technician
4. Speech Therapist

DUTIES & RESPONSIBILITIES:

A. Otolaryngologist:

Duties are similar to any other specialist.

1. To take history, examine and treat diseases of the ear, nose, upper pharynx, larynx, oral cavity, and other head and neck structures.
2. To patiently listen to patients' complaints.
3. To make a provisional diagnosis.
4. To advice various diagnostic tests as needed.
5. To establish the nature and severity of the disorder, and prescribe medications or conduct surgery.
6. To self-perform a test if required.
7. To perform surgeries as per requirement.
8. To treat sleep disorders.
9. To work closely with other consultants of same department or specialists of other departments to solve various medical issues.
10. To actively participate in different national and international workshops in various capacity like delegate, speaker and/or organizer.

B. Audiologist

1. Will be working with ENT consultants.
2. Shall be working as an assistant to ENT consultants in OPD.
3. Shall be in proper uniform as prescribed by the hospital.
4. Shall be responsible for hearing testing and screening programs.
5. Will evaluate hearing and balancing disorders.
6. Shall carry out various hearing tests on patients with the available diagnostic equipment such as Audiometers, Tympanometers, Impedance meters etc.
7. Shall perform other special tests on patients with hearing disorders.
8. Shall ensure proper functioning, maintenance and calibration of such equipment.
9. May be asked to help ENT surgeons in the OT during their surgery.
10. Shall keep records of (log book) maintenance and calibrations.
11. Shall counsel patients before taking up any test.
12. Shall explain/demonstrate the test before actually taking it up.
13. Shall also be responsible for demonstrating wearing of hearing aids. Will train the patient in wearing such aids.

14. Shall ensure safe and healthy working environment.
15. Shall respect patient rights of safety and privacy.
16. Shall monitor patients' progress undergoing treatment in this department.
17. Shall maintain and update patients' records.
18. Shall be taking care of all operated patients during their hospital stay.
19. Shall maintain and update all records and registers as required by the hospital.
20. To ensure confidentiality of all information obtained from the patient during the course of examination/treatment.
21. Shall perform other administrative work of the department.
22. Shall indent and receive supplies from the market/stores.
23. Shall be carrying out other duties as asked by seniors.

C. ENT Technician:

1. To be punctual on duty.
2. To be in proper attire while on duty.
3. To perform various diagnostic tests such as Pure Tome Audiometry, Impedance Audiometry, Evoked Potential Audiometry etc.
4. To evaluate hearing and balance disorders.
5. To develop and perform/supervise hearing testing sessions.
6. To advise special hearing devices and train patients in its usages.
7. To perform, assist in speech therapy.
8. To perform other special tests of this department.
9. To assist ENT surgeons in their surgical procedures.
10. To assist ENT Surgeons in conducting their OPD.
11. To perform basic nursing duties.
12. To perform administrative work such as documentation, maintenance of records & inventory etc.
13. To keep record of all tests and procedures conducted in his/her department.
14. To organize and conduct various screening programs.
15. To ensure confidentiality of all information.
16. To maintain all equipment in working condition. Troubleshooting and minor repair of devices should be undertaken by him/her and assisting in major repairs undertaken by respective engineers.
17. To indent various supplies required for this department.
18. To participate in meetings when called for.
19. To perform any other task given by seniors.

D. Speech Therapist:

1. Duties are very much similar to that of an Audiologist.
2. Their duty is to identify, evaluate, treat and prevent congenital or acquired speech and hearing problems.
3. They work under direct guidance of departmental head.
4. To identify and assess the nature of problem (slurring, delayed speaking, harsh voice and swallowing disorders etc.) and its cause.
5. To use available equipment and instruments to diagnose and evaluate patient's hearing & speech impairment.
6. To help and train patients with cleft lip and cleft palate, facial paralysis and similar neurological disorders.
7. To identify a suitable treatment plan and execute it.

8. To assess and impart training to patients with hearing and speech problems.
9. To teach patients about methods of speaking to improve their speech.
10. To review and improve/modify plan as per improvement in patient condition.
11. To help in reducing the disability.
12. They may also teach patients alternative communication methods (sign language).
13. To counsel patient and relatives about the problem and possibilities of outcome.
14. To prescribe suitable artificial devices to overcome problems.
15. To prepare reports and maintain confidentiality.
16. To maintain proper records of all patients who attend this clinic.
17. To liaise with doctors, physiotherapist and family members.
18. To impart training to assistants.
19. To maintain inventory of equipment available in this department.
20. To be responsible for upkeep of instruments and equipment available in this department.
21. To complete other paper work as required by hospital policies and procedures.
22. To carry out any other duty assigned by departmental head.

STANDARD OPERATING PROCEDURES (SOP):

A. OPD Services Procedure:

Similar to any other OPD

1. Registration of the patient at central registration counter.
2. Escorting the patient to the OPD chamber.
3. Examination by the doctor.
4. Referring the patient to diagnostic departments for investigations as advised.
5. Patient consults the doctor with reports.
6. Consulting the doctor
7. The doctor advice treatment based on his examination and reports.
8. Patient is given appointment for surgery, if required.
9. Follow up date is given to the patient
10. The patient goes home

B. IPD Procedure:

Again, it is similar to any other admission procedure.

1. Central registration.
2. Preparation of IPD case sheet after proper counselling and deposit of advance
3. Patient is escorted to the ward.
4. Ensure that informed consent has been taken.

C. Preoperative Preparation:

1. General:
   a. Ensure Informed Written Consent is done.
   b. Ensure all documentation is complete (e.g., PAC, Investigation results etc).
   c. Follow all preparation instructions of surgeon and anaesthetist.

2. Ear Surgery:
   a. Ensure hair is washed properly.
   b. Shaving where indicated.
3. Tonsillectomy
   a. Nose should be decongested with nasal decongestant pack for smooth nasal intubation.
4. Nose Surgery:
a. Nose should be decongested with nasal decongestant pack prior to sending to OT.

D. Miscellaneous:

1. Infection control measures should be followed as per the guidelines.
2. All emergency drugs and equipment should be kept ready and available at all times to combat any emergency during admission/surgery.
3. Patients' rights of privacy should be maintained at all times.
4. If suspect an MLC, inform hospital administration immediately.
5. Disposal of BMW must be as per hospital protocol.
6. Patients file documented by the Doctors and Nurses should be kept as confidential.
7. Ward should be kept clean and tidy; silence and visitor control should be observed before ward round.

CHECK LISTS:

1. Checklist ENT Equipment – OPD:

SN	Item	Qty
1	Audiometer, Pure tone	1
2	Aural Syringe	1
3	BP Apparatus	1
4	Bull's Eye Lamp	1
5	Diagnostic Set	1
6	Endoscopy Unit is a desirable item in today's ENT clinic	1
7	ENT Examination Chair/ENT Workstation	1
8	Epistaxis Catheters	3
9	Fibreoptic Head Lamp - Head Mirror with Head Bans	1
10	Hartmann's Aural Forceps	1
11	Impedance Audiometer	1
12	Jobson Horne Probe with Ring & Curette	1
13	Kidney Tray	2
14	Laryngeal Mirrors	4
15	Laryngoscope Hopkins, 0 degree	1
16	Nasal Foreign Body Hook	1
17	Nasal Speculums Thodicum, set of 6	4
18	Nasopharyngeal mirrors	4

SN	Item	Qty
19	Rechargeable Auroscope, Aural Speculums	4
20	Siegle's Pneumatic Speculum	1
21	Slow Suction Apparatus	1
22	Steriliser	1
23	Stethoscope	1
24	Tilley's nasal Dressing Forceps	1
25	Tongue Depressors (Disposable)	
26	Tuning Fork (216, 532, 1024 Hz)	1
27	Wax Curette	3
28	Wood Carrier	2

2. Checklist ENT Surgical Sets:

Following surgical instruments sets should be made available:

a. **Major Sets:**
   1. Tonsillectomy and adenoidectomy set
   2. Set for nasal bone fracture
   3. Septoplasty set
   4. Caldwel luc set
   5. Antrostomy set
   6. Rhinoplasty Set
   7. FESS set
   8. Direct laryngoscopy set
   9. Micro laryngoscopy set
   10. Tympanoplasty set
   11. Mastoidectomy set
   12. Stapedectomy set
   13. Oesophagoscopy set
   14. Bronchoscopy set
   15. Tracheostomy set

b. **Minor Sets:**
   1. Antral wash set
   2. Direct laryngoscope set

c. **Operating microscope**

ENT INSTRUMENTS SETS DETAILS:

A. **Instruments for Tympanoplasty/Mastoidectomy:**

Self-Retaining Mastoid Retractor	Micro Motor Drill System
Burrs: Cutting 7, 6, 5, 4, 3.1, 2.3, 1.4 mm	Burrs: Diamond 6, 5, 4, 2.7, 1 mm
Circular Glass Slides x 2	Farabery Periosteal Elevator

Canal Wall Elevator	Meenen's Cell Seeker with Curette
Suction Catheters with adopter, Size: 18, 14, 20	Aural speculum
Drum Curette	Graft Knife & Graft Press
Mallet & Gouge	Mastoid Seeker
Malleus Head Nipper	

B. **FESS/Septoplasty:**

Gauze and Mallet	Curved Suction
Through cut Forceps, Straight & Up turned	70 mm, 0 Degree Telescope
Bayonet forceps	Killians Nasal Speculum
Freer Elevator	Ballenger's Swivel Knife
Takahashi Forceps	Retrograde Punch

C. **Tonsillectomy/Adenoidectomy:**

Boyle's Davis Mouth Gag, Paediatric & Adult- 4 sizes	Tonsil Holding Forceps
Tonsil Anterior Pillar Retractor with Dissector	Waugh's Tenaculum
Negus Long Artery Forceps	Eve's Tonsil Snare
St. Thompson's Adenoid Curette with Guard	Bipod
Burkit Artery Forceps	Yankauer oropharyngeal suction tip

D. **Direct Laryngoscopy & Biopsy:**

Negus Anterior Commisure Laryngoscope with 15 Degree telescope	Long Suction Forceps x 2
Lighting System for Laryngoscope	Long Biopsy Forceps
Foreign Body Removal Forceps	Laryngeal Suctions

E. **Tracheostomy Set:**

Needle Holder	BP Knife Handle
Ribbon Right Angled Retractors	Curved Artery Forceps
Straight Artery Forceps	Cricoid hook
Tracheal Dilators	

3. Checklist ENT Surgery:

A. **Sign In (Patient is wheeled in)**

1. Patient has verbally confirmed his/her name.
2. Patient has verbally confirmed name of the procedure and site of procedure.
3. Patient has given written consent?
4. Patient has been asked about any known allergy.
5. Anaesthesia safety check done, if anaesthesia is required.

6. Intubation articles are available.
7. Patient vitals are being monitored.

B. **Time Out (Before Incision)**
1. All team members know each other by name.
2. All team members once again confirm the procedure.
3. Required investigation results are displayed.
4. Concern, if any, is discussed.
5. Required equipment (scopes) are available.
6. Required drugs and consumables are available.

C. **Sign Out (Before patient leaves the procedure table)**
1. Procedure details are recorded. (Medical records completed)
2. Specimen, if any, is correctly labelled and sent to lab for examination.
3. Post procedure concern, if any, is reviewed with recovery nurse.
4. Post procedure medication has been discussed with the patient. (If the patient is conscious otherwise discuss with the recovery nurse)

4. Check List ENT Surgery Patients

A. **Before Surgery**
1. No anti-coagulants (not even aspirin, vitamin E) for 2 weeks before the surgery
2. Come without any facial make-up on day of surgery.

B. **After Surgery**
1. Keep your head elevated during sleep.
2. Take liquid and semi solid diet.
3. Do not blow your nose/do not cough violently.
4. Increase your activity level as per your comfort level.
5. Keep area of surgery as clean as possible.
6. Keep your mouth and teeth clean. (Gargling with Betadine)
7. Consult the surgeon immediately if you notice anything unusual.
8. Follow surgeon's instructions.

KEY PERFORMANCE INDICATORS: Specific to ENT

1. **Percentage of patients waiting time in OPD more than the benchmark**

   Benchmark: 30 minutes

   Measuring Frequency: Monthly

   Formula:

   Total number of patients who waited for more than 30 minutes in a given period divided by total OPD attendance in that period multiplied by 100 (one hundred)

2. **Percentage of patients whose hearing improved after myringoplasty:**

   Benchmark: Should be more than 70 percent

   Frequency: Monthly

   Formula:

   Total number of patients who improved divided by total myringoplasty surgeries undertaken in that period multiplied by 100 (one hundred)

3. **Incidence of Haemorrhage after tonsillectomy surgery:**
   Benchmark: Should be less than 3 percent
   Formula:
   Number of patients reporting haemorrhage after the tonsillectomy in a given period divided by total tonsillectomy procedures performed in that period multiplied by 100 (one hundred)
   Note: More set of KPIs for ENT department can be developed as per policy of the hospital. Other KPIs are same as that of any surgery and inpatient.

TOPICS FOR CME/CONFERENCES:

1. Allergic Rhinitis
2. Paediatric ENT
3. Endoscopy in ENT
4. Workshop of Rhinoplasty
5. Workshop on Sleep Apnoea

FUTURE PLANS:

1. To start endoscopic surgeries.
2. To start cochlear implant
3. ……

STATIONARY FORMATS:

1. Audiogram:

Hospital Name

Date: …………………

Patient Name: ……………………………………………… Age/Sex: ………………………

PATIENT NAME………… AGE………… SEX…………

1964 ISO

TEST	Right Ear (Red)	Left Ear (Blue)
AIR	0-0	X-X
AIR OPP EAR MASKED	Δ-Δ	□-□
NO RESPONSE	↓	↓
BONE	<	>
BONE OPP EAR MASKED	[	]
HEARING EVALUATION		
AVE P.T.		
SRT		
PB% CORRECT		
MCL	NO	

VALUES 125 250 500 750 1k 1.5k 2k 3k 4k 6k 8k 10k 12k HZ

-10 0 10 20 30 40 50 60 70 80 90 100 110 120

Hearing Threshold Level in dB

TEST	Right Ear	Left Ear
RINNE		
WEBER		
ABC		
SPECIAL TEST		
RECRUIT-MENT		
SISI		
T.T.S.		

Remarks :

Signature

2. ENT Case Sheet for IPD Patients:

Page-01

Hospital Name

DEPARTMENT OF OTORHINOLARYNGOLOGY

INDOOR CASE SHEET

Surgeon In-charge: UHID No.:

Name of Patient: Ward/Bed No.:

Age/Sex: Date and Time of Admission:

Occupation: Date and Time of Discharge:

Address: Date of Operation:

Result:

Summary of the Case:

Diagnosis:

Signature of Surgeon:

Signature of Anaesthetist:

Signature of OT Technician/Nurse:

Page-02

(Back of Page-01)

Complaints with Duration:

1. …………
2. ……………
3. ……………

Past Illness:

Family History:

Personal History:

History of Present Illness:

Page-03

A. General Examination: Temperature:

General Condition Pulse:

Conjunctive: Respiration:

Nail: B.P.:

Teeth and Gums: Lymph nodes:

Examination of the Face & Neck:

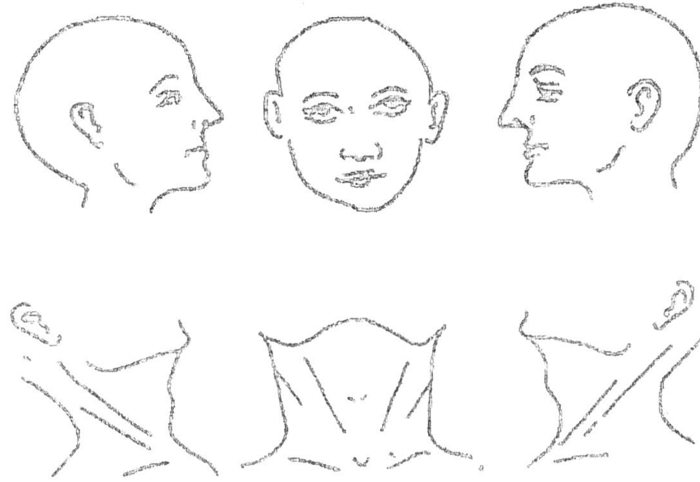

B. Systemic Examination:

C.V. System

Respiratory System

G.I. Track

Nervous System

C. Local Examination:

Oral cavity & Oropharynx

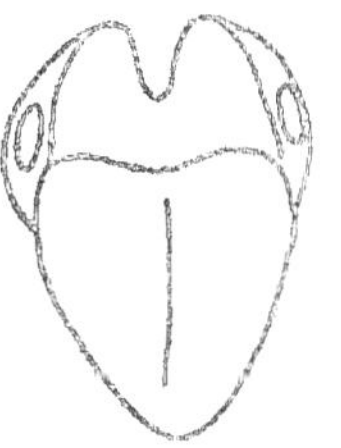

Page-04

(On the back of P-03)

Larynx and Hypopharynx

Indirect Laryngoscopy Examination

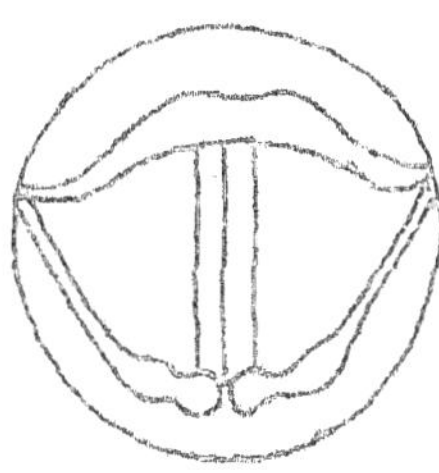

Inspiration

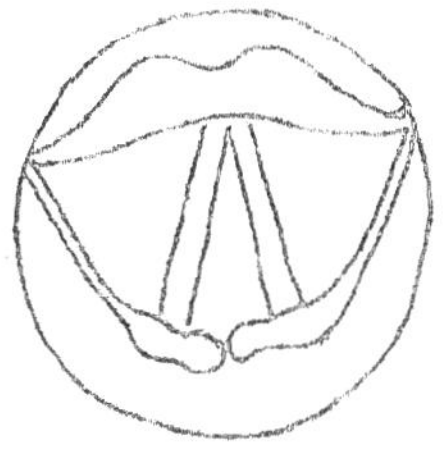

Phonation

Nose and Nasopharynx

External Examination:

Anterior Rhinoscopy:

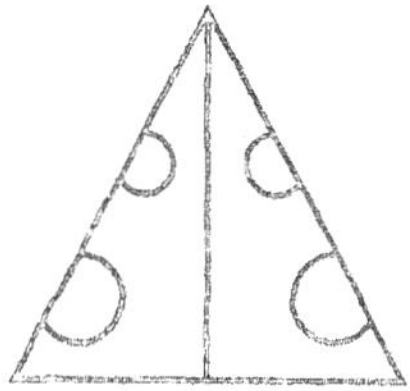

Posterior Rhinoscopy:

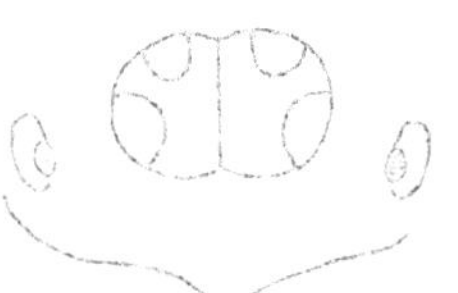

Page-05

EAR

Examination	Right Ear	Left Year
1. Pinna 2. Post and Pre-auricular Region 3. External Auditory Meatus 4. Tympanic Membrane		

Nystagmus

Fistula test

Eustachian Tube Patency

Cranial Nerves

Tuning fork tests

Test	Right Ear	Left Ear
Rinne's Test		
Weber's Test		
Absolute bone conduction		

Page-06

(On the back of P-05)

Investigation:

Caloric Test:

Rt./E 30°C

Lt./E 44°C

Audiogram (Pure Tone)

Preoperative Postoperative

	125	250	500	1000	2000	4000	6000	8000	125	250	500	1000	2000	4000	6000	8000
10																
0																
10																
20																
30																
40																
50																
60																
70																
80																
90																
100																
110																

Audiogram (Impedance) Right Left

Ipsilateral Reflexes

Contralateral Reflexes

Investigation Reports:

Blood:

Hb%

T.L.C.

D.L.C.

E.S.R.

G.B.P.

B.T. & C.T.

F.B.S.

S. Urea

S. ALK. Phosphatase

Urine – Exam. Alb. Sugar M/E

Swab for culture and sensitivity

Biopsy

X-Rays

Any other special investigations

Clinical Diagnosis & Proposed line of Management

Page-07

Operation Notes

Surgeon: .... Assistant Surgeon/Technician: ....

Name of Operation:

Site:

Anaesthetist:

Date of Operation:

Anaesthesia:

Operation Steps:

Page-08

(On the back of P-07)

PROGRESS REPORT

Date	Findings	Treatment

BIBLIOGRAPHY, REFERENCES & ACKNOWLEDGMENTS:

1. Indian Public Health Standards (IPHS)

   Guidelines for District Hospitals (101 to 500 Bedded) Revised 2012 Directorate General of Health Services Ministry of Health & Family Welfare, Government of India
2. "Standard Operating Procedures SOP For Hospitals 2nd Edition" by Dr. Arun K. Agarwal
3. "Duties & Responsibilities of Hospital Staff" by Dr. Arun Kumar
4. "Checklists for Hospitals" by Dr. Arun K. Agarwal
5. Standard Operating Procedures (SOPs) for (JDW/NRH), Quality Assurance and Standardization Division , (QASD) Ministry of Health, Thimphu: Bhutan

Chapter – 13

DEPARTMENT OF GASTROENTEROLOGY

INDEX

INTRODUCTION:

Gastroenterology in general, has grown very rapidly all over the world and has already started branching into further sub-specialization such as hepatology, pancreatology, functional bowel disorders with motility studies, therapeutic endoscopy and endoscopic ultrasound.

Gastroenterology focuses on the entire digestive system which includes the oesophagus, stomach, intestines, colon, pancreas, gall bladder, bile ducts as well as the liver and anus. The disorders afflicting all these organs from top to bottom are so extensive that it requires comprehensive diagnosis and treatment.

The department is equipped to offer a comprehensive range of services including diagnosis and management of GI, Digestive& Liver diseases through medication and minimally invasive procedures. The department of gastroenterology has state-of-the-art diagnostic and therapeutic facilities. The department has latest models of video-endoscopes.

Services offered include comprehensive high-end clinical care and emergency services to patients suffering from disorders of the digestive tract, liver and pancreato-biliary system including both basic and advanced endoscopic diagnostic and therapeutic procedures.

Endoscopy means looking inside and typically refers to looking inside the body for medical reasons using an endoscope, an instrument used to examine the interior of a hollow organ or cavity of the body. Unlike most other medical imaging techniques, endoscopes are inserted directly into the organ.

[Endoscopy; From Wikipedia, the free encyclopedia. https://en.wikipedia.org/wiki/Endoscopy. Assessed on 4-3-2016]

Practically endoscopy is done to visualise inside the patient's body without performing a surgical (invasive) procedure. The procedure is also common to obtain biopsies or removing foreign bodies.

OVERVIEW:

1. Patient care - High quality, state-of-the-art, evidence based
2. Affordable - Treat all patients however sick or poor
3. Quality training of GI Residents
4. Research - Finding Indian solutions for Indian problems

AIMS, VISION & MISSION:

1. To focus on the individualised care of patients to cater to their needs with the best care and support we can offer to them.
2. To make use of various specialities available in the hospital including radiology and cardiology to work as multidisciplinary team as per patient needs.
3. To provide value added innovative, consistent, and continuously improving health and medical care to sustain and further improve clinical outcomes, patient safety, & patient satisfaction.
4. To evolve as a benchmark in quality healthcare available to one and all.
5. To ensure accessible and affordable quality healthcare by compassionate medical professionals to all.
6. To be the centre of excellence for medical research and academics.
7. To cultivate an environment of trust, honesty, mutual respect, equality, and ethics.
8. To take initiative in increasing awareness among general public in preventive aspects of gastrointestinal and liver diseases.

INFRASTRUCTURE:

The Department in this hospital is located on the ground floor. Gastroenterology OPD service are conducted in the main OPD block of the hospital.

The hospital does not have any dedicated beds in its indoor facility as such patients. These patients can be admitted in any room, ward or ICU.

The department does have a separate dedicated endoscopic theatre for all procedures. The operation theatres are common and other OPD facilities are shared with other patients.

EQUIPMENT:

Endoscopes are both "RIGID" and "FLEXIBLE".

Following endoscopes are commonly available. These scopes have names as per their usages.

1. Gastro Intestinal Fiberscope
2. Oesophago Fiberscope
3. Duodeno Fiberscope
4. Colono Fiberscope
5. Flexible Nasopharyngo Laryngoscope
6. Very thin Paediatric Upper GI Endoscope
7. Gas Insufflator, Automatic
8. Electro Surgical Units
9. Endoscope Washer
10. Leakage Tester
11. Endoscopic Disinfection System
12. Endoscopic Photographic Equipment
13. Lecture Scope
14. Xenon Cold Light Source
15. Hand Instruments
    a. Veress Needle, spring loaded, small (120mm)
    b. Sheath/Cannula, 5.5 mm & 11mm with automatic flap valve & also manual control,
    c. Trocar, SS, 11mm with safety guard
    d. Trocar with pyramidal tip, 5.5 mm
    e. Reducer Sleeve with silicon latch (11mm to 5.5mm)
    f. Maxigrip Grasping Forceps, 5mm, with double action, insulated, autoclavable, rotatable
    g. Dissecting Forceps, curved, Maryland, 5mm, insulated, autoclavable, rotatable
    h. Fenestrated Grasper, 5mm, insulated, rotatable dismantlable, autoclavable, double action jaws
    i. Metzenbaum, Curved Scissors, 5mm, Insulated rotatable, dismantlable, autoclavable, double action jaw
    j. Claw Forceps, 2x3 teeth, single action jaw, non-rotatable
    k. Unipolar connection cable
    l. Suction-Irrigation cannula, trumpet type, 5mm
    m. Clip Applicator (for medium large clips), rotatable with flushing channel,
    n. Hook Electrode, 5mm
    o. Aspiration Needle
    p. Stone Basket & Graspers
    q. Etc.

SERVICES OFFERED/AVAILABLE:

All the services are available round the clock, seven days a week.

Medical Gastroenterology:

It offers both diagnostic and therapeutic facility (Medical Gastroenterology), namely;

Diagnostic Services:

1. Upper GI Endoscopy: for the diagnosis of Peptic Ulcers, Polyps and gastric bleeding.
2. Colonoscopy: for Colon bleeding, polyps and colitis
3. Liver Biopsy

Therapeutic Services:

1. Endoscopic Sclerotherapy,
2. Endoscopic Variceal Ligation
3. Endoscopic Glue Injection for GI Bleeding Cases,
4. Endoscopic Removal of Foreign Bodies,
5. Endoscopic Dilation of Strictures Both Benign and Malignant Type,
6. Therapeutic ERCP For Removal of Common Bile Duct Stones
7. Placement of Stent in Bile and Pancreatic Duct in Cancer Patients.
8. Pneumatic balloon dilatation of Achalasia Cardia
9. Argon Plasma Coagulation
10. Percutaneous endoscopic gastrostomy (PEG)

Surgical Gastroenterology:

Surgical technology has been refined and treatment of benign and cancerous diseases of the digestive tract has evolved alongside it as a super speciality. Rapid advances in the field of surgery namely "Minimal access surgery" or "Keyhole surgery" and organ transplantation are very closely associated with abdominal surgery further widening the horizons of Surgical Gastroenterology.

Following surgeries are performed by this department in this hospital.

The Surgeries performed routinely are:

1. Oesophagus:
   a. Cancer Oesophagus - Esophagectomy
   b. Management of Corrosive Strictures
   c. Lap management of Achalasia Cardia
   d. Lap management of GERD
2. Stomach:
   a. Malignancy-D2 Gastrectomy
   b. Surgery for GIST
   c. Bariatric Surgery
3. Small Bowel:
   a. Lap and Open Enteric Surgeries
4. Large Bowel:
   a. Surgery for Malignancy-Anterior Resection (Lap/Open)
   b. Surgery for Inflammatory Bowel disease (Open/Lap)
   c. Surgery for Familial Polyposis
5. Perianal Surgery:
   a. VAFT for recurrent Fistula In Ano,
   b. Complex Pilonidal Sinus.

6. Liver:
   a. Hepatic Resection
   b. Lap Hydatid Surgery
   c. Liver Trauma
   d. TACE/RFA for HCC
   e. Liver Transplant
7. Biliary System:
   a. Bile duct Strictures
   b. Hilar Cholangio Carcinoma
   c. Stone disease
8. Pancreas:
   a. Management of Acute Pancreas
   b. Pancreatic Necrosectomy
   c. Whipple's Surgery (pancreaticoduodenectomy)
   d. Distal Pancreatectomy (Open/Lap)
9. Lap Splenectomy
10. Surgery for Portal HT: Shunt Surgery/Devascularization

SPECIALITY CLINICS:

1. Liver clinic
2. Hernia Clinic

OPD Services:

OPD functions as per OPD schedule of the hospital.

The procedure is same as that of any other specialist's OPD

STAFFING/MANPOWER:

The team of specialist in this hospital is highly experienced and trained in the field of Gastroenterology.

They offer best services by using state of art equipment available in this hospital.

DUTIES & RESPONSIBILITIES:

A. Gastroenterologist:

Gastroenterologists are the one type of physician specialized in the field of the digestive tract.

Duties are of a similar nature as that of any specialist.

1. The doctor should be well experienced in performing various endoscopic procedures on patients such as colonoscopies, and endoscopies.
2. To consult with patients and examine them to understand their health concerns.
3. They must develop and implement a comprehensive treatment plan, which may include surgery or other interventions such as chemotherapy, radiation therapy, or palliative care.

4. Medical Gastroenterologists must be expert in his field as patients come to them for proper diagnosis and relief from the problems that are plaguing their health.
5. They may perform tests or may prescribe medication, as the treatment plan for each patient is as unique as each condition
6. A Surgical Gastroenterologist should carry out surgical interventions to manage acute and chronic conditions, as well as providing comprehensive care before and after surgery.
7. A Surgical Gastroenterologist must perform necessary surgeries that are required to fix any problems within this area of the body.
8. They may work closely with other healthcare professionals, such as anaesthesiologists, radiologists, and medical gastroenterologists to ensure coordinated care.

B. Endoscopy Technician:

1. Will perform his/her duties under the supervision of a Gastroenterologist.
2. Will attend all phone calls and will schedule appointments.
3. Will assist clinicians during an endoscopy procedure.
4. Will ensure cleanliness of the department.
5. Will check all instruments for proper functioning before start of the procedure.
6. To check for any leakage with the help of testing instruments.
7. Will prepare the endoscopy trolley and crash cart.
8. Will ensure that all used supplies are replenished in the crash cart.
9. Will position the patient on the table.
10. Will ensure patient's dignity and privacy.
11. Will carry out the checklist (identification of the patient and the procedure) before start of the procedure.
12. Will receive pathological specimens (body fluids and biopsy specimens) from the clinician and process it to send to laboratory for examination.
13. Will monitor vital parameters of the patient before, during and after the procedure.
14. Will be responsible for maintenance of various endoscopes available in the department.
15. Will also be responsible for rental instruments; their receipt and proper return.
16. Will clean, disinfect and store the scopes and other instruments.
17. Will indent and receive supplies required for endoscopy procedures.
18. Will adhere to the infection control measures like hand wash etc. Will take standard precautions which include use of personal protective equipment (PPE) such as eye shield, face mask, gloves etc, while cleaning the scope and dealing with potentially infectious materials.
19. Will be responsible for safe upkeep of all instruments.
20. Will ensure safe disposal of biomedical and other waste as per norms.
21. Will maintain confidentiality of all information gathered during the course of treatment.
22. Will ensure recording of the procedure details by the clinician.
23. Will update all registers and records of the department as per hospital policies.
24. Will carry out other assignments allocated by seniors.

FEW CONDITIONS WHEN ENDOSCOPY IS RECOMMENDED:

1. Inflammatory bowel diseases (IBD), such as ulcerative colitis (UC) and Crohn's disease
2. Stomach ulcer
3. Chronic constipation

4. Pancreatitis
5. Gallstones
6. Unexplained bleeding in the digestive tract
7. Tumours
8. Infections
9. Blockage of the oesophagus
10. Gastroesophageal reflux disease (GERD)
11. Hiatus hernia
12. Unusual vaginal bleeding
13. Blood in your urine
14. Other digestive tract issues

Endoscopy is Used to:

1. Determine the cause of any abnormal symptoms the patient is having
2. Remove a small sample of tissue, which can then be sent to a lab for further testing; this is called an endoscopic biopsy
3. See inside the body during a surgical procedure, such as repairing a stomach ulcer, or removing gallstones or tumours.

RISKS OF AN ENDOSCOPY:

Though there are no major risks to an endoscopy procedure, still it may cause following signs and symptoms in few individuals:

1. Chest Pain
2. Damage To organs, including Possible Perforation (
3. Fever
4. Persistent Pain in the area of the Endoscopy
5. Vomiting & Difficulty in Swallowing after Upper GI Endoscopy
6. Redness and Swelling at the Incision Site
7. Dark coloured stools after Colonoscopy
8. After Capsule Endoscopy, there is a small risk that the capsule can get stuck somewhere in the digestive tract. The capsule may then need to be surgically removed.

AUDIT

Every week the departmental performance is evaluated in a comprehensive audit meeting, which is documented as an annual audit.

The elective and emergency operations performed in the previous week are discussed in this meeting.

This audit is undertaken to improve the care of patients and to consider whether current management policies need to be changed.

CHECK LISTS FOR ENDOSCOPIC SERVICES:

A. Checklist Endoscopic Suite:

SN	Check	Yes	No	Remark
1	The department has following sections; • Patient hold and examination room. • Endoscopy room. • Toilet facility. (Required when colonoscopy is done) • It will be further better if one recovery cum post endoscopic observation room is provided for at least 2 patients (2 beds). • Wait area for relatives. • Longue for staff.			
2	Common or dedicated support facilities are available? • Clean & Dirty utility rooms • Change rooms • Stores • Nurse station/Reception • Administrative area			
3	The main endoscopy room is about 200 square feet in size. One table (procedure area) is allocated about 150 to 200 sq. ft.?			
4	Each endoscopic table is having adequate patient's privacy provisions? (Curtain partition, if there are more than 1 table)			
5	Wheel chair can be wheeled up to the endoscopic table?			
6	Ceiling height is not less than 7'-10"? (2388 mm)			
7	It is recommended to have a toilet attached with colonoscopy procedure room.			
8	The endoscopic suite has 6 air changes per hour? The attached toilet will be having at least 10 air changes per hour.			
9	Space provided around the table is about 3 feet on each side?			
10	Hand washing facilities are available?			
11	Minimum 10 eclectic sockets of 16 amp are provided?			
12	Firefighting arrangements are as per local law?			
13	Biomedical waste is disposed as per law?			
14	Central medical gases have been provided?			

B. Checklist Endoscopic Procedure – 1:

1. Endoscope along with 'light source' and 'carbon-di-oxide insufflator is available?
2. Hand instruments are available and are disinfected/sterilized?
3. IV fluids are available?
4. All required drugs and consumables are in place?
5. Patient has identified himself/herself?
6. Patient has confirmed the name of the procedure & procedure site?
7. Informed consent is on record?

8. If anaesthesia is to be given, "Pre-anaesthesia Checklist" completed as per safe surgery checklist?
9. All team members know each other by name?
10. If there is specific concern, it has been discussed?
11. All patient monitoring equipment are functional?
12. After procedure;
    a. Specimen - if taken - is correctly labelled and sent to lab?
    b. Procedure details have been documented?
    c. Post procedure medical care instructions given to recovery nurse?

C. Checklist Endoscopic Procedure – 2: Based on WHO safe surgery checklist

1. **Sign In (Patient is wheeled in)**
    a. Patient has verbally confirmed his/her name.
    b. Patient has verbally confirmed name of the procedure and site of procedure.
    c. Patient has given written consent?
    d. Patient has been asked about any known allergy.
    e. Anaesthesia safety check done, if anaesthesia is required.
    f. Intubation articles are available.
    g. Patient vitals are being monitored.
2. **Time Out (Before insertion of the scope)**
    a. All team members know each other by name.
    b. All team members once again confirm the procedure.
    c. Required investigation results are displayed.
    d. Concern, if any, is discussed.
    e. Required drugs and consumables (Endoclips etc.) are available.
3. **Sign Out (Before patient leaves the procedure table)**
    a. Procedure details are recorded. (Medical records completed)
    b. Specimen, if any, is correctly labelled and sent to lab for examination.
    c. Post procedure concern, if any, is reviewed with recovery nurse.
    d. Post procedure medication has been discussed with the patient. (If the patient is conscious otherwise discuss with the recovery nurse)

D. Audit Checklist for Endoscopy:

	Audit Checklist for Endoscopy		
Location: ______________ Date: ______________			
SN	**Audit Point**	**Yes**	**No**
1	Is the sedation policy documented and implemented by the staff?		
2	Check who gives sedation and who monitors patient. Is the person administering and monitoring sedation different from the person performing the procedure?		
3	Is the patient monitored after sedation and whether the same is documented?		
4	Are the equipment and manpower available to manage patients who have gone into a deeper level of sedation than initially intended?		
5	Is the informed consent for administration of moderate sedation is obtained?		

	Audit Checklist for Endoscopy		
Location: ______________________ Date: ______________			
SN	**Audit Point**	**Yes**	**No**
6	Does the Informed consent include information regarding the procedure, risks, benefits, alternatives and as to who will perform the requisite procedure in a language that patient can understand?		
7	Are emergency medications available all the time and replenished in a timely manner when used?		
8	Does the organization adhere to cleaning, disinfection and sterilization practices?		
9	Is the Sterilized sets expiry dates and storage conditions monitored?		
10	Are the Sterilization/disinfection activities being performed as per the guidelines?		
11	Is the adequate hand washing facilities and disinfectants solutions available?		
12	Is the instruction for proper hand washing displayed and followed by the staff?		
13	Are the adequate PPE like gloves, masks available and used by the staff?		
14	Are all the equipment periodically inspected and calibrated?		
15	Are the equipment inventoried and proper logs maintained as required?		
16	Is the preventive maintenance done for the equipment?		
17	Service labels on Equipment and calibration records present?		
18	Storage of oxygen cylinders proper?		
19	Condition of Humidifiers?		
20	Is the documented policy for CPR available?		
21	Is the staff trained in BLS/ALS?		
22	Are the events during CPR recorded?		
23	Is a post-event analysis of all CPR done by a multidisciplinary committee and whether the same is been documented?		
24	Are the medication orders written in a uniform location and are clear, legible, dated, timed, named and signed?		
25	Does the documented policy and procedure on verbal orders present and implemented?		
26	Is a written order for high-risk medication done?		
27	Do the policies and procedures guide the monitoring of patients after medication administration?		
28	Is the medication administration documented?		
29	Staff interview on the methodology of administration - (whether patient, medication, dosage, route and timing verified prior to its administration)		
30	Is the patient monitored after medication administration?		
31	Knowledge to pick adverse drug events and reporting of the same?		
32	Is the Segregation of bio-medical waste done as per the guidelines?		
33	Is the instruction for the management of biomedical waste displayed?		
34	Patient interview		
35	Staff interview		
	Signature of Auditor:		

KEY PERFORMANCE INDICATORS (KPI):

1. Percentage of medication Errors
2. Percentage of Adverse drug Reaction
3. Percentage of medication Charts with error prone abbreviations
4. Percentage of UGI endoscopies performed within 24 hours of admission.

   Formula: Total number of UGI Endoscopy performed in cases who presented without complications within 24 hours of admission during one month divided by total number of UGI endoscopies performed without complications during that month multiplied by 100.
5. Percentage of patients with adverse reaction/complications after UGI Endoscopy.
6. Incidences of complications after gastrointestinal surgery.

DATA COLLECTION REGISTERS:

Indicator: % of medication Errors, % of admissions with Adverse drug Reaction, % of medication Charts with error prone abbreviations:

SN	Date	Patient Name	UHID No.	Diagnosis	Department Name	Medication Errors	Dispensing Errors	Dispensing Errors	Prescription Errors	Adverse drug reaction	Reason for adverse drug reaction	Medication chart with error prone abbreviations	Signature

STATIONARY FORMATS:

1. Colonoscopy Report Format:

Hospital Letterhead

COLONOSCOPY REPORT

Patient Name: .... Age/Sex: ....

Referred by: .... OPD/IPD No.: ....

Provisional Diagnosis: .... Date: ....

Procedure performed under: .... (I.V. Midazolam injection)

External Examination: ....

(Example: No fissure/fistula/haemorrhoids present)

Rectum: ....

(Example: Normal Mucosa/No hyperaemia/ulceration/growth seen)

Sigmoid Colon: ....

(Example: Normal Mucosa/No diverticula/polyp/growth seen/No hyperaemia/ulceration present)

Descending Colon: ....

(Example: Normal Mucosa/No hyperaemia/ulceration/growth seen/No diverticula/polyp present/ Splenic flexure normal)

Transverse Colon: ....

(Example: Normal Mucosa/No hyperaemia/ulceration/growth seen/No diverticula/growth/polyp present)

Ascending Colon: ....

(Example: Mucosa covered with liquid faecal matter/whatever Mucosa seen was normal/No growth seen/ Hepatic flexure normal)

Caecum: ....

(Example: Normal Mucosa/No hyperaemia/ulceration/growth seen)

IMPRESSION: ....

(Example: Normal study till Caecum)

Biopsy: Taken/not taken

Dr._______________

(Consultant Gastroenterologist)

2. UGI (Upper GI) ENDOSCOPY REPORT:

Hospital Letterhead

Upper GI Endoscopy Report

Patient Name: .... Age/Sex: ....

Referred by: .... OPD/IPD No.: ....

Provisional Diagnosis: .... Date: ....

Procedure performed under: .... (2 % local xylocaine anaesthesia with Olympus GIF E II Endoscope)

Oesophagus: ....

(Example: Mucosa is normal/No evidence of growth, web or diverticula/Oesophageal motility is normal/No food residue seen/Gastroesophageal junction present at ... cm from incisors and is normal/No hiatus hernia/esophagitis present)

Stomach:

Fundus: ....

(Example: Lot of food residue seen/however whatever Mucosa seen is normal/No hyperaemia/ ulceration/growth seen)

Body: ....

(Example: Normal Mucosa/no hyperaemia/ulcer seen)

Antrum: ....

(Example: Mild hyperaemia present/No ulcer/haemorrhage seen/Pylorus and incisura are normal)

Duodenum: ....

D 1: Mucosa normal. No ulcer/erosions/haemorrhage seen

D 2: Normal duodenal folds

Impression: ....

(Example: Mild antral gastritis)

Biopsy: Taken/not taken

Dr.________________

(Consultant Gastroenterologist)

BIBLIOGRAPHY, REFERENCES & ACKNOWLEDGMENTS:

1. "Standard Operating Procedures SOP For Hospitals 2nd Edition" by Dr. Arun K. Agarwal
2. "Duties & Responsibilities of Hospital Staff" by Dr. Arun Kumar
3. "Checklists for Hospitals" by Dr. Arun K. Agarwal
4. Batra Hospital, New Delhi
5. Seth GS Medical College and KEM Hospital, Mumbai, India
6. Dr. D. Y. Patil Medical College, Hospital & Research Centre, Pune, India.
7. Sir Ganga Ram Hospital, New Delhi, India

Chapter – 14

DEPARTMENT OF MATERIALS MANAGEMENT (STORE)

INDEX

1. Introduction
2. Definition
3. Planning
4. Objectives
5. Importance
6. Functions & Responsibilities
7. Process Flow
8. Staffing/Manpower
9. Organogram
10. Duties & Responsibilities
    a. Marketing Manager
    b. Procurement Manager/Purchase Manager/Materials Manager
    c. Store Supervisor
    d. Store Keeper
    e. Linen Keeper
11. Purchase Department
    a. Objectives
    b. Functions
    c. Purchasing Ethics
12. Standard Operating Procedures
    a. Purchase Procedure
        i. Guidelines for Purchase
        ii. Monthly MIS from Purchase Section
    b. Procedure in Store
    c. Linen Procedure
    d. Issue of Gate Pass
    e. Condemnation of Stores
        i. Condemnation Committee
    f. Disposal of Scrap
    g. Pest Control
        i. Minimum Requirement for Pest and Animal Control
        ii. Pest Control Plan
        iii. Measures for Mosquito Free Environment

13. Issue of Material on Loan
    a. For Departments
    b. For Staff
14. Key Performance Indicators
15. Data Collection Format for Analysing KPI
16. Check Lists
    a. Checklist Hospital Stores Planning
    b. Checklist Store Management (Materials Management)
    c. Checklist Material Purchase
    d. Checklist Material Receipt
    e. Checklist Purchase Department
    f. Checklist equipment Acceptance Report
17. Stationary Formats
    a. Demand Book
    b. Bin Card
    c. Material Receipt Report/Master Register (MRR)
    d. Material Inward Report (Daily)
    e. Stock Register
    f. Purchase Order (Sample)
    g. Gate Pass – Non-Returnable
    h. Gate Pass Returnable
    i. Equipment Log Card
    j. Material Issue Register
    k. Dhobi Book/Laundry Register:
18. Bibliography, References & Acknowledgments

INTRODUCTION:

Materials management is a process of management which co-ordinates, supervises and executes the tasks associated with the flow of materials to, through and out of the hospital in an integrated fashion. The Materials Department is a centralized procurement unit which procures, receives, stocks and distributes the material to the user department as per their need in a scientific and systematic way. This includes large equipment to small consumables **other than** drugs and medicines needed for the institution.

The usual practice of storing large quantities of commodities and supplies in every service area is a wrong trend. This compromises the space needed for the delivery of clinical services and maintaining infection prevention protocols in various service areas.

Store is the main department, which fulfils all the requirements of this hospital, necessities pertaining to maintain the various goods (Equipment, Durables, Consumables, etc.) for hospital of each department. Departments like Dialysis, Cath Lab, General OT, Cardiac OT, Maintenance etc. place their particular demand/order by writing in the 'Indent Book' and after appropriate approvals their demand of goods/material is fulfilled.

All stationary items i.e., receipts, different types of Vouchers, Registers, Copies, Envelopes of all kinds etc. are checked and verified by the Store In-charge and distributed accordingly.

All electric material like switches, plugs, bulbs & tubes checked & issued by Store for the maintenance department of this Hospital.

DEFINITION:

Materials management includes all activities of material from stage of forecasting requirements to procurement, storage, distribution, utilization to final disposal. Materials Management, to be effective and efficient, should aim to optimise utility of available resources.

PLANNING:

General Stores should have vehicular accessibility and ventilation, security and firefighting arrangements. Hospital shall have standard operating procedure for local purchase, indent management, storage preparation of monthly requirement plan and Inventory analysis.

The hospital should have adequate and spacious stores located away from patient traffic with facilities for storing drugs, consumables, linen, furniture, equipment, and sundry articles. Based on the nature and number of items, the main store may be divided into sub-stores such as medical and drug stores, surgical stores, furniture, and equipment, general, linen, and stationery stores.

Stores should be designed in such a way that spoilage, damage and other losses are minimised. Compactor system as compared to conventional racks may be used. Buffer stocks should be kept in separate spaces or cupboards in the drug store and basic principles like 'first expiry, first out' for drugs and vaccines should be followed. Stored materials should be periodically inspected, to prevent moisture, termite, and insects passing up the material, should be 45 cm high for outside stacks built on the ground, and 30 cm high for stacks on floors. Depending on the volume of items requiring temperature control during storage, an adequate number of refrigerators/walk-in coolers should be available. A separate inspection and stock holding section/area should be provisioned for so that there is no chance of mixing old and new stocks.

The department consists of three units:

1. Purchase,
2. Receiving Section (it is store at many hospitals)
3. and Store

OBJECTIVES:

Stores will stock all consumables/supplies material which are frequently and commonly used by various users.

1. To procure material at the lowest possible price without compromising on quality and ensuring continuity of supply.
2. To receive, inspect, document and deliver the ordered material to the user departments in time.
3. To stock optimum inventory to meet the needs of users ensuring uninterrupted supply of materials.

IMPORTANCE:

1. **Criticality:** In hospital environment, with respect to the criticality of the procedures undertaken, dependency on material (medicines & consumables) becomes greatly highlighted
2. **Expense:** Material management is capital intensive. Materials on an average amount to almost 30 to 40% of hospital's financial expenditure; containment of material cost therefore has a tremendous potential in making the hospital cost bearable to patients
3. **Revenue:** Pharmacy (retail & store) features as one of the top most revenue spinners for a hospital

FUNCTIONS & RESPONSIBILITIES:

Main functions are;

1. Receipts of goods from any source.
2. Inspection of goods.
3. Identification and storage of goods as long as they are not required for use.
4. Maintain record of all goods.
5. Distributing/issuing goods to needy section of the hospital.

Responsibilities of this department are;

1. Planning of material
2. Estimation the correct demand
3. Inviting offers
4. Finalising order after proper negotiations that is 'Purchasing'
5. Inventory management
6. Safe Keeping (Storing)
7. Quality control
8. Dispatching

Thus, it is a custodian of hospital goods which are in transit. They are responsible for safe custody and preservation of goods received.

The hospital should have separate Stores and Purchase Sections under this department, each one headed by separate officers.

Store & Purchase both combined is known as "Materials Management"

PROCESS FLOW:

1. Indent Placed from the user department
2. Indent is approved by administration (MS)
3. Checked in store for availability
4. If available the item is issued
5. If not available, a note is sent to the MS who approves it for purchase
6. Purchase following all the protocols places order
7. Material is received in the stores.
8. It is checked with the purchase order for correct quantity and specifications.
9. The representative of the user department is called to inspect and approve the item.
10. After approval; is given, it is entered in the computer (register), and GRN is generated and kept in the store for onward issue.

STAFFING/MANPOWER:

1. Procurement/Purchase Manager
2. Manager/Supervisor Store
3. Storekeeper
4. Linen Keeper
5. GDA (Helper)
6. Housekeeper

STORE ORGANISATION CHART (Organogram):

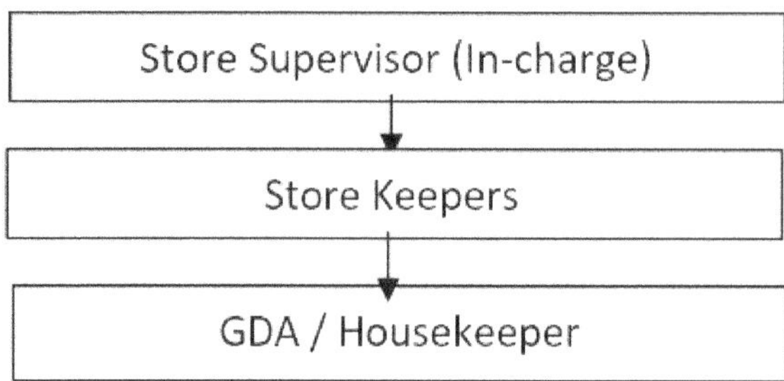

Duties & RESPONSIBILITIES:

A. Marketing Manager:

Main aim of the marketing executive is to make the public aware of the available hospital services and thus increase the demand of hospital services in the community and thus increase the profitability.

1. To develop, plan, implement and coordinate marketing plans and campaigns.
2. To carry on market survey and gather data to find out potential market which will help them in developing marketing strategies.
3. To find out the demand of the services provided by the hospital and its available competitors.
4. To regularly monitor activities of nearby hospitals and modify their plans accordingly.
5. To finalise the area where they want to do vigorous marketing.
6. They should have complete knowledge of services provided by the hospital and should know the applicable charges.
7. They are also responsible for developing and maintaining web site of the hospital and for using other social sites to the hospital's benefit.
8. They organise onsite and offsite camps and other events (CME, Talks etc).
9. To design/help in designing promotional materials such as posters and handbills.
10. They should be able to build and work in a team and should develop a network of contacts in the area of their work.
11. To regularly communicate with the audience of their area.
12. Should be able to work alone in an individual capacity also.
13. To guide in determining the rate list of the services offered by the hospital.
14. To guide the hospital in ways of improving its services depending on their market survey.
15. They are responsible for communicating people outside the hospital and presenting a positive picture of the hospital.
16. They shall be analysing about the results obtained by their marketing efforts.
17. They should be monitoring and controlling expenses of this department that is management of financial resources.
18. To prepare a good database of all corporate and companies in the catchment area.
19. To find out new catchment areas.
20. To help in empanelment of the hospital with various TPAs (Medical Insurance Providers).
21. To tie ups with companies and offer them various plans suitable to both parties.
22. To explore and collaborate with various practicing doctors to develop referrals from their clinics to hospital for specialised treatment and or tests.
23. They should have good rapport with all the people involved in generating business for the hospital.

BIBLIOGRAPHY/REFERENCES/FUTURE READING:

https://job-descriptions.careerplanner.com/Marketing-Managers.cfm (Retrieved 16 May 2018)

B. Procurement/Purchase Manager/Materials Manager:

He/she will supervise the day-to-day management of the Stores. He/she will be responsible for the stores of the hospital and will arrange for their safe custody and also for the maintenance of accounts, inventories and correct returns in respect of the same, in the manner laid down by hospital. He/she will conduct physical verification of the Stock during routine/random surprise checking. Any discrepancy, fraud or negligence, that may be detected, should be duly recorded and steps should be taken for their rectification. Any Such case(s) having serious magnitude should immediately be reported to the MS forthwith along with action taken report.

1. To be punctual on duty.
2. To organise and manage manpower of purchase department.
3. To recruit, train, motivate and evaluate performance of junior staff.
4. To develop and implement purchasing strategy, **S**tandard **O**perating **P**rocedures.
5. Will handle all equipment, consumables and other supplies required for efficient functioning of the hospital. It includes procurement, receipt, storage, accounting and distribution of supplies.
6. Will be carrying out all administrative work related to above duties.
7. Will plan and oversee all materials movement from and in the hospital.
8. Will work in cooperation with storekeeper.
9. Will coordinate with doctors and other departmental heads to acquire best and cost-effective product.
10. Will identify and receive the demand from hospital departments and stores.
11. Will coordinate with indenter to understand correct specifications and quantity of the material sought.
12. Will raise inquiry, prepare a techno-commercial comparison of offers received, recommend their vendors to the purchasing committee after proper negotiations.
13. Will be an active member of Purchase Committee.
14. Will be responsible for buying a best item at lowest price.
15. Will draft and issue purchase orders.
16. Will ensure that material received is of correct specifications and quantity.
17. Will ensure timely receipt of required items.
18. To receive bills against purchase orders issued and send them to accounts department after verification by;
    a. Purchase Manager (himself).
    b. Store in charge.
    c. Ordering Department
19. Will ensure adequate availability of supplies in the hospital.
20. Will verify bills before sending them to accounts for payment.
21. Will be responsible for proper bookkeeping, which is maintenance of all records and registers as per hospital policies.
22. Will maintain a database of prospective vendors.
23. Will follow prescribed procedures.
24. Will suggest improvements in the existing purchase policies.
25. Will execute other orders given by seniors.

Summary:

Will be responsible to procure

1. The right quality & quantity.
2. At the right time
3. At the right place
4. At the right cost.

C. Store Supervisor:

Store Supervisor maintain bills, stock of all goods, indent of different departments, entry of stock by bill & by indent is all done by Store Supervisor. Checking of stock & stock register of different departments is done by him.

1. He is responsible to Hospital Administrator for receipt and issue of material.
2. He should be a computer literate and will have to handle all correspondence related to stores and will be making computer entries.
3. He will be responsible for overall maintenance of stores for hospital to have availability of necessary supplies.
4. They will work in close coordination of hospital administration.
5. He will supervise and coordinate all activities of the store.
6. To allocate duties, evaluate work performance & efficiency of staff under him.
7. He will be responsible for the training and efficiency of staff placed under him and will participate in training programs.
8. To ensure proper and updated record keeping.
9. He will assign work to all staff placed under his subordination.
10. He will supervise all purchases in the absence of a full-time purchase manager.
11. He will be cooperating/dealing with periodical audit of the store. He will have to answer all queries/observations raised by such audit team.
12. He will help in developing and implementing standard operating procedures.
13. He will be responsible for financial management of the store.
14. To organise training programs for the store staff.
15. To help in recruitment of staff required in this department.
16. He will be responsible for good housekeeping of the area.
17. He will be responsible for all losses, pilferages and breakages.
18. Will be responsible for strict implementation of security and fire orders of the hospital.
19. He should be handling unusual circumstances and will be solving problems in store management.
20. He will carry out duties of a store keeper whenever required.
21. Will be attending meetings with vendors and suppliers.
22. To perform other related work as assigned.

D. Store Keepers:

1. He is responsible to Hospital Administrator for receipt and issue of material.
2. He will be responsible and in charge of proper provisioning, ordering, receiving, inspecting, returning, packing, labelling, storage, issue, accounting, safety, condemnation, repair and replacement of expandable and non-expandable stores.

3. Will receive all purchased goods, inspect them/get it checked by user department, will make entry in the bill of receipt of correct quantity and quality of goods. Such bills will be sent to accounts department via Hospital Administrator for payment.
4. Will unload/help in unloading materials from transport vehicles by hand or with hand operated or motorised equipment.
5. Short supply should be mentioned on the copy of 'challan'/bill given to the vendor and one that is sent to accounts. If there is any deviation in the quality, material may be out-rightly rejected.
6. Vendors should be given receipt of goods with the comment 'Received but not Checked', if so.
7. Report of all pending bills will be prepared every week and will be sent to Hospital Administrator for his follow up action. It happens when the material is received on 'challan' and bill is not sent along with the material.
8. He should know how much inventory is in store and what are required to be replenished on the basis of consumption.
9. He will be responsible for safe keeping of stores and its quality & quantity.
10. He will be responsible for issue of correct quantity against authorised requisition slips (indents).
11. He will be responsible for correct accounting of all stores under his charge.
12. He will be responsible for compliance of security and fire orders in his department.
13. He will coordinate with minor repairs.
14. He will report any untoward incident to the administrator immediately verbally and in writing.
15. He will be responsible for physical verification of stock every 3 months.
16. Correct and up-to-date inventory has to be maintained.
17. Inventory of fixed assets is to be maintained by him. Fixed assets are also to be physically verified every three months.
18. He will maintain all registers and records as per hospital policy.
19. He will be responsible for replenishment of stocks and condemnation and disposal of damaged, outdated stock.
20. He will also be responsible for sale of scrap material (empty cartoons, plastic bottles etc) accumulated in the store or anywhere in the hospital.
21. He will maintain and update database of vendors of various services and will maintain good public relations with them.
22. He will handle all correspondence related to this department.
23. He may be asked to participate in selection, training and supervision of his subordinates.
24. He will not allow any unauthorised entry in the department.
25. He will be responsible for other correlated duties.
26. To carry out any other duties as per his skills assigned by his seniors.

E. Linen Keepers:

Just like a store keeper, a linen keeper in employed if there is separate store for hospital linen.

He is responsible for indenting, purchasing, storing, distributing and condemning the linen and uniform in the hospital.

1. To keep record of all hospital linen and its distribution.
2. To ensure sufficient stock of all types of linen as per 3/5 linen per bed policy.
3. To ensure that all linen material bears hospital identification mark.
4. To put an issue date in the corner of the linen with non-washable ink, whenever new articles are issued to user department. This helps in finding out the age of that article.

5. To receive soiled linen from user departments.
6. As per hospital SOP, linen keeper will exchange all linen brought from user department immediately. If this is the policy a proper inventory has to be maintained by the linen-keeper.
7. To confirm that linen such received conforms to the issue details.
8. To check for any damaged item.
9. To send repairable items for repair to tailor. To discard un-repairable items.
10. To negotiate, fix and keep record of tailoring rates of various items. Revision in charges should be done only after proper approvals.
11. To sort linen items according to 'how they will be washed'.
12. To arrange for supply of clean & washed linen to user department as per policy of the hospital.
13. To arrange for washing of soiled linen so that the user departments do not suffer.
14. To negotiate and fix washing charges, if the laundry is outsourced.
15. To record all linen transactions with the laundry in the *'DHOBI BOOK'*/Laundry book
16. Will be responsible for exchanging of soiled hospital curtains of various departments and sending them for washing.
17. Will be responsible for exchanging and washing of staff uniform as per hospital policy.
18. To have record of linen given and received from the laundry.
19. To check washed stock for any damage done during washing or not washed properly.
20. To return the clothes not washed up to the mark for rewashing free of cost.
21. To have record of received and issued linen to user department.
22. To have some control over in-house laundry or on outsourced vendor.
23. To have correct inventory of issued linen to different departments.
24. To mark all linen with hospital name by a non-washable ink so that it does not mix up with private linen.
25. To physically check the inventory of all user departments once in 3 months.
26. To physically verify his own stock every 3 months.
27. To ensure that no unauthorised person enters the store.
28. To arrange for condemnation of damaged linen.
29. To issue condemned linen to housekeeping staff for cleaning/dusting purposes.
30. Will place indent to higher authorities for replacement of torn and unserviceable linen periodically.
31. To develop and implement Standard Procedures (SOPs) for this department.
32. To maintain and update all records, registers and ledgers as per hospital policy.
33. To segregate and arrange clean linen from soiled articles so as to minimise chances of infection.
34. To carry out any other work assigned by seniors.

Summary:

He receives, segregates, counts, records, stores, get it washed and issues linen and uniforms in the hospital.

PURCHASE DEPARTMENT:

Objectives:

1. To ensure efficiency, economy and transparency.
2. To ensure uninterrupted/timely flow of materials, equipment & services of goods of required quality to meet and support hospital services.
3. To buy competitively and wisely authorized supplies to desired specifications from approved/ reliable sources at the available reasonable prices within the time schedule.

4. To ensure that fair open and uniform purchase practices are followed to develop healthy and long-term relationship with suppliers.
5. To ensure timely formulation and commitment of purchase budget.
6. To ensure that investment made on inventory is at an optimum level and continuously strive for reduction in material costs, Capital costs and Overhead expenses.
7. Develop sources of supply to maintain competition and sustained supplies.
8. To keep management appraised of the likely shortfalls in purchase performance by introducing appropriate reporting systems with a view to seek management's intervention in time.

Functions:

1. Creation of a comprehensive and regularly updated directory of selected reliable vendors.
2. Maintenance of vendor evaluation and rating records.
3. Carry out Market surveys with a view to establishing/developing new reliable and better sources of supply and keep updated with information on latest developments.
4. Arranging negotiations with Vendors, when necessary.
5. Issue of Purchase Orders in time.
6. Follow-up of Purchase Orders till the arrival of materials and acceptance by the hospital.
7. Maintaining a library of product catalogues and manufacturers/Distributor's price lists
8. etc.
9. Maintaining up to date information regarding sales tax, excise and custom duty-rates etc.
10. Ensure timely payments to suppliers.

Purchasing Ethics

1. Honesty:
   Be straight forward in all dealing.
2. Integrity:
   Behave like a professional. Conduct business openly and fairly.
3. Flexibility:
   Be flexible in discussions.
4. Knowledge:
   Be ready to learn. Don't think that you know everything.
5. Views:
   Listen to other person's views. Respect his/her differences with that of yours.
6. Rules & Regulations:
   Always adhere to prevailing rules of the country, city and your hospital. Be aware of legal trade practices.
7. Relationship:
   Try to maintain a balanced relationship with the vendor. Business is finalized when it is win-win situation for all. Promote positive vendor client relationship.
8. Competition:
   Encourage competition among vendors.
9. Cost:
   Try to get maximum value of every rupee sent.
10. Refuse all gifts and gratitude from vendors.

STANDARD OPERATING PROCEDURES:

A. Purchase Procedure:

After approval by hospital authorities (MS) for purchase, the demand is sent to the PURCHASER.

He then floats enquiries; identify appropriate suppliers with best price.

Purchase department will co-ordinate with all the user departments and the suppliers with regard to any issues/queries arises on placing orders and complaints during warranty period.

The purchaser will also ensure that payments are settled as per the agreed terms

Guidelines for Purchase:

1. No one is authorised to purchase any item directly without following the prescribed procedure.
2. All the departments will forward their requisition/indent on weekly basis. They will forward their requisition to the STORE MANAGER.
3. Complete details must be furnished in the requisition/indent, giving technical details, description and specifications, if any, in clear handwriting. They will also indicate details of the alternate item, so that in case a particular item is not available in the market, the Purchaser can procure alternate item.
4. The Store Manager, after receipt of indent duly approved by the approving authorities, will check the availability of the item in the stores.
5. If available he will issue the required material to the department.
6. If not available, the same will be documented in the indent and will be sent back to hospital authorities for further action (purchase).
7. As far as possible, the purchases should be made from the manufacturer/authorised dealers directly.
8. Sufficient time should be given to the purchaser to enable him to bargain and purchase the item at concessional rates.
9. No one is authorised to make any changes in the indent once it is approved, without the written approval from MS.
10. No order will be placed on any supplier without indent and sanction by authorities.
11. The purchaser shall place order for store items, based on maximum – minimum levels prescribed and shall ensure that reasonable quantity is always stocked and at the same time shall ensure that no over-stocking is made. For this he will be in constant touch with the Store Manager.
12. The purchaser shall not keep any item pending, especially those which are marked urgent and very urgent. In case the item is not available in the market, he must bring it to the notice of the person who is ordering it. Efforts shall be made to procure from alternate sources.
13. Every effort should be done to avoid as far as possible requisitioning/indenting items on urgent or very urgent basis frequently.
14. The purchaser shall make efforts to purchase items at the lowest possible competitive prices and at the same time ensuring that the quality does not suffer.
15. He should obtain maximum discount, wherever possible.
16. In case the item procured does not tally with the requirement or specifications given, it is responsibility of the purchaser to return the rejected items to the supplier after a proper gate pass is issued by store manager.
17. The purchaser shall obtain minimum three quotations before preparing Purchase Order for comparison of rates. In case order is placed based on one or two quotations, justification for the same shall be given.

18. The purchaser shall settle the rates before purchasing and shall not purchase first and settle rates later, which may result in un-necessary avoidable issues.
19. While making the purchase and before accepting the material, the purchaser shall verify the expiry date & if less than six months, he should not purchase.
20. For any shortage beyond the above permissible limits, the store manager shall be held responsible.
21. All the issues from the stores shall be made on first in, first out basis.
22. Store Keeper will count all the purchased items before taking into stocks. Similarly, all persons who are physically checking the items shall count the items in stock.
23. The item shall not be procured continuously from one source. If such a situation arises, the purchaser shall bring this to the notice of MS for their making enquiries/investigations.
24. The accounts department shall procure price list from various suppliers and keep the same on record for verification by bill passing and checking persons. Whenever any changes are affected, revised price list shall be obtained for record.
25. Items, which are easily available in the market, should not be stored.
26. All purchased items must be received in the Store Department and must not be received directly by the indenting department. Only once entries are made in the stock register after proper checking by the storekeeper, items will be issued.
27. Replacement of a broken/condemned item will be obtained on demand from the main Medical Stores. Such demands will be supported by breakage book, loss statement, and board proceedings duly approved by MS.
28. Regular items should be purchased on returnable basis, if not approved by indenting department/ doctor.
29. One copy of the demand will be retained by the storekeeper and one will always remain in the book. If there is another copy available (3rd copy), it will be given to the person concerned for purchase.
30. Stock will be held in accordance with the authorized scale already prepared. The scale will be reviewed periodically by a committee of specialists and brought up to date. Stocks will be held in the proportion in which they are authorized in these scales. Surplus/deficiency will be supported with documentary authority. The standard store accounting procedure using vouchers, inventories, ledgers, expense books and tally cards will be carried out.
31. Stock verification will be carried out as under;
    a. Annual stock verification – all items.
    b. Quarterly stock verification – Expensive and controlled items as ordered by the MS.
    c. Monthly stock verification – Short life items.
    d. Random verification – any item/s as desired by the MS or his authorized representative.
32. All such verifications will be recorded, signed and dated by the officer carrying out the verification.
33. Lastly check whether 'Performance bank guarantee' is required from the vendor for particular equipment or not.

Monthly MIS from Purchase Section:

1. Total purchases with price of material divided as Capital and Non-capital items
2. List of total stock. (Inventory)
3. Expenditure on items divisible as SI and NSI
4. Expenditure on Scheduled and un-scheduled Purchases
5. Expenditure on Scheduled Purchases divisible as those through Annual Contract, through Standing Order and Consignment based purchase

6. Expenditure on Un-Scheduled Purchase divisible as those made in Cash, Credit, Local Purchase and Repeat PO
7. Expenditure on Import Purchase/Foreign Supplier
8. List of Amended POs with Amendment Reports
9. Income through Sale of Assets (working) and Condemn Capital Items
10. Income through Scrapping of Sundry items and condemn of multiple use items Depending upon the requirements the MIS shall be generated quarterly, bi-annually and annually

B. Procedure In Store:

1. When demand of material arises (non-medical & general items) is given to hospital administrator on Indent-Cum-Order form by store.
2. For departments like General OT, Cardiac OT, Cath Lab, CT, Path Lab the demand is given to Medical Superintendent on Indent-Cum-Order Form.
3. After sanctioning/pass the order, order is placed by the Purchase Officer or Store Supervisor to already approved vendors on official order form (PO).
4. When supply comes, these are checked by Security Supervisor on Main gate and the challan/bill is entered in his inward register.
5. After signing & stamping the Bill/CHALLAN, material & bill is forwarded to store.
6. Quality & quantity of items/packets etc are checked by Store Supervisor along with their expiry dates.
7. After proper checking, supply is put it in/on appropriate place in the store for further issuing.
8. Balance materials of last supply are issued firstly to the departments i.e., on First come Last serve basis.
9. Stock entry is made in stock register & rate of each item is also verified by Store Supervisor. Then stock entry & bill verified & checked by the Hospital Administrator.
10. Issue of stock to different departments by Indent & that Indent Number, date & quantity mentioned in stock register. This register is also checked on daily basis.
11. Maintaining of bills, stocking of all goods, indenting to different departments, entry of stock by bill & by indent is done by Store Supervisor.
12. Checking of stock & stock register is also done by Store Supervisor.
13. Consumable items will be demanded by user department on weekly basis.
14. Non-consumable items will be held on charge by wards/departments on inventories. Changes in the quantities so held and replacement of losses/breakage/condemned items will be countersigned by hospital authorities (MS)
15. Condemnation of any store, because of any reason, will be done only by "Condemnation Committee". MS/MD and administrator will be an integral part of this committee. Reasons for condemning the store should be clearly mentioned.

C. Linen Procedure:

1. There will be a centralised linen store (may be combined with general store) in the hospital and one linen keeper will be in-charge of that.
2. All transactions should be processed through this store & through linen keeper only.
3. The management of Linen department should be efficient and smooth, clean and adequate. This is necessary not only from the point of view of maintenance of hygiene and aseptic conditions in the hospital, but is also required to carry out hospital procedures properly and to ensure patient satisfaction.

4. The line keeper should estimate the requirement of the linen for the entire hospital for bedding, clothing to the patients, operation theatres linen & uniforms to staff members etc. on the basis of certain norms and ratios. In order to ensure sufficient stock and as linen is always subject to considerable wear and tear, the total stock should be calculated on the basis of ration per bed + 30% extra.
5. Linen will be washed by outside contractor on prefixed rates. The rates will be decided on mutual agreement on year-to-year basis.
6. It is proposed that hospital will make its own arrangement for washing of linen in the hospital premises only.
7. The management of linen department should be efficient and smooth, clean and adequate. It is essential from the point of view of maintenance of hygienic and aseptic conditions in the hospital.
8. All the departments using linen and requiring day to day change e.g., O.T., wards etc will collect all their spoiled linen and get it changed from linen room at pre-designated hours only.
9. Linen will be changed immediately and washed linen will be given in place of spoiled linen.
10. Chances of theft are reduced with the central linen service as the wards will not have too much of stock. There should be proper arrangement for preparation, distribution, washing of hospital linen and also for keeping record of receipt, stock and damage.
11. Pest control measures should be carried out in order to avoid linen from getting destroyed by insects & pests.

D. Issue of Gate Pass:

1. All the gate passes will be signed by manger/storekeeper.
2. When the material is cleared under any gate pass, security person will sign on the back with date and time and retain the copy while releasing the goods from gate.
3. All the cleared gate passes will be handed over to the accountant & in respect of materials, which are to be received back gate passes will be handed over after receipt of materials.
4. Whenever materials are received back, the security guard will sign with time and date clearly indicating materials, which are returned.
5. The accountant will check each and every copy of gate pass with bound book and sign the bound book copy for having cleared which will be handed over to MS for further checking.
6. When items are received back after reconditioning or repair, will be received first by the stores, who will issue to the concerned department after checking.
7. All GP's will be serially numbered (punched) on all copies. Besides, all the gate passbooks will be serially numbered category wise.
8. No item shall be allowed without gate pass except minor items. The gate staff (security) must keep a copy of the gate pass against each and every item going out of the gate.
9. All the signing persons should ensure that no gate pass is delayed i.e., they should immediately verify and sign the same so that work does not suffer.
10. Security department will be provided with a list of specimen signatures of concerned persons. All concerned should sign as per specimen given by them. Security staff should ensure that all signatures are genuine and verify when they have any suspicion.
11. If the materials are taken out for repair etc. and brought back and are being sent again because of any reason, in such cases a fresh gate pass will be issued and on the back of the previous gate pass, remark about having received back on "as it is" basis will be given. The same will be attached in the bound book.
12. No one including security persons will issue duplicate gate passes on any ground including that the previous one has been lost or spoiled. Signatures should be done once only and that too after having checked physically in all respects.

13. All concerned will write and sign the gate pass with ink pen or ball point pen and not with pencil.
14. In respect of material issued under non-returnable category, approval should be taken from the hospital authorities (MS)
15. MS will ensure that the gate pass procedure/clearance is followed properly. No backlog/violation. Movement of GP's will be monitored.

E. Condemnation of Stores:

1. Condemnation of equipment, medicines, disposable, records and reusable items.
2. Disposal of non-usable, beyond repair, worn out, expired, obsolete materials of the hospital.

Procedure:

STEP	ACTIVITY	RESPONSIBILITY
1.	Identify the Items.	
2.	Team of condemnation should verify and validate the materials with supporting documents or reports.	Condemnation Committee
3.	To get approval from the higher management	Administrator
4.	Consult with the relevant vendors for collection, dispose and obtain estimate.	Administrator
5.	Meeting held for destruction of materials.	Members of Medical record destruction committee
6.	Final disposal activity to be taken up by supervisor under administrator.	Supervisor & Administrator

Condemnation Committee:

Frequency of meeting:

Once in a month

Constitution:

Chairperson : Medical Supt

Members : ....

Purpose: In order to phase out scrap obsolete and unutilized items, a need is felt to formulate a committee to assess these items and take a decision on the best possible disposing options.

Scope and Functions

1. The user department will initiate the process of condemnation.
2. The items to be condemned will be identified by user department and details filled in the enclosed format.
3. The list will be circulated among the members of the condemnation committee by the last day of the month suggestive of that they can be taken up in the next month's meeting.
4. Meeting of the committee will be convened on the 10th of each month subject to items list received form a user department.
5. Reasons for condemnation are documented.
   a. Beyond Economical repair.
   b. Not repairable.
   c. Item is obsolete and there is no service provider.

F. Disposal of Scrap:

1. All departments wherefrom items would get damaged due to wear and tear or any other reason, shall have them inspected by their department heads and checked by hospital authorities from time to time.
2. After proper checking and declaration by hospital authorities of these items as scrap, these shall be forwarded to stores manager for being stored in the department at a separate place for ultimate disposal.
3. The store manager will receive all such items, have them entered in a separate register and have them stored in the specified place.
4. All disposal items like plastic cans, damaged buckets etc. which have sale, resale value shall be collected once in 3 months and parties called for disposal of these items and after negotiation of prices as per the financial guidelines, shall be disposed of by hospital authorities.
5. The store manager shall send the cloth items like torn bed sheets, curtains etc. to maintenance department to be used for cleaning purposes.
6. Whenever equipment is damaged and are declared unfit, they should also be stored in and once in 6 months, such items shall be disposed of by calling offers and after negotiations.

G. Pest Control:

Pests and animals are attracted to the hospital in search of food, water, shelter and optimal temperatures and pose a number of health threats through spreading of microbial infections and communicable diseases. Therefore, having a pest control plan and an animal and pest free environment is of utmost importance for a hospital.

Minimum Requirement for Pest and Animal Control

To ensure a pest and animal free environment, health facilities can undertake various activities which in general may include proper infrastructure maintenance, provisions of physical barriers, having a pest control plan and engagement of pest control agency. Health facility should ensure that the following requirements are met for pest and animal control:

1. Hospital should engage an external pest control agency for carrying out pest control activities including anti-termite treatment for wooden furniture and fixtures. The records of engaging such agency and pest control activities need to be maintained.
2. Hospital boundary wall should be intact (at least 2.5 metres) and cattle traps installed at all entrances and exits of the hospital to restrict entry of stray animals.
3. The windows and doors should be designed in a way to reduce or prevent entry of flying insects.
4. Hospital staff should follow and comply with best practices of housekeeping, cleaning and disinfection.
5. Staff should follow and comply with the best practices of waste management.
6. Periodic maintenance plan needs to be complied with for maintenance of cracks and holes in infrastructure and for any plumbing faults in utilities and pipes, fixing of clogs, fastening of floor drains.
7. Regular trimming of landscapes, plants, shrubs and trees also to prevent rodents from having easy access to upper levels, windows and the roof.
8. Regularly cleaning of drains and check for any drain clogs.
9. Good storage practices for materials especially food item storage in kitchens and cafeterias.
10. Coordinate with local authorities to prevent accumulation of waste around the premises of the hospital as it leads to pest infestation in and around the premises

Pest Control Plan

Health facility needs to have an effective pest control plan for ensuring a pest and animal free environment in the facility.

1. Pest control plan includes the frequency of carrying out the activities related to the pest control.
2. Besides normal frequency of carrying out these activities, such plan should also include other indications for carrying out the activities of pest control for example on incidence of pest presence (e.g., pest sightings, droppings or pest catches in monitoring traps) and when nonchemical approaches such as vacuuming, trapping and exclusion (i.e., physically blocking pests' entrance) has been unsuccessful or is inappropriate.
3. Pest control plan should also include routine inspection and monitoring for pest presence.
4. Pest control plan should also include storage conditions and methods of different materials especially for food items.
5. Hospitals can use good quality insect repellents. Tightly cover water storage containers (buckets, cisterns, rain barrels). For containers without lids, use fine wire mesh. All the septic tanks should be checked for cracks or gaps and open vent should be covered with fine wire mesh.

Measures for Mosquito Free Environment

As mosquitoes pose a major problem in India, the healthcare establishment should take some extra measures to ensure that it has a mosquito free environment. The health facility should ensure that the hospital environment is clean and all the water tanks and containers are covered.

In addition to these basic measures, the following additional measures need to be taken by the hospital to provide mosquito free environment and for patient safety:

1. Eliminate standing water in and around the hospital.
2. All the containers like coolers, buckets, planters, flower pots, trash containers should be checked for water storage and should be cleaned on weekly basis.
3. Hospitals can use good quality insect repellents.
4. Tightly cover water storage containers (buckets, cisterns, rain barrels).
5. For containers without lids, use fine wire mesh.
6. All the septic tanks should be checked for cracks or gaps and open vent should be covered with fine wire mesh.
7. Hospitals may use screens on windows and doors.
8. Use mosquito nets for patient safety, if the problem is grave.

ISSUE OF MATERIAL ON LOAN:

A. For Departments

1. In certain unforeseeable circumstances material can be lend to some other department (not transferred), so that the same is returned back later
2. In case a particular UD is in dire need of some item that is available in some other UD, the MS can ask the appropriate authority of the later department to transfer the said item to the former; this MIS will be available only through the HIS system. In case the lending department affirms, the borrowing department shall send its representative to fetch the same; stock ledgers will be appropriately updated

B. For staff (also called as Service Loan)

1. For day-to-day use of employees in the hospital (both medical and non-medical) various items are issued which are returnable to the hospital on their leaving the service of the hospital permanently (ex: Issue of stethoscope to doctors); the concerned Stores section should maintain proper records of such material loan issues
2. The store should certify receipt back of the items (in good reusable condition) to the HR Department at the time of cessation of service of the concerned employee (by NOC certification)
3. If items taken on material loan basis are lost/damaged, they may have to be redeemed for by the concerned employees

KEY PERFORMANCE INDICATORS (KPI):

1. Percentage of Items Rejected Before the Preparation Of "Goods Receipt Note" (GRN):
   Formula: (Formula for other QI can be developed in same way)
   Total quantity (Qty.) rejected divided by total quantity ordered then multiplied by 100 (one hundred)
2. Percentage of Stock Outs:
3. Percentage of variation from the prescribed procurement process:
4. Percentage of Local/Emergency Purchase:

DATA COLLECTION FORMATS FOR ANALYSIS:

1. **Percentage of Items Rejected Before the Preparation Of "Goods Receipt Note" (GRN):**

SN	Date	Name of Item	Qty.	Qty. Accepted	Qty. Rejected	Manufacturer/ Vendor Name	Reasons for Rejection	Sign

2. **Percentage of Stock Out:**

SN	Name of Item	Date of Stock Out	Nature of Item		Reasons of Stock out	Sign
			Emergency	General		

3. **Incidence of variation from the prescribed procurement process:**

SN	Date of Procurement	Purchase in which goods are purchased without three quotations	Purchase in which goods are procured without making a Purchase order	Purchase in which goods are procured by Local purchase	Any other variations	Sign

CHECK LISTS:

1. Checklist Hospital Stores Planning:

"To spend money is easy - To spend it well is hard" -Wesley C Michel

SN	Check	Yes	No	Remark
1	Analyse whether you need a 'Centralised' store or 'Decentralised' stores?			
2	Locate it on 'Service Floor' that is away from main hospital activities.			
3	Plan for different rooms for different articles. If one room (hall) create different zones for different articles.			
4	Is area allocated to 'STORE" adequate as per hospital bed strength?			
5	Goods should be stored above floor level, not on the floor. Use racks, pallets etc.			
6	Are firefighting and fire detection facilities adequate and as per regulations?			
7	Is one refrigerator planned for storing perishable items or special items requiring low temperature storage?			
8	Have you planned for some secure lockable area for controlled items?			
9	Do you have a good communication apparatus of this department with other departments of the hospital? (Communication of this department with complete hospital is very important)			
10	Provide adequate lighting and ventilation.			

2. Checklist Store Management (Materials Management):

SN	Check	Yes	No	Remark
1	Are you having documented procedures (SOPs) for various activities?			
2	Are procedures for receiving and checking articles followed?			
3	Area is not cluttered and articles are not clustered?			
4	Stock verification is periodically done?			
5	Are goods arranged in some orderly fashion?			
6	Goods are not stored just on the floor itself?			
7	Are records-maintained show important events? such as • Item name • Date of order • Date of receipt • Vendors details • Value of purchase • Expiry date, if applicable • Inspected by – usually user department (very important column) • Date of issue • Remarks			
8	Is there one master register of all types of receipts? It is called 'Material Receipt Register'			

SN	Check	Yes	No	Remark
9	Do you cross check the received material with the 'purchase order' and 'challan' sent by the vendor along with the supply?			
10	Do you maintain a register of 'discrepancies? Discrepancy = loss, damage, shortage, wrong item supplied.			
11	Do you maintain a 'Goods Return Register'?			
12	All material received from outside go to store before being issued to user/ordering department?			
13	Inventory is kept in different registers as per type of goods?			
14	Are all materials when receipt inspected for quality?			
15	Is any guideline (FIFO, LIFO) followed while issuing articles?			
16	Are 'Bin Cards' used as a tool in store management?			
17	Inflammable items are stored in separate room?			
18	Is pest control proper and adequate? Rats are not seen.			
19	Does some senior person take regular rounds of this department?			
20	Are expired and condemned goods disposed periodically?			
21	Are issues done only on authorised 'Demand Note'?			
22	Any change in consumption should be monitored.			

Note: For a good Store Management practise, answers to all checks should be in 'YES'

3. Checklist Material Purchase:

SN	Check	Yes	No	Remark
1	Justify the need of purchase for that particular item.			
2	Take permission for new purchase from concerned authorities.			
3	Write proper specifications of the items required.			
4	Get the inquiry (specifications) approved in writing by user department.			
5	Invite offers from established vendors.			
6	Prepare a techno-commercial comparison between 3 shortlisted vendors.			
7	Do compare cost of consumables used by that machine during its operation. (Sometimes a cheaper item has costly consumables)			
8	Remain impartial while making a comparison.			
9	Take opinion of existing users. Ask for list of existing installations.			
10	Discuss guarantee and payment terms in detail.			
11	Highlight delivery period.			
12	Give preference to availability of spares and service facilities for that item? Remember "**calatal ka naama gaaw.l**" the equipment is worth its cost as long as it is working.			
13	What is the cost of maintenance and servicing?			
14	Ensure that the cost is within approved budget.			
15	Issue a 'Purchase Order' highlighting all terms and conditions.			
16	Always attach the received final, negotiated offer as an annexure to the main purchase order.			

4. Checklist Material Receipt:

SN	Check	Yes	No	Remark
1	Check that entry has been made at security gate?			
2	Check that weight and/or counting is done properly and correctly?			
3	Check goods received are as per suppliers' invoice in quantity & specifications?			
4	Check that goods received are as per purchase order in quantity & specifications?			
5	Check that original packing is not tampered with? Packing is not damaged.			
6	Goods supplied are of the same make as was asked in the purchase order?			
7	Entry has to be made in 'Inward Register' (Material Receipt Register)			
8	Check that when packing is to be opened, supplier's representative is present.			
9	OR open the packing in presence of two persons and note down any discrepancy. Make a report and all should sign.			
10	Carry out visual inspection after opening the pack.			
11	Ensure that 'Quality Check' has been carried out.			
12	Prepare a summary and at least two people sign it. • Wrong item (Name & quantity of the item) • Wrong quantity (Name of item & quantity received) • Damaged/defective item (Name & Quantity) • Supplied without order (Name if known & quantity)			

5. Checklist Purchase Department:

SN	Check	Yes	No	Remark
1	Are you keeping a full database of all concerned vendors?			
2	Are you continuously updating this database?			
3	You have a separate list of approved vendors duly signed by authorities?			
4	Do you have a 'Purchase Manual'? (hospital purchase procedures)			
5	Do you keep a record of purchase orders issued and goods received or pending against them?			
6	Your purchase order Performa has been vouched by a legal expert?			
7	Do you always mention 'Place of Jurisdiction' as your hospital's city?			
8	Any changes in this Performa are duly approved by concerned authorities?			
9	Do you invite fresh offers even while placing repeat orders?			
10	Do you get your techno-commercial comparison approved and signed by concerned authorities?			
11	Do write in short reasons for placing order to this supplier on your comparison statement and get it signed by higher authorities.			

Note: A good purchase department should answer all these checks in "YES"

6. Checklist Equipment Acceptance Report:

SN	Check	Yes	No	Remark
1	Is the vendor's representative present at the time of delivery to the hospital?			
2	What are the numbers of unopened boxes?			
3	What is the condition of containers (boxes)? Whether the material was packed in a good way?			
4	What is the condition of packets after unloading? If damaged, please mention in your report.			
5	Whether all items are received as per order and are as per ordered technical specifications.			
6	Whether item has been inspected by the purchasing department at this stage or not?			

Name & Signature of the Receiver:

Name & Signature of vendor's Representative:

Note: Attach this checklist as an annexure to your 'Item Received Letter' issued to the vendor.

STATIONARY FORMATS:

1. Demand Book (Requisition cum Issue Book):

Name of the Hospital

Demand Book

To General Stores: .... Indenting Department: ....

To Medical Stores: .... Demand No.: ....

Please arrange to supply the following items: Date: ....

SN	Items	Unit	Stock In hand	Quantity Demanded	Quantity Issued	Remarks

Demanded by: Sanctioned by:

Received by: Issued by:

2. Bin Card:

Name of the Hospital

Bin Card

Name of the Item: ....

Date	Particulars	Received Qty.	Issued Qty.	Balance Qty.	Sign.	Remarks

3. Material Receipt Report/Master Register (MRR):

This register should work as master register for all purchases (A to Z) in the hospital.

Name of the Hospital

Material Receipt Report/Register

SN	L.F. No.	Date	Supplier	Item Details	Qty.	Bill No.	Rate	Taxes	Total	Issued To	Remark
Note: It is either in landscape format or both sides of the register are used.											

4. Material Inward Report (Daily):

Name of the Hospital

Daily Material Inward Report

For Date:

SN	Date	Item Description	Purchased From	Challan/Bill No	Date	Unit	Qty. As per Challan	Qty. Actual	Remark

(Storekeeper) (Checked By) (Authorized By)

5. Stock Register:

Standard stock registers are available in the market at any stationary stores.

Here is a more suitable format for inventory control

Name & Address of the Hospital

Page of register on Left

Name of the Item: ....

SN	Folio	Date	Supplier	Received	Issued	Balance	Remark

Page of register on Right

Distribution Details:

Date						
SN	Name of the Department	Qty.	Qty.	Qty.	Qty.	Qty.
	OPD					
	Emergency					
	Ward No. 1					

Date						
SN	**Name of the Department**	**Qty.**	**Qty.**	**Qty.**	**Qty.**	**Qty.**
	OT					
	CSSD					
	Etc.					

6. Purchase Order (Sample):

Hospital Letter Head

Purchase order

Ref. No.: .... Date: ....

To,

....

....

Subject: Purchase Order for ....

Dear Sir,

Please supply us following goods as per your quotation No. ...... Dated ....

This is as per our discussion with your representative Mr. ....

SN Description Qty. Unit price Total Price

1

2

Accessories:

1

2

Terms and Conditions:

1. Specifications:
   Are noted down in our order in short but specifications are as per your final quotation (Performa Invoice No. ... Dated ......)
2. Prices: are on FOR basis
   Are inclusive of all Packing, Forwarding, net for delivery at our hospital at ________________. Taxes & levies ruling at the time of delivery will not be charged separately. Also, the prices are final & prices ruling at the time of dispatch of each consignment will not be applicable.
3. Taxes & Duties:
   The GST, Excise and other state taxes are included in the order price. Any changes in taxes after acceptance of this order will not be applicable on us.
4. Delivery:
   Within 3 to 4 weeks from the date of acceptance of our order.
5. Payment Terms:
   a. Ten percent as advance. We are remitting Rs. .... as advance, as agreed, by bank draft No. ... dated ... drawn on ....(Bank) .... along with this order.

b. Fifty percent on delivery
c. Rest on installation and successful commissioning.

6. Mode of Dispatch:
By Lorry/Rail Transport under Freight paid basis. The road permit applicable to our state (Form-32) is being sent along with this order.
7. Inspection:
Inspection will be carried out jointly by your and our representative after opening of the packing.
8. Installation:
Your marketing agent/representative will come and install the items at our site, free of cost and will also provide necessary training.
9. Insurance:
You will ensure each consignment with a Govt. recognized insurance company at your cost against transit risks till destination i.e., our hospital site.
10. Warranty:
These stores will be guaranteed against any manufacturing defect or workmanship or for any defect arising during our use, except mishandling, for a period of 12 months from the date of installation.
11. Arbitration Clause: can also be added in the PO.

PLEASE QUOTE OUR REFERENCE NUMBER IN ALL YOUR FUTURE CORRESPONDENCE.

Thanking you

Yours truly,

7. Gate Pass – Non-Returnable:

Name of the Hospital

Non-Returnable Gate Pass

Gate Pass No.: Date: Time:

Supplier Name:

Bill No./Challan No.: Date:

SN	Item Description	Challan/Bill Quantity in Number or Weight	Received Quantity in Number or Weight	Returned Quantity in Number or Weight	Remarks

Store Supervisor: .... Security Officer: .... Vendor Sign: ....

8. Gate Pass Returnable:

Name of the Hospital

Non-Returnable Gate Pass

Gate Pass No.: Date: Time:

Supplier Name:

Bill No./Challan No.: Date:

SN	Item Description	Quantity in Number or Weight	Purpose of Return	Received Back (Date)	Remarks

Store Manager: .... Security Officer: .... Vendor Sign: ....

Sign of Store Manager when Received Back:

9. Equipment Log Card:

Hospital Name

EQUIPMENT LOG BOOK/CARD

Name of the Equipment: ....

Model No.: ....

Installed On: .... Warranty Starts on: ....

Description of Standard Equipment: ....

Accessories Received: ....

Pending Accessories: ....

Manufacturer's Details: ....

Dealer in India: ....

Local Contact: ....

Service Engineer Details with Telephone number: ....

Preventive Maintenance Schedule: ....

On back of this card

Columns in a landscape format to cover both Right & Left side of the register

SN	Date	Nature of Complaint	Agency informed on Date	Repair done on Date	Nature of Repair	Cost of Repair	Sign

Note:- Such card/book should be maintained for all costly medical equipment.

10. Material Issue Register:

SN	Date	Item	Qty	Issued to	Received by	Sign of Receiver	Sign Storekeeper	Remark

11. Dhobi Book/Laundry Register:

Date:				
SN	**Item Name**	**Date Given**	**Date Received**	**Remarks**

Remarks: Item not received or damaged

BIBLIOGRAPHY, REFERENCES & ACKNOWLEDGMENTS:

1. Indian Public Health Standards (IPHS), Guidelines for District Hospitals (101 to 500 Bedded) Revised 2012 Directorate General of Health Services Ministry of Health & Family Welfare, Government of India
2. "Standard Operating Procedures SOP For Hospitals 2nd Edition" by Dr. Arun K. Agarwal
3. "Duties & Responsibilities of Hospital Staff" by Dr. Arun Kumar
4. "Checklists for Hospitals" by Dr. Arun K. Agarwal
5. Johal Multispeciality Hospital, Jalandhar, Punjab, India
6. BBC Heart Care & Pruthi Hospital, Jalandhar, Punjab, India
7. Material Management By DR. I. SELVARAJ, I.R.M.S (www.pitt.edu/~super7/30011-31001/30961.ppt Retrieved 5 June 2018)
8. CMC Vellore
9. Sitaram Jindal Foundation, Manav Charitable Hospital (MCH), Bangalore
10. Purchase Manual, (ISSUE 3 – 2013), Hindustan Aeronautics Limited, Bangalore, India
11. Duties & Responsibilities of Different Employees of Health Directorate, Government of West Bengal, Health & Family Welfare Department.
12. Guidelines for Implementation Of "Kayakalp" Initiative, Ministry of Health and Family Welfare Government of India
13. https://job-descriptions.careerplanner.com/Marketing-Managers.cfm (Retrieved 16 May 2018)

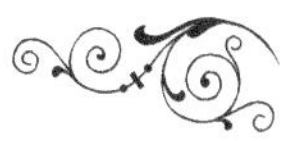

Chapter – 15

DEPARTMENT OF MORTUARY

INDEX

23. Checklists
    a. Daily Checklist
    b. Checklist Mortuary
    c. Checklist Mortuary Planning
    d. Checklist Mortuary Working
    e. Checklist Mortuary Workers
    f. Checklist Body Handing Over
    g. Checklist Mortuary Equipment
    h. Audit Checklist for Mortuary
    i. Mortuary Protocol Checklist
    j. Checklist Death Audit
24. Quality Indicators
25. Documentation
26. Stationary Formats
    a. Mortuary Register: Sample-1
    b. Mortuary Register: Sample-2
    c. Mortality Review Form
27. Bibliography, References & Acknowledgments

INTRODUCTION:

A morgue or mortuary (in a hospital or elsewhere) is used for the storage of human corpses awaiting identification or removal for autopsy or disposal by burial, cremation or other method. In modern times corpses have customarily been refrigerated to delay decomposition. [Morgue: From Wikipedia, the free encyclopedia, https://en.wikipedia.org/wiki/Morgue]

In short - it a place where dead bodies are stored prior to Autopsy, burial or cremation

Usually, the mortuary is located at far end of the facility. The facility is always under lock & key whenever it is not manned. As all hospitals do not have a well-equipped mortuary sometimes mortuary of one hospital is also used by other hospital.

In practice it has been seen that a mortuary is the most neglected area/department/section of a hospital. It is thought to be a necessary evil. Actually, it is also an important facility for any hospital of substantial size to keep the dead body and grieving relatives away from other patients. You cannot keep a dead body in the hospital ICU/ward for long time, if the relatives are not immediately ready to take it home and in such cases the body has to be shifted to such a place where it can be stored and latter disposed without any significant hindrance to hospital's normal functioning.

Though it is located away from the main hospital activities, its own importance cannot be overlooked. It is a place to provide dignified, efficient and compassionate services to the community by respectfully taking care of a dead.

Many hospitals even though they have mortuary facility, do not perform post-mortem examination. And in case of need, body has to be shifted to a government run facility for proper post-mortem examination.

When death occurs in wards and there is delay in transfer of body by next of kin, the body is immediately shifted to mortuary until other formalities of the hospital are completed.

The dead bodies can be preserved the dead bodies in the mortuary under safe, dignified and proper management and the relatives of the dead bodies can take time for funeral.

In addition to provision for holding the mortal remains, embalming services are available for long-term preservation of the mortal remains beyond 48 hours, or in order to prepare them for long-distance transport.

DESCRIPTION:

Health care workers may come into contact with recently deceased patients as part of their daily work. A number of these will have died as a result of complications of infection or infectious conditions, many of which have no immediate risk to staff handling or laying out bodies. However certain bacteria and viruses may pose a risk, if staffs are exposed to the agent or fluids/material containing those agents.

INFRASTRUCTURE/PLANNING:

The Mortuary shall be located in an area within the same building, easily accessible from the wards, emergency department and Operation Theatre. It shall be located away from general traffic routes used by public.

Facilities for proper illumination and hand washing should be available.

At least cold chamber for preservation of two dead bodies should be installed. It should be so located that the dead bodies can be transported unnoticed by the general public and patients.

Post-mortem facilities, if available then this room shall have stainless steel autopsy table with sink, a sink with running water for specimen washing and cleaning and cup-board for keeping instruments. Proper illumination and air conditioning shall be provided in the post mortem room.

A separate room for body storage shall be provided with at least 2 deep freezers for preserving the body. There shall be a waiting area for relatives and a space for religious rites.

Mortuary in this hospital is built in an area of nearly 16 x 16 feet, located near the entry gate of the hospital. It is equipped with two refrigerators having the capacity of storing three bodies each totalling six bodies at a time. No autopsy is done and mortuary is utilised only for the purpose of storage.

Appropriate temperature of the refrigerator is ensured until handing over to relatives/police.

1. The Mortuary should be located in a separate building on the ground/basement floor and must be easily accessible from any of the wards, emergency Department and Operation Theatre.
2. It should be located away from general traffic routes used by the public.
3. The post-mortem room should have stainless steel autopsy table with a sink with running water for specimen washing and cleaning and a cupboard for keeping instruments.
4. Proper illumination and air conditioning should be provided in the post-mortem room.
5. A separate room for body storage with at least two deep freezers must be made available for preserving bodies.
6. There should be a waiting area for relatives and a space for performing religious rites.
7. Separate rooms for the doctor and documentation would be necessary

Ideally it should have following areas:

1. **Cold room;** for body store for minimum of four bodies. It should have an area of about 10.5 square meters.
2. **Post mortem area**; if permitted by law. Area should be at least 14 Square meters.
3. **Store;** one room should be earmarked for storing different items. Area should be at 7 to 10 Sq. Meters.

4. Body wash and prayer room;
5. Relative waiting area with toilet and drinking water facility.
6. Doctor's Office (Autopsy Surgeon) with toilet
7. Staff room with toilet
8. Janitors closet
9. Trolley bay

Miscellaneous Requirements:

Selection of interior finishes to the area shall consider the impact on safety aspects including adequate drainage, protection from sharp edges, adequate protection against infection and other hazards.

1. **Floors:** should be hard, durable and washable. The junctions between the walls and floors should be suitably covered.
2. **Wall:** should be durable and permanent. Preferable it should have light coloured tiles up to the ceiling.
3. **Doors:** should be sliding and large enough and fly proof.
4. **Windows:** if present should allow natural light to come in.
5. **Ceilings:** must be washable, impermeable and non-porous.
6. **Lighting:** should avoid glare and should be white only.
7. **Air-conditioning:** The whole complex should be air conditioned.
8. **Safety:** should have fool proof measures for safety of the dead bodies. It should have proper firefighting arrangements.
9. **Pest Control:** proper and efficient measures should be taken for rodents, flies and mosquitoes' control.
10. **Disposal of Waste:** It should be as per hospital protocol of disposal of other BMW.

EQUIPMENT:

Please consult "Checklist Mortuary Equipment".

MORTUARY CHAMBERS:

There are two machines (Mortuary cabinets) (A and B) having the capacity for three bodies in each.

The bodies wrapped in white cloth are kept in a refrigerator having three cabins (upper, middle and lower). Numbered as 1, 2, 3.

Maximum of six bodies can be placed at a time in two of the refrigerators.

The required temperature can be regulated and is displayed on the panel/gauge on top of the refrigerator. The temperature is maintained between 2 - 5^{0}C.

The ice vendor will be called upon when the refrigerator is fully occupied and more bodies need to be kept or when the refrigerator is non-functional (happens rarely).

The address and phone number of the ice vendor is displayed at mortuary and at the security office.

Technical Specifications of a 4 Body cabinet:

1. Mortuary refrigeration system should be designed to be a reliable and durable.
2. Should accommodate 4 number of cadaver or dead body within the cabinet.
3. Temperature range: 2 to 6 degrees Celsius.
4. Double-walled with mild steel/pre-fabricated panels for outer surface and stainless steel of 316 grade (Test certificate has to be produced) for inner chamber with insulation in between.

Exterior surface should be chemically treated, antirust coated and duly finished with powder coated paint. Front opening, hinged insulated doors, door handle and lock arrangement with keys in duplicate for individual dead bodies.

5. All the doors to be fitted with high quality neoprene rubber gaskets for air tight fittings and magnetic closure fittings and lock. Washable interiors with channel for water outlet that can be plugged with rodent resistant material.
6. All stainless-steel construction completely rusts free; vapour proof incandescent lamp mounted glows on door opening Mortuary Carriage.
7. The 100 mm gap between the walls to be filled with high grade polyurethane insulation, ensuring maximum thermal efficiency.
8. Mortuary tray:

   Stainless steel Trays to carry (to accommodate a cadaver of Max. 7 ft. length) dead bodies with handles at both ends, travel on rollers fitted for easy movement.
9. Refrigeration System:
   a. Heavy duty self-contained, compact and unitary type with hermitically sealed compressors with air cooled refrigeration system and energy efficient machines capable of operation at 230 V, 50Hz, 1 PH, Ac supply. Thermostat controlled Security locks to prevent unintentional switch off.
   b. Temperature performance in range 20 to 80 degree centigrade in ambient temperature of up to 400 degrees.
   c. Refrigerant: R-22 or equivalent (Non-CFC type).
   d. Refrigeration Capacity: at 400 degrees at room temperature, 5000 BTU/Hr
   e. Control system: digital temperature Indicator – cum – controller with PT – 100 Sensors, continuously monitors and displays the mortuary temperatures.
   f. Alarm audio – visual alarm in case of temperature variation beyond limit due to power failure or any other reason.
   g. Stabilizer: of appropriate rating should be provided
   h. Rating: Input 90 V-280 V, Output: 220 V+10%
10. One trolley should be provided along with the machine.

TYPES OF MORTUARY COLD CHAMBERS:

a. **Positive temperature:**

   Bodies are kept between 2 °C (36 °F) and 4 °C (39 °F). While this is usually used for keeping bodies for up to several weeks, it does not prevent decomposition, which continues at a slower rate than at room temperature.

b. **Negative temperature:**

   Bodies are kept at between −10 °C (14 °F) and −50 °C (−58 °F). Usually used at forensic institutes, particularly when a body has not been identified. At these temperatures the body is completely frozen and decomposition is very much reduced.

   [https://en.wikipedia.org/wiki/Morgue]

FUNCTIONS:

1. This department receives dead bodies round the clock.
2. The department should normally receive dead bodies from this hospital. In some circumstances it will also receive dead bodies from other hospitals or patient home or if sent by police station for safe keeping.

3. Dead bodies-other than those mentioned above should not be collected without permission of Mortuary In-charge/hospital administration.
4. All bodies must be with identity tags.
5. Details of the case should be sent along with the body on the prescribed format. It should have UHID number, MLC number, Ward/Casualty, Name, age & address of the deceased etc.
6. Proper records should be maintained in the mortuary by the mortuary in charge/security.

Main functions of a mortuary in the hospital are;

1. Preserving dead bodies till relatives take them.
2. Keeping bodies brought by police to use mortuary facilities of this hospital as the city does not have such facilities elsewhere.
3. Keeping unclaimed bodies till disposal is arranged.
4. Keep dead bodies requiring pathological/legal postmortem.
5. Viewing and identification of dead bodies by relatives and friends.
6. For keeping dead bodies of medico-legal cases for post-mortem and then handing over.

STAFFING/MANPOWER:

Mortuary staff should be specially trained and guided to efficiently handle grieving relatives and treating dead body with respect and dignity. The end point care is as important as care in wards and ICU. If the care in mortuary (care after death) is not given properly and relatives get agitated the end result on hospital can be devastating.

ORGANISATIONAL STRUCTURE:

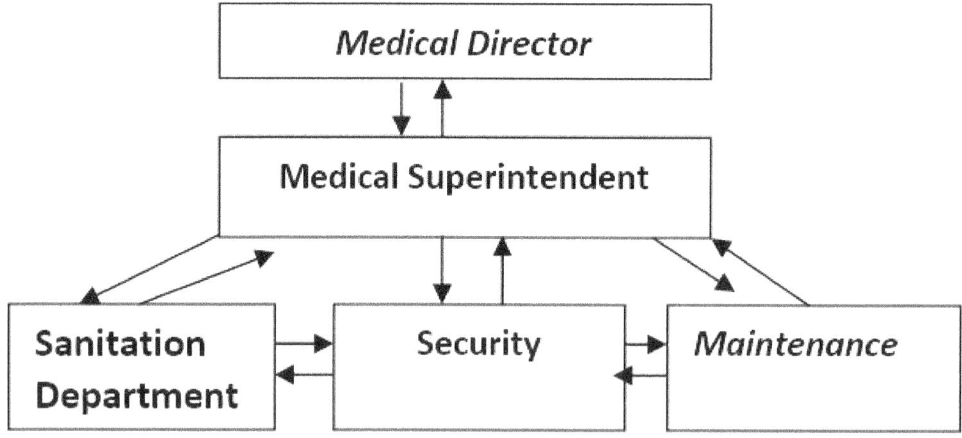

All the issues related to mortuary will be supervised and monitored by concerned officer who will be reporting to director medical as and when required.

DUTIES & RESPONSIBILITIES:

A. Duties of the Attending Physician:

1. Write death note on the case sheet.
2. Determine whether it is a normal death or unnatural death.

3. Inform police in case of an unnatural death.
4. If medico legal autopsy is requested by the police, then the body may be transported directly to Police Station or to hospital morgue.
5. Issuing of a Death Summary.
6. Obtain consent for autopsy (if requested).

B. Duties of the Attending Nurse:

1. Assisting other nursing staff, in packing and transportation of dead bodies.
2. Verify that patient ID is on body.
3. Leave all lines and tubes in place. If applicable prepare body for family viewing. Once the decision is made that there will be no autopsy, all tubes must be removed prior to release of body.
4. Release the deceased's personal belongings to relatives. It is to be documented on case sheet and should be signed by the receiver.
5. To accompany the transporting staff up to the mortuary.
6. Handing over all the documents to the Mortuary staff.
7. Transporting staff and mortuary workers should use N-95 mask.
8. She will request at least 2 Patient Care Attendants to accompany for transfer the body from the ward to the mortuary.
9. The nurse will take the signature of the relative/friend on the mortuary request form to discharge the body.
10. The nurse will enter in the register the time and date of body handed over and sign.

C. Mortuary Staff:

1. The working hours are 24 hours a day for all seven days of a week.
2. The Mortuary Key and the Register will be kept in a secured manner.
3. The Key and the Register will not be handed over to anyone except the Nurse from the respective ward or Security Supervisor.
4. The Staff Nurse will check the register for proper/correct entry of information regarding transfer and handing over of the body.

PAYMENT SYSTEM:

No fees incurred from the next of kin for utilising the facility.

Mortuary services are free. No charge incurred from the next of kin for keeping the body in the mortuary refrigerator.

STANDARD OPERATING PROCEDURES:

1. Deaths following cessation of cardio respiratory function must be confirmed in accordance with the hospital policies.
2. In case of unnatural causes of death, Police must be informed.
3. Brought Dead Cases:
   a. All brought dead patients are dealt as per MLC protocol. If EMO decides that it is a natural death, the MLC tag is removed from the patient.

b. Following patients brought dead are mandatorily treated as MLC.
   - Strangulation marks on neck
   - A woman's death within 7 years of marriage.
   - Any suspicion of foul play

   A death certificate may be issued to the relatives, if desired, specifying in bold "Brought Dead"

c. Mortuary facility may be provided if asked for.

4. Death report to be given by the resident only after lapse of an hour of pronouncing death.
5. Copy of the death report will be sent to the local authorities within prescribed time limit. In many states it is to be done online.
6. The nearest relative of the patient will be informed of the death by nurse or the resident promptly either through a messenger or by phonogram.
7. Managing Brought Dead
   1. A patient shall be declared 'Brought in Dead', if on examination;
      a. Patient is not breathing.
      b. Bothe pupils are dilated and are non-reactive to light.
      c. No Pulse, No Heart Beat.
      d. ECG is taken immediately – it is a straight line.
   2. CPR is to be carried out immediately.
   3. If there is no response, the patient is declared 'Brought in Dead'.
   4. Registration is done in the Emergency register and case sheet is prepared documenting initial examination details, CPR details and the flat ECG is attached with it.
   5. If the body is not immediately taken by relatives, it is shifted to mortuary.
   6. If needed, police have to be informed and then body is handed over to police personnel.
   7. A certificate mentioning that the patient was brought in dead may be issued.
   8. Now all case papers are filed and sent to MRD for further storage.
8. Handling of Death & Release of dead body:
   1. All deaths in the hospital are handled with utmost care.
   2. Counselling is done of next of kin. Behaviour of all concerned staff should be helping and sympathetic.
   3. All help is extended to the next of kin in shifting the body from the hospital.
   4. Required certificate is issued and acknowledgment of receipt of body is obtained on the case papers. All case papers are filed and sent to MRD.
9. No dead body will be kept in the mortuary without any identity tags.
10. In cases of stillborn and neonates less than 28 days old, relatives may take the body directly to their home.

A. End of Life Care:

In the last phase of life people seek peace and dignity. To help realise this, every person should be able to fairly expect the following elements of care from physicians, health care institutions, and the community.

1. Respect the dignity of both patient and caregivers.
2. Be sensitive to and respectful of the patient's and family's wishes.
3. Use the most appropriate measures that are consistent with patient choices.
4. Encompass alleviation of pain and other physical symptoms.
5. Assess and manage psychological, social, and spiritual/religious problems.

6. Offer continuity (the patient should be able to continue to be cared for, if so desired, by his/her primary care and specialist providers).
7. Provide access to any therapy which may realistically be expected to improve the patient's quality of life, including alternative or non-traditional treatments.
8. Provide access to palliative care and hospice care.
9. Respect the right to refuse treatment.
10. Respect the physician's professional responsibility to discontinue some treatments when appropriate, with consideration for both patient and family preferences.

Policy:

1. To provide skilful nursing, gentle handling and utmost reverence to the body after death.
2. Consideration must be shown to individuals' personal preferences, identity, spiritual, faith and cultural values. Patients may have one or more cultural beliefs or personal wishes relating to death and dying; these must be respected. There should not be any discrimination in treatment of the body in any form, to ensure that the dead body is properly preserved and handled irrespective of religion, region, caste, gender, etc.
3. No physical exploitation: Any form of physical exploitation of the body of the dead violates the basic right of the deceased person.
4. No defamation after death: The deceased person should not be defamed by any kind of statement or visible representation, made or published intending to harm his/her reputation.
5. No breach of privacy: The deceased person has the right to privacy, i.e., the right to control the dissemination of information about one's privacy.
6. Infection risks do not increase after death. Take transmission-based precautions to minimise any risk of cross-infection.
7. If the family is not present at the time of death, they must be informed by a professional with appropriate communication skills.
8. Death in hospital may necessitate by law the involvement of the registrar/legal authority.
9. It is important that healthcare workers comply with legislation, the wishes of patients/relatives and continue to follow Standard Precautions and where necessary.

Identify the following:

1. If the patient has any cultural or religious beliefs which necessitate alternative procedures to nurses undertaking Last Offices. If this is the case then follow the instructions for the specific religion guidelines.
2. If the body of the deceased is likely to leak after death, a body bag will be required.
3. If any special requests made before death, e.g., the keeping on of jewellery, clothes to be worn.
4. If the eyes have been donated for corneal grafting.
5. If there are any radiation precautions still in force.

B. Procedural Steps:

1. Condition of the dead body is to be verified and recorded properly, before keeping the dead body inside the dead body bag.
2. Physical Preparation of Dead Body should be carried out afters sometimes have elapsed after declaring the death.
3. Family members may be offered to assist in body preparation if they so desire.
4. All valuables which are on the body of the deceased should be handed over to the relatives and same must be documented in the IPD case sheet under receiver's signature.

5. On the death of a patient, who has no known next of kin, any cash or valuables such as keys, bank cards, money, jewellery or mobile phone must be deposited with the hospital authorities under two witnesses.
6. The deceased patients' property must be returned to the family sensitively.
7. Any preparation for sending the dead body to the mortuary should be done after relatives have viewed the dead, if they are easily approachable.

Preparation of Dead Body:

1. Eyes should be closed immediately as in sleep. If relatives have consented to it.
2. If the eyes are for donation, gently tape close the eyelids using micropore tape
3. Body to be straightened with arms by the sides.
4. Mouth should be closed immediately.
5. Remove all support equipment.
6. Give thorough sponging to the patient.
7. Change patient clothes.
8. Keep the head & chin in position.
9. Bandages may be used if necessary.
10. Plug nose and ears with cotton plug.
11. Cover the patient with new white bed sheet/mortuary sheet.
12. Attach an identity card to the dead body having name & IP No.
13. Allow the relatives to be with the body for a while. Arrange to meet the religious rites if possible.
14. Primary Nurse to follow the routine discharge procedure as per discharge policy.
15. Primary Nurse to arrange for dead body van, if required.
16. If the deceased has dentures ensure they are in right place as per their faith
17. Attach identification bands to a wrist and the opposite ankle of the deceased.
18. Both identification bands should contain the following information: deceased's Name, hospital UHID, date of death, ward.
19. If the lower jaw drops down significantly, consider putting on a chin support by applying bandages.
20. Place an adult incontinence pad/diaper under the deceased.
21. If the deceased is to be viewed by relatives on the ward ensure there is no blood or body Wrap the patient carefully in a sheet and fasten with tape.
22. Close all the orifices of the body with cotton plug.
23. If there is any radiation expected from the body (Once a patient has been administered with a radioactive material for diagnostic or therapeutic purposes, they will remain radioactive until the radioactive material is excreted and/or has decayed), attach a sticker "RISK OF IONIZING RADIATION" to the outside of the shroud.
24. If the deceased person has any cardiovascular implanted electronic devices (CIEDs), it should be deactivated or advice from the Cardiologist must be taken. Some devices may have risk during cremation.
25. Place the deceased in a body bag if the body is likely to leak, or if the patient has an infection/alert organism.
26. Remove gloves and plastic apron and wash hands. (Use new gloves for any additional clearing procedures to prevent direct contact with blood or body fluids or equipment contaminated with blood or body fluid).

27. If there is a risk of leakage or infection the porters will use gloves regardless of whether the body is in a bag. The attendees will wash their hands after handling a wrapped body. Complete nursing documentation.
28. AFTER CARE Ensure all notes, laboratory reports and X rays are gathered together.

C. Receiving a Dead Body:

Mandatory Documents

1. Death Certificate or a certificate that states the cause of death from Panchayat Member/Hospital/Doctor.
2. Police verification if it is MLC.
3. Mortuary Request Form.
4. Identity card of the deceased – Aadhaar Card/Voters ID Card.
5. Identity card of a person who brings the dead body- Aadhaar Card/Voters ID Card.

Mortuary Request Form – Sample-1

Name: .... Age/Sex: .... UHID/IP Number: ....

Ward/Bed Number: ....

Whether MLC or Not

Attached: Death Certificate — Original, Police Verification if it's MLC.

I am fully aware of the terms and conditions of the mortuary Services. I hereby declare that the above-mentioned information is true to the best of my knowledge and belief.

Name & Signature of Relative (while keeping the body): ....

Name & Signature of Relative (while receiving the body): ....

Mortuary Request Form – Sample-2

Hospital Name & Address

REQUEST FOR KEEPING THE BODY IN MORTUARY

TO;

EMO cum Mortuary Officer

Dear Sir/Madam

I wish to keep the body of .... S/O, D/O, W/O ....

resident of .... in the mortuary of .... (Hospital Name) for transient body custody.

I have the following declarations to submit:

1. That Hospital will not be responsible for any medico- legal issued which remain unresolved.
2. That I am the Lawful custodian of the dead body at present.
3. That the death has been duly certified and the death is without any foul play.
4. I understand that hospital does not take responsibility to any damage to the deceased body due to circumstances like prolonged power failure, theft, physical damage or any other unforeseen damage.
5. That the hospital will take all possible precautions to keep body safe but do not guarantee anything. I am keeping the body purely at my own risk.

6. That we have been explained about hospital mortuary charges and do agree to pay the amount as per the policy.
7. That the body has no valuables on itself and same has been checked by me.

Considering above undertaking please do accept my request for temporary storage of the body.

Regards,

Signature of the custodian: .... Date: .... Time: ....

Name of the custodian:

Contact no:

Address:

Please attached an identity proof of the custodian and of the deceased with this application form

Items Required

1. Dress of the deceased.
2. Artefacts to be kept along with the body.
3. Hospital reserves the right for admission. Applicants need to fill in an application form and follow the rules and regulation as mandated by the hospital.

D. Viewing of Dead Bodies by Relatives:

1. Relatives viewing bodies in the mortuary must be accompanied and the viewing of the body will be coordinated by the mortuary technician.
2. Relatives who have had physical contact with a body must be encouraged to wash their hands before leaving the mortuary.
3. Mortuary staff must advise relatives as to whether there may be any health risk for them if they wish to touch the body. If the risk of infection is significant then relatives must be discouraged from touching the body.
4. If relatives insist on seeing the body in a high risk of infection case, they may be allowed to see the face only. They must be strongly discouraged from kissing or touching the body.
5. Mortuary technician is responsible for ensuring the viewing room is maintained in an appropriate state of cleanliness at all times.

E. Issue of Dead Bodies:

1. Dead bodies preserved in the mortuary are issued after the verification of the same person who signed in the mortuary register by the mortuary in charge.
2. Signature of the receiver is obtained in the specified column of the register and the dead body is issued to him/her.
3. The mortuary cabin is disinfected, washed, and dried by the house keeping personal.
4. Dead body of an MLC case is handed over to the Police only.
5. In case of death that occurred in our hospital and is to be taken home within one or two hours are kept outside the cold cabin in a trolley along with the details noted.

STANDARDS:

1. Services are available round the clock.
2. Dead bodies are kept till the relatives take over the bodies.

3. Unclaimed bodies are kept until disposal is arranged.
4. Departmental signage's are available in local language & English.
5. Religious and cultural preferences of deceased and relatives are taken in to consideration while handling over the body.
6. Privacy and confidentiality of HIV and suicidal cases is maintained.
7. Behaviour of staff is empathetic and courteous to deceased relatives.
8. Availability of telephone and Intercom Services is ensured.
9. Floors of the Mortuary are thick, durable and can be easily cleaned.
10. Floors of the Mortuary are non-slippery and even.
11. Fire Extinguishers that are Class A, Class C type or ABC type are installed in mortuary.
12. Infection control and hand hygiene is maintained.
13. The mortuary machines are covered under AMC.
14. There is adequate illumination at morgue.
15. Hospital ensures that unauthorised entry into mortuary is not permitted
16. Hospital has sound security system to manage overcrowding in Mortuary.
17. Availability of power back in mortuary is ensured.
18. Mortuary technician maintain full records of body brought to mortuary.
19. Mortuary has system to provide identification tag/wrist band for each stored dead body.
20. All bodies sent to mortuary are accompanied with copy of death certificate issued by hospital.
21. There is procedure for immunization of the staff.
22. The department has written SOPs about its various procedures.

PROCEDURAL STEPS SUMMARISED:

1. In case of death of a patient, the concerned attending consultant is immediately informed.
2. Death should be declared to attendant in a very polite and subtle manner by the consultant
3. Preferably the treating unit consultant should visit to console and explain the cause of death to the next of kin or attendant
4. Body should be packed immediately in case of infectious cases special packing with plastic material should be done.
5. Return all the unused consumables and medicines and file sent to billing for financial clearance
6. Billing to generate two clearance slips one to the nursing staff and the other to the security
7. Death certificate, death form and death summary to be filled and written by the resident doctor
8. The file should be sent to the MRD within 48 hrs after death
9. Death certificate and death summary along with investigation reports to be handed over to the relatives while handing over the body
10. Signature of the relatives taken in the case sheet
11. All deaths are reviewed in the "Death & Morbidity Committee"
12. The Police must be notified after consultation with the Hospital Administration in all cases where;
    - Death is due to violence
    - Death results from non-natural causes within 24 hours of admission.
    - The cause of death is unknown or uncertain.
    - The patient is certified "Dead on arrival".

- When an MLC patient expires, the police will be notified immediately and no death certificate will be issued to the attendant. Body will be kept in the mortuary until the police arrive and the DC will be handed over to them.

13. In case of an MLC:
    a. No original documents to be handed over to the relatives
    b. Death certificate and body handed over to the police
    c. All the documents handed over to the police (I.O.), a copy of the same should be maintained after getting it signed from the police for hospital record
    d. Death summary should also be handed over to the police

INFECTION CONTROL:

Health care workers may come into contact with recently deceased patients as part of their daily work. A number of these will have died as a result of complications of infection or infectious conditions, many of which have no immediate risk to staff handling or laying out bodies. However certain bacteria and viruses may pose a risk, if staffs are exposed to the agent or fluids/material containing those agents.

1. In some cases, the body of a deceased person may present a risk of infection because of an active communicable disease or carrier status. This may have been confirmed or undiagnosed.
2. Where it is known that the body of a deceased person may constitute an increased risk of infection, staff should follow the guidance of Infection Control set by the hospital.
3. Adequate provision for hand washing must be made.
4. There should be provision of appropriate cleaning, waste storage and waste disposal.
5. Make provision of safety shower and eye wash or eye/face wash within the mortuary if body washing by family members is allowed.
6. Antiseptic hand rub must be provided.
7. The staff must wear the PPE while handling the body.
8. The mortuary will be cleaned after removal of body with 1% Chlorine solution.
9. The Infection Control Nurse (ICN) will be responsible for supervising the same.
10. **Hospital Infection Control Committee** should look into the control measures provided in the mortuary.

Contact with whole or part human remains carries potential risks associated with pathogenic microbiological organisms that may be present in human blood and tissue.

Infectious conditions in the recently deceased include;

a. Blood borne pathogens such as Hepatitis viruses such as HBV, HCV, HDV, HEV and the HIV
b. Tuberculosis
c. Gastrointestinal organisms
d. Group A streptococcal infection
e. Possibly meningitis and septicaemia

Autopsies are not handled at the Hospital premises. Even so, a single exposure may cause infection. The primary ways to protect personnel who handle human remains against infectious diseases are;

a. Use of PPE
b. Observance of safety, hygiene, and infection control practices
c. Proper handling and disposal of medical waste

Recommended Immunization for Staff:

1. Hepatitis-B
2. Tetanus

OCCUPATIONAL HAZARDS:

The commonly occurred occupational hazards at mortuary are

1. Accidental injuries, musculoskeletal injuries during handling of dead bodies.
2. Incised and cut injuries due to sharp instruments are also common.
3. The blood-borne and air -borne infections are also common in mortuary like mycobacterium tuberculosis infection.
4. To prevent these blood-borne infections regular vaccination in every 6 months is given to the mortuary staff.

QUALITY CONTROL:

1. The mortuary chambers have panels with digital display which will display the set temperature and the actual temperature.
2. Double checking of the temperature is done using a thermometer kept inside, once a day.
3. When the temperature is not at the expected range the maintenance personnel will be informed (the respective company personnel may be called by Maintenance Department for further action to be taken.)

CLEANLINESS MEASURES:

1. Cleaning of the chambers and the premises maintained and monitored by sanitary inspector.
2. Disinfection: The premises being cleaned thrice daily and as and when required using recognised disinfectants for washing and wet mopping of the floor.
3. Hand mopping of the outer surfaces of the cabinets is also being carried out and the cabins are cleaned each time after body being taken out using a disinfectant.
4. Housekeeping staff are advised to wear face mask and gloves while working.

PEST CONTROL MEASURES:

1. The work has been assigned to a private agency (as appointed by Hospital authorities) and is monitored and recorded by sanitary inspector.
2. Spraying of herbal pesticides is done once a week.

BODY IDENTIFICATION PROCEDURE:

At the site of death, body is covered in white cloth. Body will have identification tag and labelling done using cotton plaster, which is pasted, on the pectoral area. The label contains the following information: Name, age, sex, IP number, and date of admission, date of death, time of death, ward number, doctor's name, diagnosis and MLC status. Required information is written on the death (Mortuary) register including the cabin (upper, middle or lower). Security personnel is always present while receiving and handing over the body. He double checks the information required.

TRANSPORTATION:

1. To maintain the dignity of the deceased person and ensure the safety of personnel, staff must identify any risk factors prior to requesting transfer. This will ensure that the staffs have the appropriate equipment and number of personnel required for transfer.
2. No protective clothing to be worn by staff while transportation
3. Bodies are transported using Hearse Service which is outsourced to a private agency.
4. In case of excessive leakage of fluid from, the transportation of cadaver is to be stopped to mortuary.
5. If body is to be transferred to the mortuary, it should be done on a dedicated (separate) trolley.
6. Mortuary staff must be alerted prior to transportation of any infection risk bodies.
7. Hospital ambulances are not used for the same.
8. The security personnel checks and ensures final bill paid and death certificate before handing over the body to the next of kin.
9. He also takes the signature of kin while being handed over to them.
10. Relatives can arrange for the conveyance on their own.
11. In case of Medico Legal Cases (MLCs) bodies are handed over to the concerned police.
12. The unclaimed bodies are taken by Hearse brought by Police.
13. When there is a delay from police, enquiry is done either by CSO/ASO or by Deputy Medical Superintendents from time to time by calling on to the respective police station.
14. After transportation, proper hand washing to be followed by staffs.

MAINTENANCE:

During breakdown of the mortuary cabinets, maintenance department supervisor on duty will be called immediately. Ice vendor will be called to supply ice blocks when required/till corrective measures are taken. The contact person's name and phone numbers are displayed on the refrigerator and also at the security office. The record is maintained regarding the problems and corrective action taken by Maintenance Department and security personnel.

Any maintenance done is monitored by concerned administrator and maintenance department.

TRAINING:

Mortuary staff should be specially trained and guided to efficiently handle grieving relatives and treating dead body with respect and dignity. The end point care is as important as care in wards and ICU. If the care in mortuary (care after death) is not given properly and relatives get agitated the end result on hospital can be devastating.

Training should be given regarding handling the body, behaviour and infection control to the concerned personnel by the concerned authorities. (HR/CSO/Quality Executive).

All staff that is responsible for caring of the dead should be trained appropriately in their roles.

PROCESS FLOW:

1. Body is received in the mortuary.
2. Entry is made in the concerned register.
3. Check for MLC status.
4. Body is kept in one designated tray/bin,
5. Temperature of the cabinet is checked and constantly checked.

6. While handing over the body to next of kin:
    a. Check for payment of final bill.
    b. Check that DC is issued.
7. Security signs the Register and DC handed over to next of kin/police
8. Body transported in Hearse on contract or to the relative's vehicle
9. Security personnel will inform the police when there is death of MLC patient in the hospital.
10. He will play a key role in each step from the time of receiving the body till the handing over of body to police (next of kin or/and police) and must accompany the police while Death Certificate being issued by the sister concerned after bills are cleared.

Dead bodies with labels are received from various departments of the hospital (casualty, ICU, wards etc) when the patient party is not taking the body immediately. Bodies are also received when the death has occurred outside the hospital but have brought to avail the refrigeration facility provided at hospital. This requires permission from the Director Medical or Additional M.S. or D.M.S.

CHECK LIST:

A. Daily Checklist:

Checks	Frequency	Department
Temperature of the refrigerator when body is kept	Every hour	Security
Cleanliness of the refrigerator cabin	Whenever body is removed	Sanitation
Cleanliness of the premises	Thrice a day (also, as & when required)	Sanitation
Working condition of the exhaust fans (Two in no.)	Once a day	Security
Working condition of the tube lights (Two in no.)	Once a day	Security

B. Checklist Mortuary:

SN	Check	Yes	No	Remark
1	Is mortuary located in a separate building? Or if in main building, it should be in the basement with direct approach.			
2	Is it located away from main services of the hospital?			
3	Is it easily approachable by a heavy vehicle?			
4	Can main gate of the mortuary be assessed without crisscrossing normal traffic of the hospital?			
5	Is the size of this department proportionate to the expected arrival of dead bodies?			
6	Is signage displayed in both local & English language?			
7	Does it have adequate waiting area?			
8	Has planning done for adequate facilities of drinking water and wash-room?			
9	Are mortuary windows meshed to stop insects and flies?			
10	Are fire detection and firefighting arrangements as per norms?			
11	Is body fluid spillage immediately taken care off?			
12	Are hand wash facilities available?			
13	Have you catered for backup power supply?			
14	Is security of the area good?			
15	Is mortuary area well ventilated?			

SN	Check	Yes	No	Remark
16	Check availability of body cabinets.			
17	Proper record is maintained of receiving and disposal of bodies?			
18	Is a licence required to have a facility of mortuary in your State?			

C. Checklist Mortuary Planning:

SN	Check	Yes	No	Remark
1	Mortuary has minimum following 4 sections; (1) Reception Room (2) Body storage area (3) Post mortem room (only if a teaching hospital) and (4) Support services			
2	Main body room has refrigerated body boxes, having facility for storing 2 to 4 bodies (depending on size and nature of the hospital) at a time?			
3	There is an attached toilet for staff?			
4	There is one Post-mortem doctor's room of about 14 x 20 feet for police/relatives to have meeting with the doctor?			
5	Hand washing facility in main body room and in post-mortem room?			
6	Preferably an office cum computer room of about 12 x 12 feet?			
7	Preferably a separate store room of about 10 x 12 feet?			
8	Change rooms for staff?			
9	Separate record room? Records can be kept in the hospital's MRD (Medical Record Department), if the mortuary is attached with a hospital?			
10	Toilet for general public?			
11	Drinking water for general public?			
12	Sitting place for general public?			
13	If the mortuary is separately located and is not inside the hospital premises, then it should have a security lockable gate?			
14	Autopsy room has a raised platform for doing post-mortems?			
15	The floors are of non-porous nature and walls are tiled for easy and effective cleaning?			
16	Telephone/Intercom should have been provided?			
17	Computer with LAN for integrating it with hospital HMS (Hospital Management System Software)			
18	If a teaching hospital, provision of viewing gallery around autopsy room?			
19	Parking place for vehicles of relatives and staff?			
20	Doors and windows are fly proof?			
21	The whole area is well lit?			

D. Checklist Mortuary Working:

SN	Check	Yes	No	Remark
1	It has got proper refrigerated body boxes.			
2	Dead body is handled with proper respect and dignity?			
3	The deceased person is never left naked on the trolley at any time?			

SN	Check	Yes	No	Remark
4	Mortuary staff is informed well in advance before sending a body there?			
5	Body is always sent along with the death certificate or a written request on hospital letterhead.			
6	Special precautions are undertaken while handling bodies suspected of harbouring infectious disease.			
7	The person in-charge maintains full record of all dead bodies brought in? • The arrival and disposal of a dead body is well documented and all movements are well recorded? • All procedures from the receipt of a dead body to its handing over are properly documented? • Body is released only after proper identification? • Body handing over receipt is always obtained?			
8	An ID tag (Identification tag or a tag on great toe) is put on all bodies?			
9	Valuables are recorded and handed over to next of kin in writing? Valuables are removed from the body only after consent of family members?			
10	Mortuary has documented SOPs (Standard Operating Procedures) for various departmental activities?			
11	In case of a death of a medico-legal case, body is handed over to the police only?			
12	The staff deployed is properly vaccinated & is courteous and sympathetic?			
13	Staff is provided with PPE (Personal Protective Equipment) to prevent staff from coming in contact with blood and other body fluids?			
14	Staff recognises and respect individual cultural and religious practises?			
15	Mortuary staff does not discuss medical issues with the bereaved family or individual? E.g., cause of death etc. Mortuary staff is not allowed to speak to the public or press.			
16	A complaint cum suggestion box is available in this department?			
17	Entry to mortuary is restricted to authorised personnel only?			
18	Temperature of the mortuary cabinets is monitored? Power supply is maintained 24 x 7?			
19	Staff washes their hands with antiseptic soap before and after handling a dead body?			
20	The floor of the mortuary is always kept clean?			
21	Colour coded waste bins are available as per biomedical waste disposal norms?			
22	Hospital administrator takes daily round of the facility?			

E. Checklist Mortuary Workers:

SN	Check	Yes	No	Remark
1	Staff wears PPE (Personal Protective Equipment) all the time while working in a mortuary?			
2	Staff does not wear outside clothing in the mortuary?			
3	Staff washes hands before and after entering the mortuary?			
4	Staff wears face mask & gloves while entering inside the body storage area?			
5	Mortuary staff is properly vaccinated against Tetanus, Hepatitis A, Hepatitis B?			

SN	Check	Yes	No	Remark
6	Staff undergoes regular health check-up?			
7	Cuts and abrasions, if any, on the body of staff are properly covered with bandages and dressings?			
8	Mortuary staff is aware of the diagnosis of the deceased?			
9	Staff does not eat/drink inside the body storage area?			

F. Checklist Body Handing Over:

SN	Check	Yes	No	Remark
1	Body has been identified.			
2	Check if any legal papers required.			
3	Person authorized to receive the body has signed the mortuary register?			
4	Staff person who hands over the body has also signed in the register?			
5	Check that personal property has been handed over.			
6	Religions obligations are taken care of as per the faith of the deceased?			
7	Check that body tray of the refrigerated cabinet is cleaned and disinfected before returning it to body cabinet.			

G. Checklist Mortuary Equipment:

Equipment for Autopsy

SN		Check/Item	Qty	Remark
1	Basin, 12″		1	
2	Weighing machines		3	
	a	Whole body weighing scale	1	
	b	Balance to weight 100 gms to 10 kg	1	
	c	Balance to weigh 0.2 gms to 10 gms	1	
3	Cutting instruments-stainless steel:			
	a	Skull cutter (electrical)	1	
	B	Organ knife 10′ blade, solid forged	1	
	c	Organ knife 6″ blade, solid forged	1	
	d	Caltin solid forged		
	e	Cartilage knife 5-1/2″ blade solid forged	2	
	f	Rib cutter	1	
	g	Cartilage knife 4″ blade/solid forged	2	
	h	Brain knife 10″ blade, solid forged	1	
	i	Resection knife 3″ blade, solid forged	2	
	j	Scalpels, BP Handle with blades	1 set	
	k	Bistoury, probe pointed solid forged	1	

SN		Check/Item	Qty	Remark
4	Scissors (stainless steel):			
	a	Scissors; blunt sharp 8″	1	
	b	Scissors; blunt/sharp 6″	1	
	c	Scissors; dissecting 5″ with one probe point for coronary artery	1	
	d	Scissors; bowel, Bernard 11″		
5	Forceps (stainless steel):			
	a	Bone cutting forceps 10″ straight	1	
	b	Bone cutting forceps 10″ angled	1	
	c	Rib-shears 9-1/2″	1	
	d	Dissecting forceps 6″	1	
	e	Dissecting forceps 8″	1	
	f	Dissecting forceps 10″	1	
	g	Toothed and un-toothed forceps	6 each	
6	Post-mortem Scissors:			
	a	Saw, Bernard 11″ stainless steel Blade	1	
	B	Saw, Bernard 9″ stainless steel Blade	1	
7	Straight and curved Enterotome, viscrotome		1 each	
8	Miscellaneous:			
	a	Coronet stainless steel	1	
	b	Needles, post-mortem half curved & double curved	1 dozen	
	c	Probes silver with eye 10″	1	
	d	Chisel, straight 3/4 ″ blade	2	
	e	Chisel, spine with locating point (stainless steel)	1	
	f	Gouge, 3/4″ blade, stainless steel	1	
	g	Hammer with wrench stainless steel	1	
	h	Measures 12″ stainless steel	1	
	i	Mallet, boxwood with metal bands	1	
	j	Small table 20″ × 24″ × 12″ for dissection of organs	1	
	K	Measuring jug (one litre)	1	
	l	Metal/steel scale	2	
	m	Magnifying glass	3	
	n	Instrument trolley	3	
	o	Cabinet	1	
	p	Wooden boards	3	
	q	Rubber gloves	Adequate quantity	
	r	Aprons	Adequate quantity	

SN	Check/Item	Qty	Remark
9	Suction Pump & Aspirators	1 each	
10	Body Scale	1	
11	Repairing materials like: Thread white, cotton wool (absorbent), wool waste, a variety of discarded clothes, malleable wire, Polythene bags, Gloves, Masks, and Aprons etc.		
12	Plastic Bins: For fixing large specimens		

This is as per the recommendation of Survey Committee Report on Medico-legal Practices in India, 1964)

CHEMICAL AND ARTICLES:

SN	Check/Item	Qty	Remark
1	Bleaching powder for cleaning mortuary table floors, etc.		
2	2% Glutaraldehyde for cleaning instruments.		
3	Formative for sending specimens needing his to pathology.		
4	Rectified and Methylated spirit	As preservative	
5	Thymol crystals		
6	Common salt		
7	Sodium fluoride		
8	Potassium oxalate		
9	EDTA vials and tubes		
10	Sterilized glass tubes (plain).		
11	Sterilized glass tubes with swabs		
12	Liquid paraffin		
13	Sealing wax etc.		
14	Big size envelopes, plain papers etc.		

H. Audit Checklist for Mortuary:

SN	Audit Checklist for Mortuary	Remarks
	Date:	
1	Mortuary facilities present?	
2	Cold storage and back-up power available?	
3	Staff safety and personal protective equipment available?	
4	Disinfection activities followed?	
5	Maintenance plant of machinery present?	
6	Electrical safety practices	
7	Staff awareness on safety practices	
8	Monitoring of T & C in case this activity is outsourced	
	Signature of Auditor:	

I. Mortuary Protocol Checklist:

MORTUARY PROTOCOL CHECK LIST

Patient Name: .... Age/Sex: .... DOA: ....

UHID No.: .... Ward/Bed: .... Department: ....

SN	Check	Remark
a. To be completed by the Medical Officer:		
1	Date & Time of Death?	
2	Death due to? Communicable/Infectious diseases?	Yes/No
3	If yes; relatives and attendants explained about the communicable disease, care of the body and precautions to be taken?	Yes/No
Name & Signature of the MO:		
b. To be completed by the Nursing Staff:		
1	Bleeding sites present?	Yes/No
2	If yes, are they covered?	Yes/No
3	Secretion present on the body?	Yes/No
4	Excretion on the body?	Yes/No
5	All orifices covered?	Yes/No
6	Universal Precautions followed by everyone handling the body?	Yes/No
7	If infected, deceased packed in body bag?	Yes/No
8	If infected, patient dress disposed of in yellow bag for Incineration?	Yes/No
Name and signature of the staff nurse:		
c. To be completed by security:		
1	Body adequately covered with cloth?	Yes/No
2	Body handed over to family?	Yes/No
	Name & Signature of the Family Member: Relation with the deceased: Date:	

J. Checklist Death Audit

Following information should be available on the deceased medical case sheet:

1. Name, age, sex and complete address.
2. Date and time of admission.
3. Admission through OPD/Emergency, Planned or unplanned.
4. Present history and examination findings.
5. GC (general condition) of the patient on arrival in the hospital.
6. Were family members informed about poor GC, if this was the case?
7. Date and time of informing consultant by casualty medical officer.
8. Date and time of first examination by treating consultant.
9. Details of immediate treatment.

10. What investigations were ordered?
11. When the reports were ready?
12. Was the prognosis explained to the relatives at the time of admission?
13. Did consultant/physician who were present at the time of death put death notes?
14. Opinion of the auditor about appropriateness of treatment.
15. Any other action//suggestion by auditor
16. Name and signature of the auditor

QUALITY INDICATORS (KPI):

1. Proportion of non-MLC cases.
2. Occupancy rate of body cabinets for dead bodies.
3. Mean storage time of dead body in the mortuary.
4. Down time for mortuary (body cabinets cooling system) equipment.

DOCUMENTATION:

1. Mortuary Register
2. Consent

STATIONARY FORMATS:

1. Format of a Mortuary Register: Sample-1

Date	Time In	Cabinet A or B (1,2,3)	Name	Ward	Home Address.	Final bill no.	Death Cert.	MLC No.	Reg. No.	Sign. Next of kin	Vehicle No.	Driver name and Sign.	Date	Time out	Security Sign.

These books are maintained by the security personnel and kept at security office.

2. Format of a Mortuary Register: Sample-2

Date	Name of Deceased	MRD/ID number of the deseeded	Age/Sex	Cause of Death	Date & Time of Death	Date & Time of receiving body in the mortuary	Identification Mark & Finger Impression	Details of next-of-kin	Post mortem done or not; if yes write details	List of valuables removed from the body	Sign of mortuary technician	Name of person (next-of-kin) receiving body	Signature of receiver	Remark

3. Mortality Review Form:

MORTALITY REVIEW FORM

Name of patient: .... Age/Sex: ....

Name of the Consultant: ....

Date of Admission: .... Date of Death: ....

Diagnosis: ....

Department: ....

Summary of Events:

Root Cause Analysis:

Corrective Action Taken:

Recommended Preventive Action:

Prepared By:

Sign of Committee Presiding Officer:

Sign of Chair Person:

BIBLIOGRAPHY, REFERENCES & ACKNOWLEDGMENTS:

1. Indian Public Health Standards (IPHS)
   Guidelines for District Hospitals (101 to 500 Bedded) Revised 2012 Directorate General of Health Services Ministry of Health & Family Welfare, Government of India
2. "Standard Operating Procedures SOP For Hospitals 2nd Edition" by Dr. Arun K. Agarwal
3. "Duties & Responsibilities of Hospital Staff" by Dr. Arun Kumar
4. "Checklists for Hospitals" by Dr. Arun K. Agarwal
5. Planning And Designing Of Modern Mortuary Complex In Tertiary Care, IIJFMT 4(1) 2006
   By: Dr. Sanju Singh, Dr. U.S. Sinha, Dr. A.K. Kapoor, Dr. S.K. Verma, Dr. Dalbir Singh, Dr. Susheel Sharma
   http://icfmt.net/journal/vol4no1/designing_of_modern_mortuary_complex.htm
6. Compendium of Norms for Designing of Hospitals & Medical Institutions, July 2019
   Published by Directorate General: Central Public Works Department, New Delhi
7. BBC Heart Care & Pruthi Hospital, Jalandhar
8. Death in Hospital Procedures, NHS Lothian,
   https://policyonline.nhslothian.scot/Policies/Procedure/Death%20in%20Hospital%20Procedures%20(Combined).pdf
9. Design and Layout of Mortuary Complex for a Medical College and Peripheral Hospitals; by Basant Lal Sirohiwal*, Paliwal PK, Luv Sharma and Hitesh Chawla, Department of Forensic Medicine, Pt. B.D. Sharma Postgraduate Institution of Medical Sciences, University of Health Sciences, Rohtak, Haryana, India
10. Hospital Manual, DGHS, MoHFW, GOI
11. Capital Hospital –Bhubaneswar, (Health & F.W. Deptt., Govt. Of Odisha)
12. National Quality Assurance Standards

Chapter – 16

DEPARTMENT OF NEPHROLOGY

INDEX

INTRODUCTION:

Nephrology is defined as study of kidney and kidney related diseases.

This department of the hospital boosts for having state-of-art equipment and facilities to diagnose and treat simple as well as complex kidney related ailments.

The department focuses on ensuring normal kidney functions by treating conditions that damage kidney.

AIM, VISION & MISSION:

1. To address all kidney related diseases in a holistic manner
2. To provide comprehensive treatment to patients visiting this department.

3. To provide most modern services in various fields of nephrology to patients at an affordable cost.
4. To create research material of national and international standard and publish them.
5. To provide all services under one roof.
6. To create standards comparable to national and international standards.

INFRASTRUCTURE/EQUIPMENT:

OPDs are located on ground floor while the Dialysis department is located on first floor of this hospital.

Wards are on 3rd floor while ICU is on 5th floor of the hospital.

1. Haemodialysis Machines.
2. Clinical Laboratory
3. Endoscopic Equipment and instruments.
4. ABG machine
5. CT, MRI, Ultrasound
6. Ventilators

DISEASES TREATED IN THIS DEPARTMENT:

Following are few conditions that are treated in the department of Nephrology of this hospital.

1. Presence of urea, protein, sugar, blood, casts, and crystals in urine in excess amount,
2. Acute and chronic Renal Failures,
3. Renal damage (Damaged kidney filtration system),
4. Kidney diseases associated with systemic disorders such as Hypertension, Diabetes etc when renal functions are affected,
5. Inflammations of Kidney (nephritis, Glomerulonephritis),
6. Tumours of Cancers of the kidneys, bladder, and urethra,
7. Infections of Kidney, bladder and urethra,
8. Renal vascular diseases,
9. Autoimmune diseases,
10. Electrolyte or acid-base imbalance
11. Hydronephrosis, Nephrotic Syndrome,
12. Dialysis department is a part of this department,
13. Some diseases related to kidney functions such as anaemia,
14. Renal Transplantations.
15. Hereditary renal disorders
16. Kidney Trauma

COMMON SYMPTOMS & SIGNS IN KIDNEY RELATED CONDITIONS:

1. Swelling in the legs, ankles, or feet
2. Consistent headaches
3. Swelling and stiffness of joints
4. Unexplained blood pressure problems
5. Muscle cramps, numbness, or weakness

6. Blood in the urine (haematuria)
7. Reduced urine output
8. Undefined loss of appetite

FACILITIES/SERVICES AVAILABLE/OFFERED IN THIS DEPARTMENT:

1. OPD consultation (On daily basis)
2. Casualty Services
3. Dialysis (both haemodialysis and peritoneal dialysis)
4. Renal Transplant
5. Ultrasound required for Guided Biopsies
6. Support services of CT, X-Ray, MRI for Intravenous urography, IVP, Renal angiography etc
7. Fully equipped pathology Laboratory
8. OT for various diagnostic and therapeutic endoscopic procedures.
9. Ambulatory Blood Pressure monitoring
10. Robotic Surgery

PROCEDURES PERFORMED IN THIS DEPARTMENT:

1. Haemodialysis and peritoneal dialysis.
2. SLED, CRRT
3. Kidney and prostate Biopsy (Endoscopic Procedures)
4. Permcath Insertion.
5. Preparing AV Fistula.
6. Renal nutrition Therapy.
7. Renal Transplant.

OPD:

1. Outpatient consultation for age group of patients.
2. Diagnose, prevent and treats such ailments with medication without admission
3. Follow up of such cases after indoor/surgical treatment.

SPECIALTY CLINICS:

1. Paediatric Nephrology
2. Renal Transplant
3. Dialysis Clinic
4. Diabetic Nephropathy Clinic

STAFFING:

The department is headed by well qualified and experienced Nephrologists assisted with a team of trained support staff.

1. Nephrologists
2. Psychologists

3. Nurses
4. Technicians, (OT and Dialysis Technicians)
5. Urologists to advice
6. Dieticians

HIGHLIGHTS OF THE DEPARTMENT:

1. Quality care at affordable price.
2. Qualified faculty and support staff.
3. Modern Dialysis Unit with 10 haemodialysis machines.
4. Kidney and prostate biopsies under ultrasound guidance.
5. A dedicated renal ward and renal ICU

DUTIES AND RESPONSIBILITIES:

A. Duties of Nephrologists:

1. Consulting, examining and advising proper treatment to patients in OPD, IPD and Casualty.
   This would include taking medical history, blood and urine tests, kidney ultrasound, biopsy, etc., depending on the condition.
2. Referring patients to urologists as per need.
3. Taking care of patients after a surgical procedure even if performed by a urologist.
4. Performing skilled procedures and operations.
5. Providing pre and post operative care.
6. Charting right treatment plan, monitoring and administering medication.
7. To keep all medical records, update as per NABH requirements.
8. To continuously monitor quality indicators (KPI).
9. Responsibility of specialist medical care.
10. Accountability of clinical outcomes.
11. Maintaining proper and complete medical records.
12. Other normal duties as Disposal of BMW, taking care of hospital acquired infections (infection control) etc.
13. To take part in committees meeting whenever called for.
14. To keep himself abreast with modern techniques by attending seminars and conferences.
15. To undertake studies and research.
16. To interact with other departments whenever required.
17. Will visit the department regularly (daily or at-least twice a week).
18. Will be responsible for overall functioning of this department.
19. Will assess each patient before start of first dialysis and will give instruction of dialysis.
20. Will take and ensure that infection control measures.
21. Will evaluate the dialysis technician and other dialysis staff.
22. Will provide round the clock coverage to this department in this hospital.
23. Will regularly review the patient's undergoing dialysis.
24. Will supervise/guide the in-house doctor who is responsible to this department (Dialysis doctor - JR).

B. Duties & Responsibilities of a Dialysis JR (Dialysis Doctor):

1. Will be responsible for day-to-day management of patients.
2. Will assess the patient before start of each dialysis session for hemodynamic status, recent surgery, vascular access, bleeding disorders etc.
3. Will be involved with dialysis technician in patient management during dialysis.
4. Will handle any emergency situation with the patient.
5. Will be in-charge of this department for day-to-day operations.
6. Will be responsible for updating/answering patient/relatives' queries.

STATIONARY FORMATS:

1. AUDIT REPORT FORMAT OF NEPHROLOGY

AUDIT REPORT FORMAT OF NEPHROLOGY

(Especially for transplant section)

AS PER ISO 9001:2008, ISO 14001:2004 & OHSAS 18001

Date of Audit: ....

Auditors: a) ....

Auditee: a) ....

S.N.	Observations	Remark
1	SOPs to be reviewed for adequacy?	
2	List of records/activities are maintained in the department?	
3	Quality policy and objectives are not known to staff?	
4	Document and data control procedure is implemented?	
5	Register for client's complaint/CAPA needs to be maintained. (Sentinel events/ADRs to be maintained)	
6	There is general awareness for standard/quality manual?	
7	Key indicators for process performance are maintained in the department. Trend analysis to be maintained.	

Quality Indicators (KPI):

1. Percentage of patients undergoing dialysis after renal transplant:
   Formula:
   Number of patients undergoing dialysis after renal transplant divided by total number of renal transplants undertaken in that period and then multiplied by 100
2. Percentage of patients undergoing pre-emptive dialysis before taking up renal transplant for any medical reason:
   Formula:
   Number of patients undergoing pre-emptive dialysis during a period divided by total renal transplants in that period multiplied by 100

3. Incidence of Hospital Associated Infection in Renal IPD/ICU:
   Formula:
   Number of patients reporting HAI divided by total admissions in wards & ICU during same period multiplied by 100
4. Mortality rate after renal transplant:
   Formula:
   Number of patients died within 1 month of renal transplant surgery divided by total renal transplants performed during same period then multiplies by 100
5. Patients waiting time in OPD/Dialysis
6. Patents satisfaction level.

RENAL TRANSPLANT:

1. Kidney transplant is a good and effective treatment option for a patient with "End Stage Renal Disease".
2. The transplant surgery can be performed by availing a live donor kidney or cadaveric Donor.
3. The hospital follows Transplantation of Human Organs Act 1994.
4. As far as possible only related donors are accepted.
5. Un related donors must have previous authorization from a special committee
6. The live donor nephrectomy is performed both by open surgery and by laparoscopic method.
7. The transplant surgery is done in a dedicated operation theatre.
8. Post surgery the patient is kept in isolation to prevent any cross infection.
9. The patient is discharged after complete stabilization.
10. The hospital has conducted about ...... transplants in last year.

Conditions Leading To Renal Transplant:

When the kidneys stop working, the condition is referred to as ESRD ("end-stage renal disease"). Toxic waste products accumulate in the body and either dialysis or a kidney transplant is required to sustain life.

The most common causes of kidney failure include:

1. Diabetes
2. Hypertensive nephrosclerosis
3. Polycystic kidney disease
4. Glomerular diseases
5. Renovascular and other vascular diseases
6. Congenital, familial and metabolic disorders
7. Tubular and interstitial diseases
8. Neoplasms

AREAS OF RESEARCH:

1. Autoimmune diseases of kidney.
2. Complications of Chronic Renal Diseases.

BIBLIOGRAPHY, REFERENCES & ACKNOWLEDGMENTS:

1. "Standard Operating Procedures SOP For Hospitals 2nd Edition" by Dr. Arun K. Agarwal
2. "Duties & Responsibilities of Hospital Staff" by Dr. Arun Kumar
3. "Checklists for Hospitals" by Dr. Arun K. Agarwal
4. Standard Operating Procedures (SOP) For Hospitals In India: Complete with Stationery Formats Used in Various Departments in a Hospital– 19 July 2022 by Arun K. Agarwal
5. Indian Public Health Standards (IPHS)

   Guidelines for District Hospitals (101 to 500 Bedded) Revised 2012 Directorate General of Health Services Ministry of Health & Family Welfare, Government of India
6. Hospital Manual. DGHS, Ministry of Health & Family Welfare, GOI

Chapter – 17

DEPARTMENT OF DIALYSIS

INDEX

1. Introduction
2. Definition
3. Services
4. Department Planning
5. Some Facts
6. Typical Layout of a Dialysis Unit
7. Equipment Planning
8. Specifications in a Haemodialysis Machine
9. RO Water Plant
10. List of Consumables in Dialysis Department
11. Electrical Load of Various Machines
12. Water Quality Standards for Haemodialysis
13. Types of Dialysis
14. Infrastructure
15. Staffing (Personnel Planning)
16. Organogram
17. Operational Timings
18. Duties & Responsibilities
    a. Dialysis Technician
    b. Dialysis Nurse
19. Procedure
20. General Instructions
21. Starting of Haemodialysis Process
22. Complications during Dialysis
23. Disinfection of HD Machines
24. Quality Indicators of Dialysis Unit (KPI)
25. Check Lists
    a. Checklist Dialysis Technician
    b. Checklist Dialysis Centre (Planning)
    c. Checklist Dialysis
    d. Checklist Infection Prevention in Dialysis
    e. Checklist Disinfection of Dialysis Machine & Area

f. Checklist Dialysis Procedure
g. Checklist Dialyser Reuse/Reprocessing
h. Checklist Daily Reporting (MIS)
i. Dialysis Unit Audit Checklist

26. Stationary Formats
    a. Consent for Dialysis
    b. Haemodialysis Record Booklet
    c. Master Register
27. Records to be Maintained
    a. Relating to Patient care
    b. Incident and Accident Record: (KPI Record)
    c. Water treatment Record
    d. Staff Vaccination Status
28. List of Legal Requirements
29. Bibliography/References/Future Reading

INTRODUCTION:

Dialysis is a process for removing waste and excess water from the blood and is used primarily as an artificial replacement for lost kidney function in people with kidney failure.

Dialysis may be used for those with an acute disturbance in kidney function (acute kidney injury, previously acute renal failure) or progressive but chronically worsening kidney function—a state known as chronic kidney disease stage 5 (previously chronic renal failure or end-stage renal disease). The latter form may develop over months or years, but in contrast to acute kidney injury is not usually reversible and dialysis is regarded as a "holding measure" until a kidney transplant can be performed or sometimes as the only supportive measure in those for whom a transplant would be inappropriate.

[From Wikipedia, the free encyclopedia; https://en.wikipedia.org/wiki/Dialysis]

Dialysis s required when our normal kidneys are not able to perform to its capacity

Dialysis allows patients with kidney failure a chance to live productive lives.

It is also called as RRT – Renal Replacement Therapy.

The department of dialysis in this hospital is equipped with world class machines and other facilities.

DEFINITION:

Dialysis is a type of renal replacement therapy which is used to provide an artificial replacement for lost kidney functions. There are two main forms of dialysis, Haemodialysis and Peritoneal Dialysis, both of which are life support treatments; but dialysis does not treat kidney diseases. Dialysis may be used for patients who have recently lost kidney functions (acute renal failure) or for patients who have permanently lost kidney functions (chronic or end-stage renal failure).

SERVICES:

The dialysis department is located on .... (basement) of this hospital. It is spread in about 100 Sq. Meters. It has got four dialysis machines. One is reserved for Hepatitis B+ patients.

The department is equipped with 4 state-of-the-art machines. The reverse osmosis plant is located on the terrace which supplies RO water to these four machines as well as two another two dialysis locations in MICU/SICU.

The department also takes care of pre-operative dialysis of the patients who are advised so.

We can easily accept up-to 8 patients per day.

It is a professionally managed unit, equipped with highly skilled Nephrologists and Urologists who are available round the clock.

Hepatitis patients are provided dialysis on a separate machine in a separate cubicle.

The unit also has dialysis chairs to provide treatment in sitting positions so that patients can also read newspapers etc. The department has one TV also for entertainment of patients during the treatment process in an air-conditioned atmosphere.

DEPARTMENT PLANNING:

1. The location should offer easy access for outpatients.
2. Accessibility to the renal dialysis centre from parking and public transportation shall be a consideration. The location of a renal dialysis facility shall offer access from parking and from public transportation, if available.
3. At least one examination room should be provided with clear floor area of approximately 100 Sq. Feet. – 11' x 10' (10 Sq. Meters). It should have a wash basin and a counter for writing purposes.
4. Waiting/reception area should be approximately 200 Sq. Feet.
5. Head side of each treatment bay (Machine) should have stable power supply of about 3 sockets (6 pin sockets) of 5/15 ampere, Oxygen and suction outlet, RO water inlet and an outlet (drainage point). UPS should be provided with a backup of at-least 30 minutes. The haemodialysis machine should be on UPS, even if internal battery is provided with the machines.
6. The temperature of treatment area should be maintained at 21-22 degree Celsius and Rh should be maintained at 55 to 60%.
7. The treatment area should be separate from waiting areas and it should have cubicle partition for providing privacy to each patient.
8. Each cubicle should be about 80 Sq. Feet. There should be a space of about 4 feet between two dialysis beds/chairs.
9. The nurse station should be inside the treatment area so as to provide visual observation to each cubicle.
10. There should be a separate bay for Hepatitis –B positive (HBsAg +) patients, again within visual contact with nurse station. If separate machine is not available, the normal machine after use will be decontaminated by cleaning all external surfaces with soap and water followed by application of a disinfectant (according to manufacturer's directions) prior to use on another patient.
11. There should be one clean supply room. (Area about 100 Sq. Feet)
12. It will be better if one dirty utility is also provided to store soiled items. It should have wash basin, work counter, storage cabinets and soiled linen hamper. It should have a floor area of 50–80 Sq. Feet.
13. The department should have parking area for wheel chairs, stretchers etc.
14. There should be one change room for staff to change before entering in the treatment area.
15. There should be a toilet attached or nearby the treatment area. Approximate size should be 50 Sq. Feet.

16. There should be one Dialyser reprocessing (dialyser wash) room. This room should have proper ventilation arrangements.
17. Separate plumbing should be done for RO water supply at each machine station.
18. RO water machine should be housed in a separate area. It has a pumping mechanism to supply water at a required pressure. If so one switch should be provided in the treatment area near dialysis technician place so that he can start and stop the pump from inside the treatment area.
19. The overall ambience of the treatment area should be cheerful and not dull.
20. The entry door should be 1.21 meter wide to facilitate easy movements of beds & equipment.
21. Beds may be mechanical or electrical with detachable/collapsible side railings.
22. Air-conditioning: The temperature should be maintained at 22 to 24 degrees Celsius with 55 to 60% humidity.
23. Plumbing & Drainage: All treated water pipelines should be stainless steel grade 316 or medical grade PVC. There should be minimum bends & blind loops should be avoided. All drainage should be connected directly to the main drainage line. There should be no bends or blind loops.

SOME FACTS:

1. 150 litres of De-ionized water is required per patient.
2. 30 litres per hour De-ionized water is required per machine.
3. Artificial Kidney can be used 4 to 5 times depending on the Brand.
4. Artificial Kidney is washed by locally made equipment – called DIALYSER REUSE SYSTEM – by cleaning solution (Bleaching Powder + H_2O_2 + H_2O)

Typical layout of a Dialysis Department:

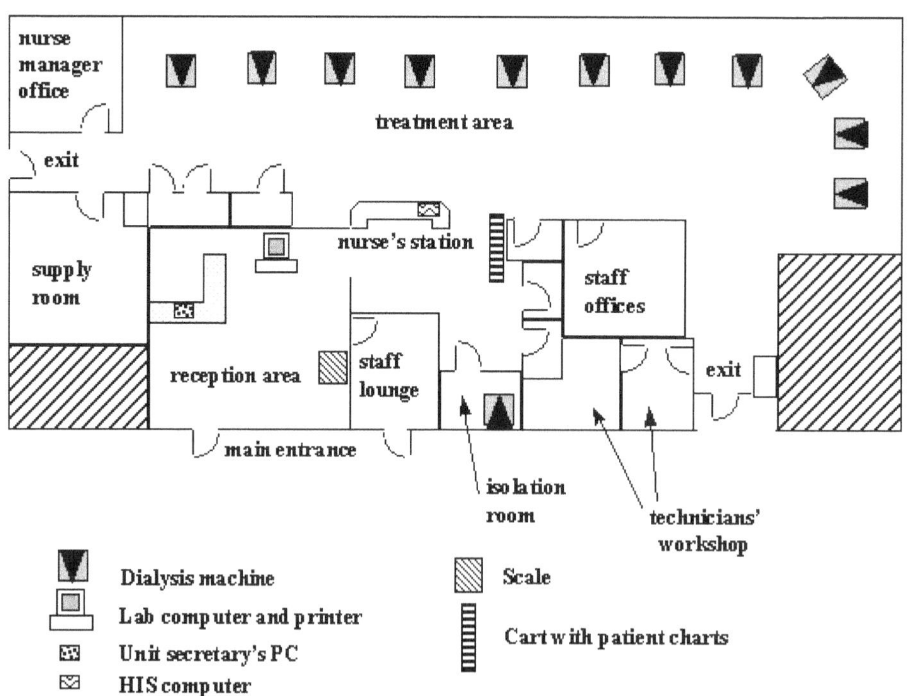

Typical planning of one treatment cubicle:

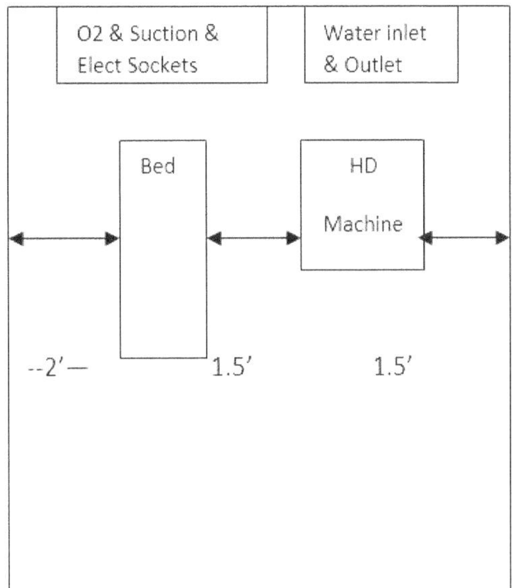

EQUIPMENT PLANNING:

For 4 Dialysis Machines:

Dialysis Room

SN	Equipment	Qty		SN	Equipment	Qty
01.	Haemodialysis Machine (for both Acetate & Bicarbonate)	4		02.	Bed, Fowler	4
03.	IV Stand	4		04.	Television	1
05.	ECG Monitor with SpO2 & NIBP	4		06.	Central Oxygen Outlet	4

Nurse Station

SN	Equipment	Qty		SN	Equipment	Qty
01.	X-Ray View Box	1		02.	Table (or Counter)	1
03.	Chair, on castors	1		04.	BP Apparatus, dial type	1
05.	Torch, 2-cell	1		06.	Notice Board	1
07.	Wall Clock	1		08.	Emergency Trolley, c/w all medicines	1
09	Bin, disposal, Bio-medical waste, 3 colours	03		10.	Defibrillator	1

Relative Wait

SN	Equipment	Qty		SN	Equipment	Qty
01.	Television Set	1		02.	Sofa Set, 3-seater	2
03.	Sofa Set, 1-seater	3		04.	Table, Centre	1
05.	Water Dispenser/Coffee machine	1				

SPECIFICATIONS IN A HAEMODIALYSIS MACHINE:

A. **Must have:**

1. Blood pump to achieve a unidirectional flow of up to 400 ml/min
2. Heparin pump
3. Arterial line and venous line pressure monitors
4. Functional air bubble detector
5. Mixing proportion unit with bicarbonate dialysis facility, rate of dialysate delivery from 300 to 500 ml/min or more.
6. Conductivity meter
7. Functional blood leak detector
8. Dialysate temperature regulator that has a range of temperature 35 to 39 degree centigrade
9. Volumetric UF control
10. Safety devices: functioning alarms, venous blood clamp

B. **Optional:**

1. On-line blood volume monitor
2. On-line urea clearance
3. Sodium profiling of dialysate
4. Single needle dialysis facility
5. Haemodia-filtration
6. Optical detector

C. **Disinfection of a HD Machine:**

1. After any case of blood leak into dialysate
2. Regular disinfection once a week
3. If a culture shows any infection.

RO WATER PLANT:

1. For a department with 4 dialysis machines, requirement will be of one RO plant of capacity of 500 L/Hr
2. One RO plant of capacity of 500 litters per hour will require a room size of 10′ x 8′
3. The plant should be maintained as per manufacturer's guidelines.
4. The output water quality should be always tested and monitored at regular intervals.

LIST OF CONSUMABLES IN DIALYSIS DEPARTMENT:

SN	Equipment	SN	Equipment
01.	I.V. Fluids	02.	H.D. Fluids (Bicarb & Acetate)
03.	Acetic Acid	04.	Citric Acid
05.	Medicines	05.	Fistula Needle
07.	Guide Wire	08.	Dialysers & Tubing
09.	Femoral Catheter	10.	Introducer Cannula
11.	I.V. Set	12.	B.T. Set
13.	Syringes	14.	Cotton
15.	Formalin	16.	H2O2

SN	Equipment		SN	Equipment
17.	Gauze		18.	Spirit
19.	Betadine			

ELECTRICAL LOAD OF VARIOUS MACHINES:

Approximate electrical load is as follows. It may differ on the make of equipment.

SN	Equipment	Unit Load (VA)	On DG (VA)	ON UPS (VA)
1	Dialysis Unit	2000	2000	Battery is available
2	RO Plant (500 l/hr)	4000	4000	4000
3	Monitor (ECG, SpO2, NIBP)	200	200	Battery is available
4	Defibrillator	50	50	Battery is available

WATER QUALITY STANDARDS FOR HAEMODIALYSIS:

Category	Substance	Symbol	AAMI max. level (Also recommended by the RA) *	From EC ** Pharmacopoeia
1	Aluminium	Al	0.01 ppm	0.01 ppm
1	Copper	Cu	0.1 ppm	#
1	Fluoride	F	0.2 ppm	0.2 ppm
1	Nitrates	NO3	2 ppm	2 ppm
1	Sulphate	SO4	100 ppm	50 ppm
1	Zinc	Zn	0.1 ppm	0.1 ppm
1	Chloramines		0.1 ppm	
1	Free Chlorine	CL2	0.5 ppm	
1	Total Available Chlorine			0.1 ppm
2	Calcium	Ca	2 ppm	2 ppm
2	Magnesium	Mg	4 ppm	2 ppm
2	Potassium	K	8 ppm	2 ppm
2	Sodium	Na	70 ppm	50 ppm
2	Chlorides	Cl		50 ppm
3	Arsenic	As	0.005 ppm.	#
3	Barium	Ba	0.1 ppm.	#
3	Cadmium	Cd	0.001 ppm.	#
3	Chromium	Cr	0.01 ppm.	#
3	Lead	Pb	0.005 ppm.	#
3	Mercury	Hg	0.002 ppm	0.001 ppm
3	Selenium	Se	0.01 ppm	
3	Silver	Ag	0.005	#
	pH			6 8 pH

Category	Substance	Symbol	AAMI max. level (Also recommended by the RA) *	From EC ** Pharmacopoeia
	Oxidisable Substances			Nil
	Ammonium			0.2 ppm
	Heavy Metals			0.1 ppm
	Microbial Contamination		TVC < 200 per ml	TVC < 100 per ml
	Endotoxins		10.0 EU/ml	< 0.25 EU/ml

Categories:

1. Toxic substances described in Dialysis literature.
2. Non-toxic substances included in dialysis fluid.
3. Substances described as toxic in Drinking Water literature.

   * From a draft document by the Standards Subcommittee of the Renal Association.

   ** From 'Water for diluting concentrated haemodialysis solutions' Annex to the European Pharmacopoeia Fascicule 16. (Adopted by the Council of Europe)

   # included in the global limit for Heavy Metals

(Taken from "The Association for the Advancement of Medical Instrumentation (USA) 1981")

(The Renal Association, European Community 1992)

TYPES OF DIALYSIS:

1. Haemodialysis and
2. Peritoneal dialysis.

INFRASTRUCTURE:

The dialysis department of this hospital is located on first floor of the hospital. It is currently equipped with 10 haemodialysis machines with dedicated support facilities for each machine. The department has dedicated machines for patients who are HbsAg positive.

The department also has a dedicated RO plant for supply of RO water to haemodialysis machines. It is ensured that TDS and hardness of this RO water is meeting national and international standards.

STAFFING (Personnel Planning):

Counter	General Shift 9 am to 6 pm	Shift 1 8 am to 2 pm	Shift 2 2 pm to 8 pm	Shift 3 8 pm to 8 am (next day)	Reliever	Total
Nephrologist	1					1
Dialysis Doctor (JR)	1					1
Dialysis Technician	2					2
Staff Nurse	2					2
Dialysis Attendant (Ward Boy)	1					1
Housekeeper	1					1
Total	8					8

ORGANOGRAM (Organisational Structure) Dialysis Dept.:

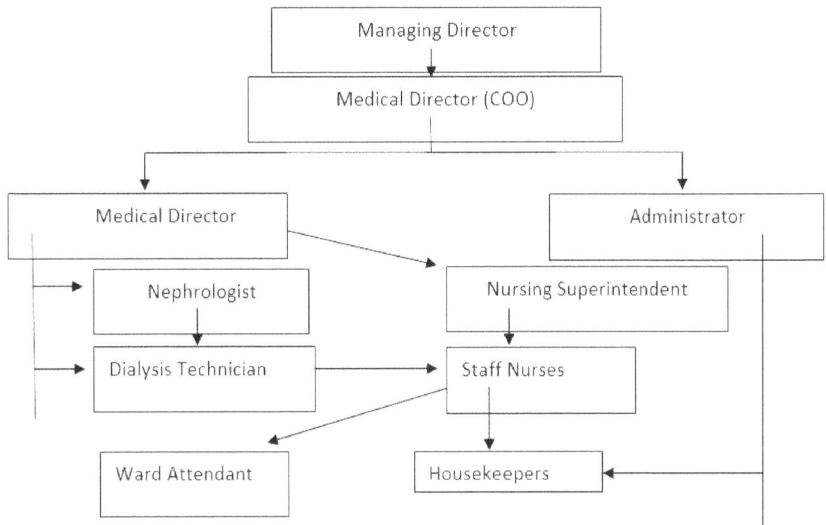

OPERATIONAL TIMINGS:

The department will work from 9.00 am in the morning till 5.00 pm in the evening with one hour lunch break.

Emergency dialysis will be undertaken at any time.

DUTIES & RESPONSIBILITIES:

A. Duties & Responsibilities of Dialysis Technicians:

1. Will always wear apron on duty.
2. Will keep the machines in working order. He should always inform the Maintenance Department/ Biomedical department and M.S., if any of the machines is not working.
3. May allow only one attendant with the patient at the time of dialysis, that too with very sick or fussy patients after the permission of the doctor in-charge.
4. Will handle all telephonic quarries regarding dialysis.
5. Will give appointments in consultation with Nephrologists/Urologists.
6. Will keep the department always under lock & key.
7. Will also be responsible for proper functioning and operation of R.O. plant and he will take care of it with the Maintenance Department (electrician on duty).
8. Will keep the RO plant under lock and the keys will be with him.
9. Will switched off lights and fans when not in use. Electricity saving is the duty of all.
10. Will use the department TV strictly for the use of the patient and should not be used for entertainment of the staff.
11. Will remember that eating and drinking (except water & tea) is not allowed for the staff. Patient can have diet as per instructions of the NEPHROLOGIST.
12. Will check the Emergency Trolley every day in the morning for medicines and other stock and will replenish any used item that is keeping the inventory of medicines and other consumables.
13. To maintain proper inventory in the 'Crash Cart' provided in this department to meet any emergency.
14. To ensure that all patients booked for dialysis are tested for Hepatitis-B and other viral markers.
15. Will identify the patient and transport him up to dialysis bed.

16. Will explain the whole dialysis process to first-timers.
17. Will respond quickly to emergency situations and patient calls.
18. Will continuously monitor the vascular access of the patient.
19. Will document patient's vitals (pre-dialysis weight, temperature, BP, Pulse & Respiration).
20. To make sure that the alarms and monitors are set as per re commendations of the manufacturer of the machine.
21. To make sure temperature, conductivity of the water is in accordance with the set protocols.
22. To explain the full procedure to the patient before starting the process.
23. To take a written 'Informed Consent' at all dialysis sessions from all patients, paid or complimentary.
24. Will maintain a register of patients undergoing dialysis and also the consumables used per patient. It will help in proper inventory keeping and in calculating the cost incurred per patient.
25. Will operate the dialysis machine. He will be responsible for their operation, cleaning, and sterilisation.
26. Will record all findings before, during and after dialysis in "Dialysis Record" of the patient, as per format printed on that.
27. As dialysis technicians work with blood, they must exercise strict safety precautions against infectious diseases such as hepatitis and AIDS.
28. Generally, procedure should be started after proper billing.
29. To carry out work allocated to 'Dialysis Nurse' in her absence.
30. Will participate in quality improvement meetings.
31. Will perform all such duties as allocated by his seniors.

B. Duties & Responsibilities of Dialysis Nurse:

Summary: A dialysis nurse is a registered nurse specialised in nephrology nursing. His/her work involves taking care of patients with impaired kidney function undergoing haemodialysis or peritoneal dialysis. The dialysis nurse must have an intricate knowledge of the machines of both types of dialysis; administer the dialysis from start to finish; discuss and explain concerns and answer relevant questions of the patient; and monitor and asses the patient's vital signs and reaction to treatment.

1. Will perform all primary nursing duties which include routine assessments, determining risks, and administering transfusions if necessary, recording chart data and information for the nephrologists to assess the patient's condition.
2. Will also educate the patient about his or her treatment.
3. Will also check and ensure the function of the machine and other necessary equipment before/ during dialysis.
4. Will keep an eye (for any oversight/mistake) on technician work and will cooperate with him.
5. Will train any new incumbent in the proper usage of the dialysis machines and safety protocols.
6. Will be responsible for inventory upkeep of consumables and non-consumables items.
7. Will check the patient for vitals before starting the actual dialysis.
8. Will check all the pathological investigation reports.
9. Will help the Nephrologists/Technician in starting the dialysis.
10. Will educate patient about his/her treatment.
11. Will start the dialysis after verifying financial clearances.
12. Will check the functioning of the machine before start of the procedure.
13. To administer medications as per advice of the nephrologists.
14. Will keep an eye on patient vitals at all times during the dialysis.
15. Will ensure comfort of the patient during the procedure.
16. Will not allow visitors inside the dialysis ward when the treatment is on.

17. Will monitor dialysis progress and
18. Will follow up with dialysis patients.
19. Will complete documentation of all patients as required by hospital policies.
20. Will replenish the depleted stocks.
21. Will deal with biomedical waste as per law.
22. Will adhere to hospital policies and procedures.

PROCEDURE:

It can simply be written in three steps.

a. Initiation (Starting)
b. Monitoring (During)
c. Discontinuation (Termination)

GENERAL INSTRUCTIONS:

1. All procedures will be done by appointment usually (Except in emergency cases or by orders of the Nephrologists). Appointment for dialysis should be taken by the patient or by the attendant of the patient.
2. It shall be the responsibility of the dialysis technician to prior inform Nephrologists regarding haemodialysis & to maintenance department to avoid power fluctuation during dialysis process.
3. On the day of dialysis technician shall get the consent form filled by the patient or by the attendant of the patient.
4. Before starting dialysis process, technician shall ensure regarding the deposit of dialysis charges at reception.
5. During dialysis it shall be the duty of technician to ensure that attendants of patient sit outside the dialysis room.
6. No person shall be allowed to enter in the dialysis room with shoes.
7. Dialysis technician must wear gloves and other protective garments at the starting of dialysis & at the termination of dialysis.
8. Technician must inform to staff nurse on duty at ICU to seek help during dialysis process. (Provided staff nurse is free)
9. All accessories in dialysis room i.e., TV, Blower, etc. shall remain switched off if dialysis is not in process.
10. It shall be the responsibility of dialysis technician to check the conductivity of R.O. water one-day before the dialysis process.
11. It shall be entire responsibility of the technician to ensure the availability of requisite stock of medicines & dialysis Material.
12. All telephonic queries about dialysis will be diverted to dialysis technician. He should handle these queries with great care.
13. The Nephrologist should immediately be informed of any booking of dialysis. In-fact all booking should be done in consultation with the Nephrologist.
14. Eating and drinking will be allowed only in specified area.
15. Hand washing is mandatory before and after each patient contact and after removal of gloves.
16. Staff having any cut or lacerations, must cover that with waterproof dressings.
17. All patients undergoing dialysis must be tested for Hepatitis-B (HBsAg testing).
18. Patients with Hepatitis-C need not be segregated and will not require a separate machine.
19. All dialysis staff should be vaccinated with Hepatitis-B Vaccine.

STARTING OF HAEMODIALYSIS PROCESS:

1. Rinse the Machine for at least five minutes. It helps in removing dust particles, any bacteria formation in the tubing.
2. Take weight of the patient to compare it with post dialysis weight.
3. Do priming of dialyser and tubing with at least one & half litter normal saline to remove the air from the extra corporeal circuit.
4. Put BP cuff on patient's hand to record BP during treatment.
5. Part preparation – Shaving of the femoral triangle or cleaning of the AV fistula or intrajugular catheter whichever is applicable.
6. Catheterisation of Vascular excess or flushing intrajugular catheter with saline as per requirement.
7. Give Heparin dose to avoid blood clotting as per the advised of the Nephrologist.

   (to be given after every hour during dialysis also)
8. Technician shall enter in the haemodialysis record book; blood pressure after every half an hour, Heparin dose, pre & post dialysis weight, weight loss, medication, complications.
9. It shall be the responsibility of the nephrologist to enter his/her comments regarding dialysis in the HD record book.
10. **Pre-dialysis safety checks;**
    a. Check water system for; Temperature, Resistivity & Residual disinfectant.
    b. Prescribed Dialyzer & Concentrate
    c. Dialysis Machine Safety for;
       - Alarms active,
       - Dialysate conductivity &/or pH
    d. Integrity of Extracorporeal Circuit
    e. If Dialyzer is Reused;
       - Check patient's name on label,
       - Perform Disinfectant residual test.
11. **Pre-dialysis Patient Evaluation:**
    a. Physical Parameters: Weight, BP (stand & sitting), Temperature, Pulse & Respiration, Complaints
    b. Evaluate Access Status;
       - Signs of infection – redness, tenderness, unusual warmth, purulent drainage
       - Patency - Graft & AVF: bruit, thrill, Catheter: easy aspiration (post disinfection)
       - Direction of flow (identify A & V)
    c. Follow Universal Precautions: Wash hands, Put Glove, Gown & Mask, Take eye protection
12. **Initiation of Dialysis:**
    a. Graft/Fistula;
       Select sites, disinfect it, anesthetise it, insert needles
    b. Catheters;
       Disinfect catheter limbs, Aspirate heparin from limbs, Evaluate patency
    c. Draw Blood Work;
       Prior to administering heparin, from arterial port, Administer heparin post draw
    d. Initiate Blood Flow to Dialyzer:
       Connect lines & Start at low BFR

13. **Post Initiation:**
    a. Calculate/Apply TMP;
    - Fluid gain/# Hours = UF vol (ml/hr)
    - UF Volume/UF Coefficient = TMP
    - TMP = V resistance + Neg pressure

    b. Set machine parameters;
    - BFR, DFR, UFR, & Alarm limits
    - Dialysate temp & Heparin Infusion rate

    c. Take Patient comfort measures
14. **Do proper charting of;**
    a. Prescribed parameters
    b. Pre & Post patient assessment
    c. Vital signs during treatment
    d. Medications given
    e. Treatment parameters - BFR, DFR, A & V pressures, TMP/UFR
    f. Patient/machine complications
    g. Put your (dialysis technician) signature on all documents
15. **During Haemodialysis Process:**
    a. Record BP every half hour
    b. Keep a check on the site (fistula/femoral needle etc) for any leakage.

Summary:

Detect complications:

A. Blood Related Complications;
   1. Air in Blood Circuit
   2. Air Embolism
   3. Blood Loss
   4. Access Recirculation
   5. Clotting
   6. Poor BFR
   7. Needle Infiltration

B. Dialysate Side Complications;
   1. Dialysate Temperature (Hypothermia, Hyperthermia)
   2. Haemolysis (Dialysate temperature, kinked blood lines, formaldehyde in dialysate lines, inadequate water treatment - chloramines, copper, zinc, nitrates
   3. Crenation (Hypertonic dialysate)

C. Patient Related Complications;

   Fatigue, Itchy Skin, Hypotension, Hypertension, Muscle Cramps, Headache, Nausea & Vomiting, Fever &/or Chills, Fistula/Graft Infection, Thrombosis, Fistula Aneurysm, Pseudo-aneurysm, Central Venous Catheter Infection, Catheter Thrombosis, Cardiac Dysrhythmia, Pericarditis, pericardial effusion, cardiac tamponade, Dialysis Disequilibrium Syndrome, First Use Syndrome, Seizures, Angina, Anaphylaxis, Pruritis, Steal Syndrome, Cardiac Arrest, Dialysis Encephalopathy (Al++)

D. Look for Extracorporeal Circuit Pressures

E. Do charting and put signature on case papers.

16. **Termination of Haemodialysis Process:**
    a. Discontinue heparin infusion
    b. Chart patient & machine parameters
    c. Draw post-dialysis blood samples
    d. Transfer the blood from extra corporeal circuit to the patient's body.
    e. Check patient's BP before disconnection
    f. Remove Catheter/needle
    g. Assess the patient
    h. Wash the dialyser and tubing by Hydrogen Peroxide & water (For reuse).
    i. Get the post dialysis weight of the patient.
    j. Enter in the haemodialysis record book of the patient; next date of Haemodialysis.
    k. Send the patient home/ward.
17. **Post-dialysis machine care:**
    a. Disconnect and rinse concentrate lines
    b. Remove dialyzer & bloodlines & dispose in biomedical waste container if not to be reused.
    c. Remove other disposables
    d. Remove & disinfect non-disposables (ex. clamps)
    e. Clean & disinfect outside of machine
18. **If Dialyser is to be reused:**
    a. Ensure that it is filled with saline or heparinised saline
    b. Ensure properly labelled with patient ID data
    c. Deposit in reuse area/cupboard within 10-15 min post dialysis

COMPLICATIONS DURING DIALYSIS:

1. Hypotension
2. Hypoglycaemia.
3. And Cramps

DISINFECTION OF HD MACHINES

The HD machine should be disinfected;

1. After an episode of blood leak in to the dialysate.
2. If surveillance cultures show high CFU or endotoxin levels
3. Regular disinfection at least once a week.
4. After each dialysis session or once a day (optional).
5. Bleach or Citrosteril (Combination of Citric, maleic and oxalic acid) or heat or a combination may be used for disinfection of HD machines.

Steps of Bleach Disinfection:

1. Bleach (Sodium hypochlorite 5%) is used for disinfecting the machine.
2. Bleach should not be heated.
3. If bleach disinfection is required for the blood leak, rinse machine for 15 minutes.
4. Ensure that power and water supply to the machine are operational.

5. Turn on the machines.
6. Press cleaning key.
7. Use up/down arrow keys to select "Cleaning (font supplied)"
8. Select Treatment/Rinse – select chemical mode – confirm.
9. Machine alarm "! Connect disinfectant" displayed.
10. Place PICKUP STICK Concentrate connectors into sodium hypochlorite at the front of the machine.
11. Press conf key, "Please Wait" displayed.
12. On completion "Mandatory rinse end" displayed.
13. Test for residual bleach using Chlorine test strips on completion of cycle.

Steps of Citrosteril Disinfection:

1. Following conditions/reminder must be fulfilled before activating the cleaning program:
   a. The dialysate lines are connected to the shunt (Rinse bridge).
   b. The shunt door is closed.
   c. The concentrate suction tubes are in the appropriate rinse ports.
   d. The optical detector does not sense blood.
2. Citrosteril should be fitted to the rear of the machine
3. Citrosteril should be heated (≥ 60 degree C) for efficient results.
4. Ensure that power and water supply to the machine are operational.
5. Turn on the machines.
6. Ensure the basic conditions/reminder (mentioned above) has been reviewed.
7. Press cleaning key.
8. Use up/down key to select the desired program- "Hot Disinfection".
9. Press conf key, "-F-HDIS- or –F-HDIS-M-HR- "displayed.
10. On completion "Mandatory Rinse End" will be displayed.
11. It is not necessary to test residual citric acid if Citrosteril is used, since it is a decaying agent which is formulated in a non-toxic solution.

QUALITY INDICATORS OF DIALYSIS UNIT:

1. Percentage of patients undergoing dialysis after renal transplant:
   Formula:
   Number of patients undergoing dialysis after renal transplant divided by total number of renal transplants undertaken in that period and then multiplied by 100
2. Percentage of patients undergoing pre-emptive dialysis before taking up renal transplant for any medical reason:
   Formula:
   Number of patients undergoing pre-emptive dialysis during a period divided by total renal transplants in that period multiplied by 100
3. Percentage of patients undergoing dialysis with AV Fistula:
   Formula: On same basis as above
4. Percentage of patients undergoing dialysis with femoral route:
   Formula: On same basis as above
5. Percentage of patency of AV Fistula:
6. One year survival rate on dialysis:

7. One year dialysis attrition rate:
8. Vascular access bloodstream infection rates in haemodialysis patients
9. Patents satisfaction level.
10. Incidence of complications.
11. Incidence of post-dialysis side effects.
12. Incidence of cross infection (should be less than 2%).
13. Post dialysis parameters (reduction in level of Urea & Creatinine up-to 65% and reduction in body weight.
14. Average number of patients treated daily.

CHECK LISTS:

A. Checklist For Dialysis Technician:

1. Each and every patient is assessed before undergoing dialysis?
2. Every patient is investigated for following every month?

Blood Urea	Serum Creatinine	Serum Sodium & Potassium
CBC	SGPT & SGOT	ECG

3. Medical records for each patient are generated and kept?
4. Female patients are taken in presence of a female attendant/employee?
5. Informed consent is taken from all patients?
6. Patients are given sufficient time to get their queries answered?
7. Measures are taken to reduce chances of hospital acquired infections?
8. A dialysis record card/discharge summary is always given to the patient at the end of each dialysis session?
9. Pre-dialysis and post-dialysis weight of the patient is monitored?
10. Blood spills are immediately taken care of?

B. Checklist Dialysis Centre (Planning):

SN	Check	Yes	No	Remark
1	The centre is registered with local authorities under "Clinical Establishment Act"?			
2	The centre has NOC from local Pollution Control Board?			
3	One dialysis cubicle is minimum 100 square feet in area?			
4	Each bed/cubicle has oxygen and suction supply preferable by central pipe line system?			
5	Each bed is having SpO2 monitoring system? Preferably basic 5 parameter vital sign monitor should be available at each bed side.			
6	Centre has a nurse Call Bell for each patient bed?			
7	Hospital has separate cubicle for handling +ve cases (Hepatitis B, C/HCV)?			
8	Cubicles for handling +ve cases have separate drainage system?			
9	Hand washing station/facility are available within the dialysis complex?			
10	Dialysers are reprocessed separately for normal and +ve patients?			
11	Dialyser reprocessing/washing area is away from main dialysis cubicles?			
12	Treated water/RO water pipeline for haemodialysis machines are of Stainless steel or of Medical grade PVC?			

SN	Check	Yes	No	Remark
13	Water supply to machines is with minimum bends.			
14	Water supply is checked for contamination at-least once in a month?			
15	A TV/piped music has been provided for patients' entertainment during dialysis?			
16	Each patient can be visually seen/watched from the central nurse station?			
17	Fire detection and firefighting controls are available within the department?			
18	A Defibrillator is available in the centre?			
19	The total environment is clean, safe and hygienic?			
20	The centre has good waiting area for the attendants of patients?			
21	Emergency drug trolley/Tray/Crash Cart are available inside the department?			
22	Biomedical waste disposal is as per government rules and regulations?			
23	Suitable power back-up is available?			
24	RO Plant membranes are cleaned and changed periodically?			

C. Checklist Dialysis:

SN	Check	Yes	No	Remark
1	Each and every patient is assessed before undergoing dialysis?			
2	Every patient is investigated for following every month? Blood Urea Serum Creatinine Serum Sodium & Potassium CBC SGPT & SGOT ECG			
3	Medical records for each patient are generated and kept?			
4	Female patients are taken in presence of a female attendant/employee?			
5	Informed consent is taken from all patients?			
6	Patients are given sufficient time to get their queries answered?			
7	Measures are taken to reduce chances of hospital acquired infections?			
8	A dialysis record card/discharge summary is always given to the patient at the end of each dialysis session?			
9	Pre-dialysis and post-dialysis weight of the patient is monitored?			
10	Blood spills are immediately taken care of?			

D. Checklist Infection Prevention in Dialysis:

SN	Check	Yes	No	Remark
1	All patients are tested for HBV, HCV and HIV before being taken for dialysis?			
2	Hands wash before starting and after ending a dialysis?			
3	Staff with any cut/abrasion in hands is using gloves?			

SN	Check	Yes	No	Remark
4	Personal protective apparels (Plastic Apron, Gloves, Eye glasses if required, etc.) are worn by staff?			
5	Staff must wear gloves before starting a dialysis?			
6	Hands are also washed after removal of gloves?			
7	Gloves are changed between patients?			
8	Blood spills are immediately taken care as per predefined protocol?			
9	The whole centre and dialysis cubicle in particular are clean and disinfected regularly?			
10	Dialysis machines are disinfected as per protocol/SOP?			
11	Machine is cleaned with a damp cloth externally after each procedure?			
12	Dialysis beds and other paraphernalia are also cleaned with soap water at the start of the day?			
13	All biomedical waste is disposed in prescribed manner?			
14	All staff is properly vaccinated against hepatitis B?			
15	Patients with communicable infections are given special care? They are asked to wear a face mask at least?			

E. Checklist Disinfection of Dialysis Machine & Area

SN	Check	Yes	No	Remarks
Before Disinfection				
1	Are there any visible sign of contamination of the machine?			
2	Check that all tubing and dialyser are disconnected and discarded.			
3	Check that waste bins are emptied.			
4	Dispose all single use items.			
5	Remove your gloves and wash your hands.			
Routine Disinfection				
6	Check that new gloves are worn			
7	Use disinfectant to all sides of the haemodialysis machine; rub it from dirty to clean side. Allow it to dry. Leave it for few minutes as per manufacturer's instructions.			
8	Wipe the machine clean.			
9	Similarly other articles of patient use (bed, bucket, etc.) should also be disinfected.			
10	Remove gloves and wash your hands.			

F. Checklist Dialysis Procedure

Based on WHO "Safe Surgery Checklist"

SIGN – IN (Before taking in Dialysis Cubicle)

1. Dialysis cubicle and HD machine is disinfected and ready to take next patient.
2. Next patient's investigations are in place.
3. Dialyser (old or new) and tubing along with dialysis solution is ready.
4. Patient's AV access is ready or need to be made.
5. Patient is not having an infection for which extra precautions (face mask etc.), may be required.

TIME – OUT (Before connecting to the HD machine)

1. Patient has identified himself/herself by name.
2. Patient history does not suggest any recent sickness.
3. Patient pre-dialysis medical examination (BP, Weight, etc.) done.
4. Duration of dialysis and other plan discussed with the patient as well as with the nurse/dialysis technician.
5. Patient consent taken.

SIGN – OUT (Before patient leaves the dialysis cubicle)

1. HD Machine detached from the patient.
2. Patient BP and weight is checked.
3. Discharge summary given to the patient with date of next dialysis.

G. Checklist Dialyser Reuse/Reprocessing:

SN	Checks	Yes	No	Remark
1	Start reprocessing of DIALYSER just after you finish the dialysis.			
2	Check the DIALYSER for any visible blood clot, cracks or any structural damage.			
3	Patient ID is placed on the DIALYSER for future identification along with the number of times it has been used.			
4	Preferably for better results an automatic DIALYSER reprocessing machine should be used.			
5	A leak test (pressure test) and blood volume test should be performed and DIALYSER is discarded if this test fails.			
6	DIALYSERS are disinfected to remove microbes.			
7	New and Reusable DIALYSERS are separately stored.			
8	Do not mix DIALYSERS of +ve patients with others dialysers.			
9	Wash and rinse each DIALYSER just before reuse.			

Note: Patients with Hepatitis B infection are generally given single use dialysers.

H. Checklist Daily Reporting (MIS):

S.N.	Parameters	Remarks
1	No. of patients on dialysis today?	
2	Consent taken from all?	
3	Any special Dialyser Used?	
4	Any complication during dialysis?	
5	All machines working?	
6	If not, BME/Company informed?	
7	Departmental TV was kept ON?	
8	Weighing machine is, OK?	
9	No expired/near expiry medicine/Consumable?	
10	A nephrologist has been the case at least once?	
11	Department is clean?	
12	Both nurse and GDA are present?	

I. Dialysis Unit Audit Checklist:

NABH Reference	Check Points
Primary Audit Check Points	
HIC 2d	1. Overall adherence to infection control 2. Re-use policy of tubes, how safely it was kept and the labelling requirement to prevent exchange/ensure patient's safety. 3. Check Adequate soap, masks, gloves and disinfectants are available 4. Quality of RO water
PRE 3e	• Policy on consent. Who can give consent when patient is incapable
FMS 3c, e	• All equipment is inventoried and log maintained/calibrated • Preventive maintenance/service labels on Equipment/calibration records
Secondary Audit Check Points	
	1. Patient interview 2. Staff interview
COP 4b	• Training in CPR – BLS/ALS
MOM 3g, h	• Emergency drug management
HIC 2d	• Sterilized sets: expiry dates, storage conditions
HIC 5a-e	1. Check hand washing facilities for staff in all care area, instructions for proper hand washing 2. Check Adequate soap, masks, gloves and disinfectants are available
HIC 8b	• Segregation of bio-medical waste

STATIONARY FORMATS:

A. Consent Form for Dialysis:

Hospital Name & Address etc

Department of Nephrology

CONSENT FOR DIALYSIS

Name: -- Age/Sex: ----------------- Registration No.: ---------------

With my physician and members of the treatment team, I have had a discussion of:

1. The technique and nature of the haemodialysis procedure;
2. The alternatives to haemodialysis;
3. The necessity for undergoing haemodialysis;
4. The risk of or from the procedure;
5. The possible side effect of the procedure, some of them can be life threatening & even fatal like heart attacks, cardiac arrhythmias, cerebrovascular accident, intractable hypotension and infection;
6. Additional & different procedure as deemed necessary to tackle any unforeseen/unknown conditions;
7. The medications that might be required during and after treatment;
8. The consequences of refusing haemodialysis treatment;
9. The advantages & disadvantages of re-use of dialyser;
10. The risks of blood transfusions;
11. The risks of getting viral hepatitis in haemodialysis unit in-spite of immunisation (where applicable) in-spite of all precaution taken by the dialysis staff;
12. The need for temporary vascular access such as femoral/subclavian, catheterization & complication thereof (e.g., local hematomas, pneumothorax etc.);

I understand these aspects of the procedure and believe that I have been well informed and given full opportunity to ask questions and receive additional information.

I hereby consent to undergo haemodialysis treatment in the Dialysis Unit of this (name) Hospital.

Signature of the Patient/Relative: --

Witness: ----------------------------

Date: -----------------------------

B. Haemodialysis Record Booklet:

HAEMODIALYSIS RECORD

(FRONT COVER of the booklet of size 1/8)

Page-1

Name of the Hospital	
LOGO	
HAEMODIALYSIS RECORD	
Patient Name:	
C.R. No.:	
Patient Address:	
Hospital Telephone Numbers:	
Please bring this card on every Dialysis	

HAEMODIALYSIS RECORD

(BACK-SIDE OF FRONT COVER of the card of size 1/8)

Page-2

Name ____________________________________

Age _____________ Sex __________

Diagnosis____________________________________

Known Allergies_______________________________

Blood Group__________________________________

Follow up on Date ___________At_________

Date ___________At_________

Date ___________At_________

Date ___________At_________

Consultant I/C	Resident_____________
Name _____________	Name _____________
Signature ___________	Signature _____________

HAEMODIALYSIS RECORD

(INSIDE LEAVES) of the card of size 1/8

Page-3

<table>
<tr><td colspan="8">Date:</td><td colspan="3">HD No.:</td></tr>
<tr><td colspan="11">Bicarbonate/Acetate:</td></tr>
<tr><td rowspan="2">Weight:</td><td colspan="10">Pre-Dialysis:</td></tr>
<tr><td colspan="10">Post Dialysis:</td></tr>
<tr><td colspan="11">B.P. Record</td></tr>
<tr><td>Timings in Hours</td><td>0</td><td>1/2</td><td>1</td><td>1.5</td><td>2</td><td>2.5</td><td>3</td><td>3.5</td><td colspan="2">4</td></tr>
<tr><td>B.P.</td><td></td><td></td><td></td><td></td><td></td><td></td><td></td><td></td><td colspan="2"></td></tr>
<tr><td>Duration:</td><td></td><td></td><td></td><td></td><td></td><td></td><td></td><td></td><td colspan="2"></td></tr>
<tr><td colspan="11">Vascular Access: AVF/ISC/SCC/FVC/AV Shunt:</td></tr>
<tr><td colspan="11">Blood Flow:</td></tr>
<tr><td colspan="11">Ultra Filtration:</td></tr>
<tr><td colspan="11">Heparin Dose:</td></tr>
<tr><td colspan="11">Complications:</td></tr>
<tr><td colspan="11">Medications:</td></tr>
<tr><td colspan="11">Comments:</td></tr>
<tr><td colspan="11">Next Dialysis On:</td></tr>
</table>

Back of Booklet:

You can mention:

1. List of Specialities/Consultants
2. List of facilities
3. INSTRUCTIONS TO DIALYSIS PATIENT
4. GUIDE MAP/HOSPITAL PHOTO

C. MASTER REGISTER:

Date	SN	Patient Name	UHID No.	Bill/Cash Receipt No.	Amount	Dialyser Type	Line: Single/Double/Triple Lumen	TPA details, if applicable	Consumption							Remarks
									IV Set	Heparin Amp	Gloves	Normal Saline	Dialyser	Fistula Needle	Misc.	

RECORDS TO BE MAINTAINED:

A. Relating to Patient Care:

1. Dialysis Record (Master Register)
2. Departmental Manual (SOP)
3. Completed Consent Form
4. Patient's Completed Dialysis Record
5. Fortnightly Culture Reports
6. Transfer/referral slip (for patients that will be transferred or referred to another health facility)

B. Incident and Accident Record: (KPI Record):

1. Complications related to dialysis procedure
2. Complications related to vascular access
3. Complications related to disease process
4. Staff/patient's hepatitis status

C. Water treatment Record:

1. Bacteriological Testing
2. Chemical Testing (TDS, PH etc)

D. Staff Vaccination Status:

1. Hepatitis B (double dose) – 0, 1,2,6 months
2. Influenza – annually
3. Pneumococcal – every 5 years

LIST OF LEGAL REQUIREMENTS:

1. Registration under Nursing Home Act/Medical Establishment Act
2. Authorisation from Pollution Control Board for BMW

3. MOU with third party for collection of BMW
4. NOC from Fire Department

BIBLIOGRAPHY/REFERENCES/FUTURE READING:

1. Dialysis Procedures. Initiation, Monitoring, Discontinuing. Susan Hansen, MBA, RN, CHT (www.hdcn.com)
2. DRAFT 2014 Guidelines for Design and Construction of Health Care Facilities
3. http://www.fgiguidelines.net/comments/draft/2014draft_3.10_Dialysis.pdf
4. © January 2007 Healthcare Information and Management Systems Society. (http://www.himss.org)
5. Guidelines for Maintenance Haemodialysis in India (www.isn-india.com/images/Image/HD_standards_Draft.pdf)
6. Chapter 316 - Dialysis Centre - Office of Construction and Facilities (www.cfm.va.gov/til/space/SPchapter316.pdf)

   Department of Veterans Affairs. VA Space Planning Criteria (316). Washington, D.C. 20402. March 2008 (SEPS Version 1.6).
7. Nephrology Deptt. & Dialysis Dr. (Lt. Col.) D. Acharya M.B.B.S.(Kolkata), M.S.(Delhi) P.G.D.H.H.M.(PUNE)
8. Checklists for Hospitals; by Dr. Arun K. Agarwal; notionpress.com, 2017
9. "Standard Operating Procedures SOP For Hospitals 2nd Edition" by Dr. Arun K. Agarwal
10. "Duties & Responsibilities of Hospital Staff" by Dr. Arun Kumar
11. Standard Operating Procedures (SOP) For Hospitals In India: Complete with Stationery Formats Used in Various Departments in a Hospital– 19 July 2022 by Arun K. Agarwal
12. Guidelines for Dialysis Centre, Directorate General of Health Services, Government of India (http://clinicalestablishments.gov.in/WriteReadData/8451.pdf)
13. Indian Public Health Standards (IPHS)

    Guidelines for District Hospitals (101 to 500 Bedded) Revised 2012 Directorate General of Health Services Ministry of Health & Family Welfare, Government of India
14. Hospital Manual. DGHS, Ministry of Health & Family Welfare, GOI

Chapter – 18

DEPARTMENT OF OPHTHALMOLOGY

INDEX

INTRODUCTION:

"World is beautiful"

'Thamasoma Jyothir Gamaya' - Lead us from darkness to Light

Ophthalmology is the branch of medicine that deals with the anatomy, physiology and diseases of the eyeball.

The department of ophthalmology is unique in this hospital as it provides the best of ophthalmology services by the most experienced & renowned doctors providing for treatment for anterior segment as well as posterior segment disorders of the eye along with well-trained opticians, spectacle shop & orthoptist.

The department provides 24 × 7 emergency services and indoor services. OPD services are provided 6 days a week and this practice caters to on an average 50 patients in a day. The eye department is supported by a competent in-house laboratory and on-call radiology services and internal cross referrals with other specialties. The ophthalmic specialties currently available in the department are general ophthalmology, anterior segment, microsurgery, Posterior segment examination & Evaluation, Medical retina, surgical retina for uncomplicated retinal detachment surgery, Ophthalmoplasty, Glaucoma & Squint evaluation & treatment, Refraction & glasses, optometry & vision testing facilities.

This department is fully equipped with latest equipment for complete examination, diagnosis, and treatment (both medically and surgically) of all eye diseases in both adult and paediatric patients.

Almost all eye disorders can be diagnosed and treated well in an ethical manner.

The Department has state of the art equipment for diagnostic and therapeutic purposes.

Presently about .... patients visit OPD every day

On an average .... surgeries are performed on monthly basis.

OBJECTIVES:

1. To extend and facilitate high class affordable ophthalmic services to all strata of society.
2. To continuously improve on departmental standards in providing preventive, curative and palliative patient care.
3. To develop ophthalmic care through subsidized eye care camps to the needy strata of society as part of corporate social responsibility.

AIM:

1. To provide highest quality ophthalmic care to all sections of the society.
2. To outreach distant community by conducting regular eye camps.
3. To treat all without any consideration of caste and creed.
4. Better eye care at affordable cost.

VISION:

1. Our vision is to restore vision.
2. The Department of Ophthalmology of this hospital is committed to be a 'CENTRE OF EXCELLENCE' by excelling in each of our core areas—patient care, research, and education.
3. Help Indian Government in all its blindness prevention and Health education programs such as The Motiya Bind Mukti Abhiyaan of the Government of Delhi.

MISSION:

The Department of Ophthalmology has the mission to combat eye disease and to reduce the prevalence of blindness through a scientific approach by providing equitable, excellent and efficient eye care to the people

1. To conduct continuing educational programs and activities to keep up with the changing trends in the field.
2. To create awareness about eye donation in the Society by conducting various programs.
3. To create awareness about glaucoma in the Society.
4. To prevent and treat blindness to the extent possible for this hospital.
5. To be actively associated with "All India Ophthalmological Society and Society for Prevention of Blindness in India".
6. To assist in the implementation of National Program for the prevention of blindness & rehabilitation of the visually impaired

BEST PRACTICES:

1. Our hospital has all the latest equipment & facilities for the benefit of patients.
2. Some cataract surgeries are done free of cost in the NPCB programme.
3. Every day a separate specialty clinic is conducted by the respective specialist doctor.
4. Some Vitrectomy as well as Keratoplasty surgeries are conducted free of cost? in our hospital (under MPJAY).
5. We conduct multiple cataract camps as well as other multi-diagnostic camps for free that give maximum benefit to the patients.

SCOPE OF SERVICES:

The department is providing all kinds of comprehensive eye care facilities, emergency services and ROP screening as well.

A. OPD Services:

1. OPD Timings: 9.00 am to 5.00 pm (as per the hospital policy)
2. Specialty clinics for Glaucoma, Retina, Squint, Cornea, Contact lens, Oculoplasty and Paediatric Ophthalmology.
3. 24 hours emergency ophthalmic services.
4. Facilities for indoor admission and care.
5. Undergraduate and Postgraduate teaching, if applicable

B. In-patient Services

1. Surgical procedures such as; Cataract surgery.
2. All Retina and Vitreous surgeries
3. Paediatric cataract surgeries.
4. Eye Banking and corneal transplant services are also available.
5. Surgical procedures for diseases of lid, Conjunctiva, Lachrymal sac, Orbit, Glaucoma and Cornea are done regularly with advanced techniques.
6. Newborns are screened for Retinopathy of Prematurity and treated with Laser & surgery.
7. All types of lasers are available for the treatment of eye diseases.

SPECIALITY SERVICES/CLINICS:

SN	Name of the Clinic	Days	Timings
1	Glaucoma Clinic		
2	Retina Clinic		
3	Cerebral visual impairment clinic		
4	Eye bank Services		
5	Squint Clinic		
6	Cornea Clinic		
7	Orbit And Oculoplasty Clinic		

SERVICES ARE AVAILABLE FOR:

1. Treatment of Superficial Infection.
2. Treatment of Deep Infections.
3. Treatment of Refractive Errors
4. Treatment of Glaucoma.
5. Eye problems following systemic disorders.
6. Cataract, Squint and Amblyopia, Corneal Blindness.
7. Foreign Body and Injuries.

8. Malignancy/Retinal Diseases.
9. And Paediatric Ophthalmology

OPHTHALMOLOGY PROCEDURES:

A. OPD Procedures

1. Refraction,
2. Syringing and probing,
3. Foreign body removal, (Conjunctival/Corneal,
4. Epilation,
5. Suture removal,
6. Sub-conjunctival & Retrobulbar injection,
7. Tonometry, Biometry/keratometry, Automated perimetry,
8. Indirect Ophthalmoscopy, Retinoscopy.
9. And ....

B. IPD Procedures

1. Pterygium excision, I & C of chalazion, Wart excision, Cauterization (thermal), Lid abscess incision & drainage (I&D), lid tear,
2. Examination under General Anaesthesia,
3. Canthotomy, paracentesis, Air injection & re-suturing,
4. Enucleation with/without implant,
5. Perforating corneo-scleral injury repair,
6. Cataract, extraction with IOL (including Phacoemulsification),
7. Glaucoma surgery (e.g., Trabeculectomy),
8. Corneal perforation/Iris prolapsed surgery,
9. Lid tumours, Conjunctival cyst, Capsulotomy,
10. Anterior chamber wash, Evisceration.
11. And ....

IMPORTANT MEDICINES

Following medicines must be available at the pharmacy of the hospital with ophthalmology services.

Acyclovir Ointment 3%	Ciprofloxacin Drops 0.3%	Gentamicin Drops 0.3%
Gentamicin Injection 40 mg/ml	Povidone iodine Drops 0.6%	Povidone iodine Drops 5%
Prednisolone Drops 0.1%	Prednisolone Drops 1%	Acetazolamide Tablet 250 mg
Pilocarpine Drops 2%	Pilocarpine Drops 4%	Timolol Drop 0.5%
Atropine Ointment 1%	Homatropine Drops 2%	Carboxymethylcellulose Drops 0.5%
Tropicamide Drops 1% (Store in a refrigerator (8 to 15°C) Do not freeze		

INFRASTRUCTURE:

The OPD is situated on the ground floor of the hospital, while operations are taken in general operation theatres.

1. Eye OPDs (General and Speciality Clinic Rooms)
2. Minor OT
3. Major OT
4. Separate Refraction Room

LIST OF OPD EQUIPMENT:

Ophthalmoscope- Direct and Indirect With 20 D Lens	Slit Lamp
Refraction Units, Near & Distant Vision Charts	Streak Retinoscope
A- Scan Biometer and B- Scan	Keratometer
Auto-Refractometer	Fundus Camera
Applanation Tonometer/Non-Contact Tonometer	OCT
Trial Lens Set With Trial Frame Adult/Children	Punctum Dilator
Lacrimal Cannula And Probes	Lid Retractors (Desmarres)
Foreign Body Spud and Needle	Colour Vision Chart
Flash Autoclave	Ophthalmic Chair
Lensometer	EXIMER Laser

LIST OF EYE O.T. EQUIPMENT:

OT Table, OT light - Ceiling Double Dome	Anaesthesia workstation	Electrical Suction
Laryngoscope with 5 Blades (LED)	Piped Medical Gases	Flash Autoclave
Defibrillator (AED plus Manual with ECG)	Surgical Diathermy – Bipolar	ECG Machine
Operating Microscope	Infusion Pump	Cryo surgery
Surgical instruments as required for each surgery	Phaco Machine	Nd Yag Laser
Essential OT Equipment		

INSTRUMENTS SET for CATARACT:

SN	Name	Specs	Size	Qty
1	Mast Pakistan Surgical Inst Cataract	Adult	L = 15 mm	2
2	Halsted Mosquito Forceps	Straight	5″	2
3	Backhaus Towel Clamps	S.S.	3.5″	4
4	Castroviejo-Kalt Needle Holder	Tungsten Carbide TC	5.5″	2
5	Castroviejo Needle Holders	Straight with Catch Smooth	5.5″	2
6	Barraquer Needle Holders	Without Catch Delicate	5.25″	2

SN	Name	Specs	Size	Qty
7	Bonn Delicate Scissors	Curved	3.5 "	2
8	Westcott Tenotomy Scissors	Blunt Tips Spring Handle	4.25 "	2
9	Colibri Corneal Utility Forceps	1x2 Teeth 0.4 mm	3 "	2
10	Dieffenbach Bulldog	Serrated Fine Straight	1.5 "	2
11	Simcoe Irrigation Cannula	Aspirating	--	2
12	Bishop-Harmon Cannula	Silicon Bulb Only	--	2
13	Ribbon Iris Scissors	Curved	4 "	2
14	Vannas Scissors	On Flat Delicate Angled	3.25 "	2
15	Vannas Scissors	Curved	3 "	2
16	Kraff-Utrata Capsulorhexis Forceps	Angled Jaws Flat Handle With Iris Stops 12mm Long Smooth Jaws 0.33 mm Tip	4 "	2
17	Castroviejo Colibri Forceps	Extra Delicate	4.25 "	
18	Barraquer Dewecker Iris Scissors	Delicate	2.25 "	2
19	Castroviejo Caliper	S.S.	3.25 '	2

OUTREACH ACTIVITIES

EYE Camps

1. Eye camps are conducted at peripheral areas of the hospital.
2. These camps are conducted as standalone and also as a part of multi-diagnostic camps.
3. School children eye health camps are also held.
4. Screening & Counselling for computer related vision problem is done regularly.
5. Public is made aware of Eye Donation.

STAFFING:

1. Ophthalmologists
2. Ophthalmic Technician
3. Optometrist.
4. Helpers and Housekeepers.

DUTIES & RESPONSIBILITIES: (to be modified as per policies of the Hospital)

A. OPTOMETRIST

1. They work under direct supervision of an ophthalmologist.
2. To assist ophthalmologists in carrying out eye examination of patients.
3. To prepare patients for examination.
4. They are responsible for recording history of the patient about his/her illness and doing refraction (anterior segment examination).
5. They are responsible for instillation of diagnostic drugs in patient eyes.

6. They are authorised to prescribe and fit various vision aids such as spectacles, contact lenses etc.
7. They will verify the dispensed optical aids, spectacles etc for correctness.
8. Cases are seen by optometrist before being referred to an ophthalmologist.
9. To prescribe vision therapy and orthoptic treatment.
10. To use equipment and instruments at disposal to find out correct type of refractive error and visual abnormality.
11. To use other diagnostic equipment as per advice of the doctor.
12. To ensure correct recording of visual acuity.
13. To cross check the refraction by means of subjective lens trial set.
14. They are also responsible for external eye examination to find out any visual abnormality in the eye.
15. To prescribe correct glasses, contact lenses etc.
16. To train the patient in wearing contact lenses.
17. They are responsible for counselling services. To guide patients about eye health and correct way of using eyes and glasses while reading and writing.
18. They are also responsible for treating binocular abnormalities with the help of a SYNOPTOPHORE.
19. To prepare patients for eye surgery.
20. To assist during surgery if asked for.
21. They are also responsible for organising 'eye camps.
22. He is also responsible for dispensing of various visual aids including glasses.
23. To help patient to perform in various eye exercises and educate them.
24. Will be responsible for safe custody and proper maintenance of equipment put under his/her control.
25. To carry other duties as per his/her skills as assigned by seniors.

B. OPHTHALMIC TECHNICIAN

1. They will be working directly under supervision of ophthalmologists.
2. They will operate ophthalmic equipment placed in the department for eye examination.
3. They will assist doctors (ophthalmologists) in their work.
4. They will prepare patients to be examined by the ophthalmologist.
5. They will collect patient's history & assist doctors during eye examination.
6. They will address patients' queries promptly and effectively.
7. They will perform certain diagnostic tests as per their skill and on doctors' instructions. They should be able to practically operate all diagnostic equipment placed in this department.
8. They also do all work of an optometrist that is refraction and operating eye exercise equipment in his/her absence.
9. They will administer topical ophthalmic medicines (eye drops) for detailed ophthalmic examination.
10. They will assist patient in inserting and removing contact lenses. Will train patients in its use.
11. They will scrub and assist doctors during eye surgeries.
12. They will do ophthalmic dressings.
13. They will guide patients about good eye care.
14. They will wash, clean and sterilise ophthalmic instruments.
15. They will maintain patient records and will maintain confidentiality of these records.
16. They will maintain other records and registers as per policies and procedures of the hospital.
17. They will be responsible for maintenance and preventive maintenance of ophthalmic equipment and their repair in case of break downs.

18. They will also do other administrative and clerical work when required.
19. In large hospitals an experienced technician is labelled as 'Chief Ophthalmic Technician' and they supervise other technician and optometrists.
20. To carry out other assignments as asked by seniors.

C. OPHTHALMIC LABORATORY TECHNICIAN

1. To use machines and tools available in the ophthalmic lab.
2. To be responsible for proper maintenance and repair of these equipment.
3. To cut eye glasses to size, polish them and fit them to a spectacle frame.
4. To communicate with the prescribing ophthalmologist or optometrist whenever required.
5. To judge the quality of the uncut glasses.
6. To verify the power of the lenses before cutting.
7. To assemble spectacle frames and repair them if required.
8. To examine optometrist prescription, broken lens pieces etc to determine specifications for the lenses.
9. To work with contact lenses also.
10. To adjust lenses and frames to correct alignment.

D. ORTHOPTIST

1. To assist ophthalmologists in performing various diagnostic ophthalmic procedures.
2. To self-carry out diagnostic ophthalmic procedures.
3. To take patient history & examine the patient for visual abnormalities.
4. To give therapy as per ophthalmologists' prescription.
5. To coordinate with doctors, technicians to prepare a suitable treatment plan.
6. To provide instructions and guidance to family members and allay their apprehensions.
7. To use and take care of various equipment under his or her charge.
8. To be present in camps to screen patients for visual disorders.
9. To train patients with visual disorders on home therapy and correct use of binocular vision.

E. OPHTHALMOLOGIST (DOCTOR)

1. To distribute duties and responsibilities to all support staff.
2. To maintain discipline, regularity and punctuality. To prepare roaster if required.
3. To monitor performance of his supportive staff.
4. To ensure availability of optimal facilities.
5. To carry out periodic stock verification.
6. To ensure that OPD and OT instruments are always serviceable.
7. To ensure proper communication with other departments.
8. To organise CMEs and lectures for training to staff.
9. Should have professional indemnity insurance of minimum Rs. 20 las.
10. To conduct a comprehensive eye test of patients and assess their vision.
11. Managing ophthalmic conditions, being responsible for both the medical and psychological aspects of dealing with patients
12. To examine anterior chamber in details.
13. To examine the condition of the retina, eye muscles and optic nerve.

14. To look for signs of cataract, glaucoma, macular degeneration, eye infection and other eye disorders
15. To prescribe eyeglasses and contact lenses to correct vision.
16. To order oral and topical medication to treat eye diseases.
17. To undertake eye surgery and treatments.
18. To make rounds of his admitted patients on regular basis.
19. To maintain all documents as per hospital policy.
20. To attend committee meetings as and when called for.
21. To suggest up gradation of methods and facilities to the management.
22. To help in prevention of HAI (Hospital Acquired Infections), Bio medical waste management.

TOPICS FOR CME:

1. Phaco Update
2. Recent updates in retinopathy of prematurity (ROP) screening
3. Fundamentals of Keratoplasty
4. Steroscopic analysis of ONH
5. Examination of Squint

KEY PERFORMANCE INDICATORS: (KPI)

Are same as that of an OPD/OT/Ward

1. **Waiting Time in Specialized OPD:**
   It is the time taken for a patient to be attended to by the doctor starting from the patient's appointment time or registration time.
   Formula:
   Number of patients seen within ninety (90) minutes in a specified month divided by Total number of patients attending Ophthalmology clinic in the corresponding month multiply by 100
   Standard: More than 90% of cases are seen within one hour
2. **Percentage of patients without ocular co-morbidity obtained visual acuity of 6/12 or better within (≤) 3 months following cataract surgery:**
   Visual acuity as a measure of good visual outcome – visual acuity of 6/12 or better following cataract surgery
   Ocular co-morbidity – pre-existing ocular problems/pathology which will influence final visual outcome.
   Inclusion: All Cataract surgeries
   Exclusion: Cases with pre-existing ocular co-morbidity that will affect the visual outcome
   Formula:
   Total number of patients without ocular co-morbidity, who underwent cataract surgery in a specified month and attained visual acuity of 6/12 or better within 3 months following surgery divide by Total number of patients without ocular co-morbidity, who underwent cataract surgery in the corresponding month multiply by 100
   Standard: More than 85%
3. **Percentage of patients developed Infectious Endophthalmitis following cataract surgery:**
   Inclusion: All patients underwent cataract surgery
   Exclusion: Traumatic cataract secondary to penetrating/perforating eye injury and Emergency cataract surgery from any cause.

Formula:

Total number of patients developing post-operative endophthalmitis within 3 months following cataract surgery in a year divide by Total number of cataract surgeries performed in that specific year multiply by 100

Standard: Less than 0.2% (2 cases per 1000 operations)

4. **Rate of Posterior Capsular Rupture during Cataract Surgery**

   Bench Mark: < 5 % (50 cases per 1000 operations)

5. **Average Frequency of Mortality/Morbidity Review being Conducted in the Department Monthly:**

   Standard: At least 1 time in 6 months

6. **Percentage of Out-patients seen by a specialist in specialty clinic per month:**

   Standard: To be decided by the hospital

7. **Waiting Time to get an appointment for First Consultation**

   Time measured from the day the patient requests for an appointment (makes a call/presents with a referral letter to the Ophthalmology Specialist Clinic) to the date of appointment for first consultation

   Total number of Diabetic patients *(who are referred for the first time to Ophthalmology clinic)* given an appointment for First Consultation within 6 weeks

8. **Waiting Time for Cataract Surgery:**
9. **Time between surgery and discharge should not be more than 2-3 days**

STATIONARY USED IN OPD:

A. OPD Record:

Name.. Age/Sex...................

Address..

Tel. No... Occupation.................................

Hospital Registration No....................................

Referring By...

Date of First Visit...

Presenting Complaints:

History of Present Illness:

Past Ocular History:

Any Eye Injury Any Eye Surgery

Medical History:

Coronary Artery Disease Asthma Diabetes

Blood Pressure Dyspepsia Gastric Ulcer Etc

Presently on any Medication?

Medicines/Dose &/Duration

Personal History:

Smoking Alcohol Tobacco Chewing

Allergy Etc

Family History:

Coronary Artery Disease	Asthma	Diabetes
Blood Pressure	Any Chronic Eye Disease in the family.	

(on Page-2)

OCULAR EXAMINATION

Vision	Left Eye	Right Eye
Without Glasses		
With Glasses		

External Examination Left Eye Right Eye

Lids

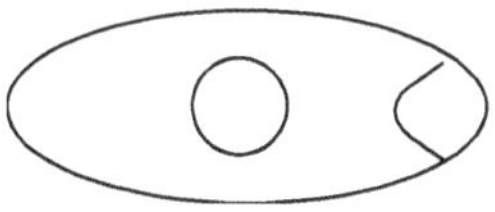

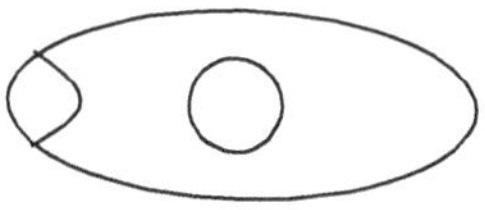

Conjunctiva

Cornea

Lens

Ocular Movements

Anterior Chamber

Pupil

Intraocular Pressure

(On Page-3)

FUNDUS EXAMINATION

Left Eye Right Eye

Disc

C/D Ratio

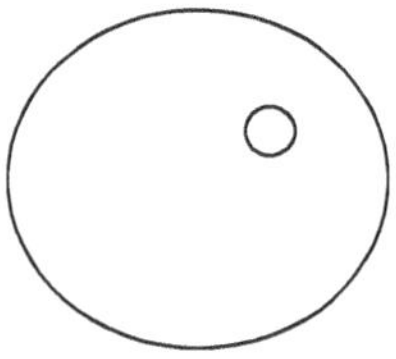

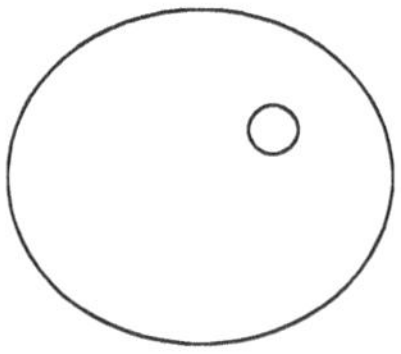

Retina

Others:

Investigations

Result

Medical Advice & Treatment

B. Ophthalmic Surgery - Operative Notes:

Page-1

Name:	Age:	Sex:	Reg. No.:

Date:

Surgeon:	Assistant:	Anaesthetist:

Pre-Operative Diagnosis:

Operation Performed:

Anaesthesia: Local/G.A.

Sterile Pre & Drapes

Exposure: : Lid Speculum: Barraquar/......

: Lid Sutures: Y/N, ...

: Superior Rectus Suture: Y/N ....

Conjunctival Flap:

: Limbus/Fornix/Nil

Entry:

: Razor Blade/B.P. Blade, ...

: Problems

Capsulotomy:

: Visilon: Y/N, ...

: Needle: ....

: Problems

Section:

: C.S. Scissors, ...

: Problems ......

12 o'clock Suture: Y/N

Use of Cautery: Y/N

Ant. Capsule Removal:

Intoto/Partially/Ant. Capsulotomy with scissors after cortical aspiration

: Problems ....

Nucleus Removal: : Vectis/Sliding/.........

: Problems

Cryo Extraction: Y/N .... Iridectomy: Y/N PISI

Partial Wound Closure: 10/0 Monofilament/......

No. ....

Page-2

Cortical Clean up: Reverse Simcoe/Automated/Classical Simcoe

Time ......

Quantity BSS

Remnants: Traces/1+/2+/......

Problems: Vitreous Prolapse/etc

Vitrectomy: Y/N Aspiration with wide bore Cannula/Weck sponges + vanas/ Automated Vitrector

Visilon/Air/BSS: Y/N Amount ....

IOL Insertion: Ac/PC

Instruments

Dialling Y/N ......

Problems: ......

Clinical Impression: In the bag/Sulcus

Wound Closure: 8-0 Silk/8-0 Monofilament

10-0 Monofilament

Total Sutures ......

Depth ......

Additional Remarks:

Drugs: Sub-conjunctival ....

Drops ......

Ointment ......

None ......

Patch & Shield ......

VARIOUS CHECKLISTS OF OPHTHALMOLOGY SERVICES:

A. Checklist Ophthalmology OPD:

SN	Check	Yes	No	Remark
1	Each patient is identified by calling his/her name?			
2	Each patient undergoes comprehensive eye examination? Coming for consultation and registering with the hospital is itself consent for OPD examination.			
3	Detailed fundus examination is undertaken for all patients?			
4	Slit lamp examination is done for each patient?			
5	Perimetry is performed for all suspected cases of 'Glaucoma'?			
6	'Objective Refraction' is done for all patients reporting in OPD?			
7	Patients with refractive error do undergo 'Subjective Refraction' after pupil dilatation.			
8	Prior to IOL surgery, power is determined by 'keratometry' and 'A-scan' regularly?			
9	Each patient is informed about the procedure and its outcome. It is called participation of the patient in the treatment			

B. Checklist Departmental Performance:

SN	Check	Yes	No	Remark
1	What is the waiting time for an OPD consultation? Should be less than 30 minutes.			
2	What is the waiting time for a cataract surgery? Should be less than 1 day.			
3	What is the incidence of post-operative infection? Should be less than 2 cases per 1000 operations (0.2%)			

SN	Check	Yes	No	Remark
4	What is the rate of operative complications? Should be less than 3%.			
5	Post operative visual acuity (after cataract surgery) is better than 6/12? Should be in more than 85% cases.			

C. Daily Checklist Eye OT:

SN	Check	Yes	No	Remark
1	Is OT cleaned, disinfected and fumigated?			
2	Are all equipment cleaned/(Cautery, Microscope, etc.)			
3	Surgical scrub container checked and replenished?			
4	Anaesthesia trolley checked? (may be required)			
5	Surgical instruments set checked for proper sterilisation? Instruments are autoclaved or sterilised by ETO. Chemical sterilisation is not to be done.			
6	Functioning of microscope & cautery checked?			
7	Linen drums (for gowning) checked and filled with fresh supply?			
8	Emergency drug trolley checked and replenished?			
9	Sheet on OT table changed?			
10	IV Fluid (RL) checked visually for clarity?			
11	UV lights, if 'ON' are put 'OFF'? UV Lights are switched ON after the end of day and are kept On during night.			
12	Culture swab taken on every Saturday before fumigation?			
13	Stock registers completed at the end of day?			
14	Surgical Checklist is followed for each surgery.			
15	Surgical instruments are not shared between cases.			

D. General Checklist Eye Surgery:

SN	Check	Yes	No	Remark
1	Eye contact procedures (Intraocular tension taking, Keratometry, A-scan etc) are done on day of surgery.			
2	Informed consent taken?			
3	RBS and BP are within limits?			
4	PAC done			
5	Pre operative antibiotic drops?			
6	Is operation microscope ready?			
7	Is ophthalmic cautery functional?			
8	Are gloves changed for each case?			
9	Is batch number of irrigating fluid recorded for each patient?			
10	Is eye prepared with 'betadine' for each surgery?			
11	Do not touch IOL and any surgical instrument without wearing gloves.			
12	Medical documentation should be full and proper for all cases.			

E. Checklist Post-Operative for Cataract Surgery:

Following checks should be performed on the next day of surgery;

1. Check vision
2. Check for IOL's stability, any dislocation.
3. Check pupil's shape and mobility.
4. Check wound for any abnormality.
5. Check vitreous and fundus
6. Do slit lamp examination.
7. Visual acuity should be >6/18.

TIPS TO SAFEGUARD VISION:

1. Wear sunglasses
2. Don't Smoke
3. Eat a healthy diet
4. Wash your hands regularly
5. Have a baseline eye exam by age 40
6. Wear eye protection when playing sports or doing home repair jobs
7. Know your family history
8. Early intervention
9. Know your eye care provider
10. Contact lens care
11. Be aware of eye fatigue
12. Take Sufficient sleep
13. When use Computer and Mobiles
    a. Keep your computer screen within 20"-24" of your eye.
    b. Keep the top of your computer screen slightly below eye level.
    c. Adjust lighting to minimize glare on the screen.
    d. Blink frequently.
    e. Take a break every 20 minutes to focus on an object 20 feet away for 20 seconds.
    f. Use lubricating eye drops to soothe irritated, dry eyes.

SOPs OF CERTAIN PROCEDURES:

A. Operation Theatre

Purpose: To operate the patient for a procedure as a routine or in an emergency in a safe and sterile environment, therefore providing highest standard of care to all patients.

1. OT sterilization to be checked and ensured by the team.
2. Patient reaches in the entry area with OT dress from the ward itself.
3. The team checks all the information of the patient's operation.
4. Necessary instruments/equipment is ready? Check.
5. The patient is operated following WHO "Safe Surgery Checklist"
6. Patient is shifted to the ward/recovery area.

7. After checkups the patient is sent home or to the ward with proper orders/discharge summary.
8. Time between surgery and discharge should not be more than 2-3 days.

B. SOP for Operating Any Equipment:

Purpose: To maintain safety of the patient as well as that of machine.

1. As a rule, do not use equipment in the presence of flammable agents.
2. Make sure that there are no naked wires and the machine is in working order.
3. Never turn the power switch off or disconnect the power without proper system shutdown.
4. Avoid concentrating the illumination output on a small area of the retina for prolonged periods of time.
5. Position the patient properly with patience.
6. Use proper appliance meant for that equipment.
7. Do not hold the power cord, but hold the mains plug to disconnect it from an outlet.
8. After measurement of each patient, wipe the forehead rest and chinrest with a clean cloth.
9. Avoid storing the device in an area with excessive heat, humidity, or dust.
10. Untrained persons should not use the machine.
11. Turn off the power and cover the instrument with a dust cover when not in use.
12. Always keep the instrument covered with a dust cloth when not in use.

C. Procedure for Vision Testing:

1. Distance between the chart and observer should be 6 meters
2. Each eye should be tested separately
3. Near vision is to be tested at reading distance
4. Glasses should provide most comfortable and sharpest vision
5. Myopia should be under-corrected and Hypermetropia should be exactly corrected
6. Now a days it is not performed in dark surroundings
7. It should not be performed when pupils are dilated
8. Spectacle prescription should not be given in case of uncontrolled blood sugar.

D. Admission Procedure/PROCESS:

1. **Registration Of Out Patient - Eye Department:**

   The eye OPD is functional between 9:00 AM to 2:00 PM from Monday to-Saturday with lunch time from 1-4 pm, the registration clerk at the OPD registration counter shall decide the specialty after hearing the complaints of the patient. The consultation fee is deposited at the same counter and the patient is directed to the eye OPD. Once the patient is examined by the consultant, relevant investigations are ordered accordingly. The reports of the investigations performed on the patient are collected the same day or the next day by the patient and reviewed by the doctor. Depending on the result of the investigations and clinical examination, patient is advised for admission or prescribed the treatment as an outpatient.
2. **Admission Through OPD:**
   1. Patient reported to OPD Registration.
   2. Registration counter clerk refer the patient to the eye consultant after registration.
   3. Patient examined and investigations ordered.

4. Depending on the reports patient is advised Inpatient/out patient management.
5. Referred to relevant consultants if patient belongs to other specialty.
6. If required admission, admit the patient as per the admission & discharge criteria.

SUMMARY

1. Depending on the results of the investigations and clinical examination, patient is prescribed medicine as an outpatient or advised admission.
2. If the patient is direct cash paying patient advance payment is deposited and admitted to either the room sharing category/Single room depending on the patient's choice and availability of bed, after completing the admission process the patient is sent to ward for further management.
3. If the patient is of insurance/corporate patient, then he is sent to the TPA section to complete the formalities and obtain the authorization. Once the authorization is obtained, the patient is admitted as per his eligibility criteria. If the authorization is denied then the patient will be treated as Cash Patient and he will go through the normal procedures.

3. **Admission Through Casualty:**

Flow Chart

1. Patient reports to casualty
2. Patient record file prepared, doctor on duty examines.
3. Medical officer examines the patient, orders investigations & inform the consultant
4. Consultant decides after reviewing the reports
5. If OPD treatment, prescribe medicines.
6. If Inpatient treatment: Admission – Follow instructions of admission & discharge criteria

SUMMARY

In case of emergency, the patient is directly taken to casualty department, where medical officer on duty informs the eye Resident who shall examines the patient, order for investigations, and start the treatment. After that he will inform the eye consultant who will decide the final decision on treatment. Patient is registered in the Casualty register. The concerned police personnel are immediately informed about any Medico legal problem like extensive injury to the eye, burns, assault, accident etc. on a prescribed Police Information Form. Those patients who do not require admission will require either Day Care facility or conservative OPD management. In case the patient requires Day Care facility then the Day Care Counter staff will prepare a Day Care file and in case the patient requires conservative OPD management then the OPD registration counter staff will prepare the Patient file.

E. PROCEDURE FOR POLICE INFORMATION:

a. In case the patient is conscious/unconscious with attendant and has severe eye injury or any other severe eye problem collect the information from the patient/attendant. In case the patient is unconscious and has no attendant, try to collect the information from the person who brought him to the hospital/any other ID proof or information available with the patient.

b. For any Medico-legal case the police information should be sent immediately to the concern police station in duplicate. The duplicate copy should be signed by the receiving authority at the police station and filed with the patient record.

F. Treatment Protocol In Ward:

1. Admission through OPD/Casualty
2. Check-up of eye: anti-segment/post. segment. Imaging/by consultant

3. Further evaluation by ophthalmic consultant
4. Treatment started
5. Morning and evening records
6. Decision on further treatment & referral if any

SUMMARY

As soon as the patient is admitted in the ward, Medical officer on duty examines the patient and writes down the clinical notes on the case sheet. The relevant investigation forms are filled and handed over to the sister who in turn gets the investigations done. If the patient requires an intravenous line, it is immediately started antibiotics and other drugs given as and when required or prescribed. The sister on duty monitors the vitals and she informs the Medical officer regarding any untoward development. The Medical officer who has examined the patient informs the consultant. The consultant than reviews the patient, his reports and prescribes the treatment required and advises the Medical officer to carry out the orders.

G. Minor OT & OPD Procedures:

1. Foreign body removal- Eye is anesthetized with topical paracaine and a spud is used to remove foreign bodies and eye is bandaged.
2. IOL power Estimation- A scan reading and keratometry is utilised for this.
3. A Scan- for IOL power and axial eye length is done after topical Anaesthesia in eye.
4. Indirect ophthalmoscopy – After dilating eye with mydroatics procedure can be done with patient in sitting or reclining position
5. Suture removal-. Using topical Anaesthesia eye sutures removal done in minor OT.
6. Syringing of lacrimal Sac – With topical Anaesthesia with paracain and punctum dilator syringe of lacrimal sac is done.
7. IOP measurement – With tonometer, with patient in reclining position the eye pressure is checked.
8. Epilation – with topical Para came anaesthesia using forceps and traction misdirected eye lashes are removed.
9. Gonioscopy – with the help of slit lamp and gonioscopy lens to assess various angles in the eye.
10. Cryo of retinal tears – with aid of indirect ophthalmoscope after pupillary dilatation the retinal is localized and cryo is carried out with patient in reclining position and topical anesthetizing of the eye.

H. Procedure For Discharge And Billing:

1. **During Normal Discharge:**

   SUMMARY

   The consultant during the round, taking into consideration of the various parameters will decide the right time for discharging the patient. The consultant informs the patient/attendants 24 hours before discharge so that they can make necessary arrangements to carry the patient back home and enable them to clear the pending bills. The patients are discharged preferably in the forenoon. The consultant gives written orders on the case sheet for the discharge of the patient. The staff nurse on duty returns all unused medicines to drug stores and sends the case sheet to cash counter for billing. The medical officer on duty prepares the discharge summary in accordance with the standard format of discharge summary. The discharge summary is then sent to the consultant for corrections and signature.

   Patient is informed about the readiness of the bill and requested to settle the same after the final bill is verified and cleared by the Admission and Discharge in charge. Cash counter staff issues the Receipt of final settlement to the attendant. The attendant shows the receipt to the ward nurse in-charge who then delivers the discharge summary to the attendant/ patient. The Medical officer explains to the patient/attendant the details in the discharge summary, medication and other follow up instructions. The ward boy ensures that the patient is transferred to the main gate of the hospital safely on a stretcher/wheel chair.

2. **Discharge Against Medical Advice/Lama**

   FLOW CHART

   1. Patient's relatives are made to sign a printed form explaining the complications and risks related to discharge against medical advice
   2. Discharge summary is made on the same lines indicating on the top:

      "DISCHARGE AGAINST MEDICAL ADVICE (LAMA)"
   3. All the investigations are also handed over to the relatives.

   SUMMARY

   For all patients leaving against medical advice (LAMA), the consultant explains in detail the consequences of leaving the hospital without proper treatment to the patient/attendants. Even if the patient wants to leave, signatures/thumb impression of the patient/attendants is taken on the case sheet and on the LAMA Performa explaining the consequences, in the presence of witness a hospital staff (nurse or doctor) who signs the documents also.

   The discharge summary for LAMA cases is prepared in the same manner as for other cases the only exception being mentioning LAMA on the top of the discharge summary. The billing process remains same as for other cases.

3. **Discharge During Night Hours:**

   Sometimes the patient needs discharge during night hours when he wants to be transferred to some other facility for further management or some other reason, and then the consultant decides the discharge. The Medical officer will prepare the discharge summary. Unused medicines are returned to drug stores. Other procedures are as per normal discharge.

4. **Discharge In Case Of Medico Legal Cases (MLC)**

   In case of Medico legal cases the discharge process and billing process remains same as for any other patient. Police clearance must be obtained before discharging any MLC case, where the police was informed at the time of admission.

5. **Day Care Admission And Discharge Procedures: -**

   The discharge slip is made and billing carried out as described previously. Once the patient is cleared for discharge, the patient is discharged with instructions to contact the consultant after going home. Day care is morning to evening only. If overnight stay is required the patient should be admitted as an outpatient. Discharge summary and discharge procedure remains same as for all inpatients.

QUALITY CONTROL:

1. Ensure accurate and reliable collection of data.
2. Develop SOPs for routine procedures.
3. Develop SOP for ophthalmological procedures.
4. Ensure that technicians adhere to the set Sops.
5. Keep equipment calibrated.
6. Keep supplied/inventory updated.
7. Prepare quality indicators (KPI) periodically.

RECORDS GENERATED:

Following records will be maintained in this department in the specified format.

1. OPD examination Records
2. Special clinic records of patients
3. Operation Register (OT Register)
4. IPD Master Register of admissions and discharges

MOBILE EYE CLINIC:

Introduction:

Blindness is a major health problem in India with the largest blind population being in India. 80 % of the blindness is due to CATARACT. Though this type of blindness can be prevented, people suffer from it because of lack of services.

Most of the services are concentrated in the cities, while 80 % of our population resides in rural areas. Also, cataract is generally a disease of old age, when the person is dependent on his family members.

Declaration of Alma Ata "Health for all by 2000 A.D. "has failed only because we could not take the Health Services to the doorstep of rural population.

Aims & Objectives:

To redeem those sufferings from curable blindness is a goal to be pursued by this Mobile Clinic.

Main aims & objectives are as follows.

1. To develop models of quality, low-cost on-going primary care in rural areas through creation of new facilities and linkage with existing facilities.
2. To extend & promote high quality eye care away from main hospitals, at the doorstep of patients.
3. To prevent blindness due to cataract through early intervention.
4. To help the base hospital to successfully attract a large number of patients.
5. To help schools in screening children for any eye disease.

Eye Camps Vs Mobile Eye Clinic:

Whenever an eye camp is held, patients are just screened for cataract operations only. Full detailed examination of the eye is not possible. It is because of lack of Medical Equipment, used for diagnosis, in the camps.

Many times, patients do not get good vision after such cataract operation, because of;

1. Poor operating conditions, and/or
2. Other underlying medical problems, which are not, diagnosed before surgery, in General Eye Camps.

All these and many more problems can be overcome, if a camp is organized after transporting required medical tools and operations are done in a planned operation theatre.

Frequent transportation of costly equipment, from the base hospital to campsite is not feasible due to many reasons.

All these problems can be overcome and the aim can be achieved by permanently mounting this equipment in a van.

Modus Operandi:

In its first phase, the mobile eye clinic will go to various villages, under the banner of the base hospital.

The task:

1. Full detailed examination of eye, minor treatment, prescription of glasses and selecting patients for operable eye problems.
2. For surgery patients will be brought or advised to come to the base hospital.
3. During second phase, another "Mobile Operation Theatre" will be commissioned and surgery will be performed at patient's door step in these vans whose Operation facilities are at par with the base hospital.

"MOBILE EYE CLINIC" is a better way of conducting eye camps in villages, though the quantum of work done is less in such clinics than in camps. It is sort of operating Satellite Unit in many villages simultaneously without having any building in each village.

The mobile clinic will visit one village a day, thus covering five villages in a week. Same villages will be visited every week for one month.

Next month again a set of 5 villages will be visited.

The doctor of the Mobile Clinic keeps One day in every week reserved for surgery at the base hospital.

The roaster can be modified as per the availability of doctors and requirements.

Suggestive Layout:

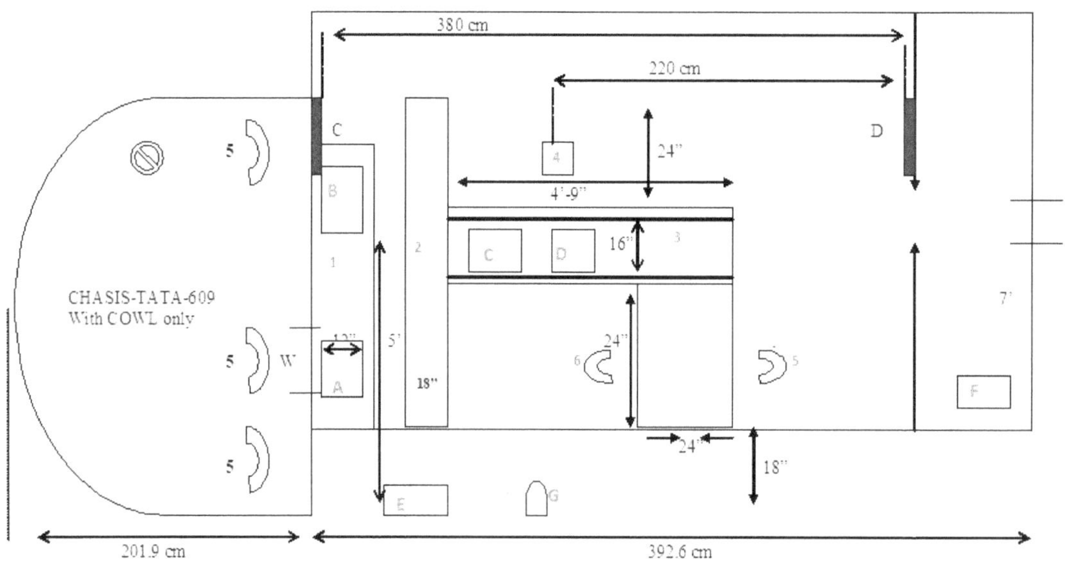

Proposed Mobile eye OPD **Drawing by Dr. Arun Agarwal**

(1) Counter 12" x 60" (2) Patient Couch 18" x 66" (3) L-shape Table 57" x 16" (4) Patient Stool (5) Attendant Chair (6) Doctor's Chair

(A) A-Scan (B) Lensometer (C) Keratometer (D) Slit Lamp (E) Indirect Ophthalmoscope (F) DG Set G = Washbasin

BIBLIOGRAPHY, REFERENCES & ACKNOWLEDGMENTS:

1. "Indian Public Health Standards (IPHS)"
   Guidelines for District Hospitals (101 to 500 Bedded) Revised 2012 Directorate General of Health Services Ministry of Health & Family Welfare, Government of India
2. INDIAN PUBLIC HEALTH STANDARDS SUB DISTRICT HOSPITAL and DISTRICT hospital, 2022, Volume-I,
   Ministry of Health & Family Welfare
3. "Standard Operating Procedures SOP For Hospitals 2nd Edition" by Dr. Arun K. Agarwal
4. "Duties & Responsibilities of Hospital Staff" by Dr. Arun Kumar
5. "Checklists for Hospitals" by Dr. Arun K. Agarwal
6. Mahatma Gandhi Institute of Medical Sciences Wardha
   https://www.mgims.ac.in/index.php/academics/departments
7. KEY PERFORMANCE INDICATORS (KPI) FOR CLINICAL DEPT. 2008: OPHTHALMOLOGY
   Section on Quality in Medical Care, Medical Development Division, Ministry of Health Malaysia December 2007
8. Aligarh Muslim University, Department of Ophthalmology [https://www.amu.ac.in/department/ophthalmology/sops]
9. Dr. Vithalrao Vikhe Patil Foundation's Medical College & Hospital, Ahmednagar. SOP For Department of Ophthalmology

Chapter – 19

DEPARTMENT OF UROLOGY

INDEX

INTRODUCTION:

Urology is a surgical speciality which deals with diseases of the male and female urinary tract and of the male reproductive organs.

The OPD of the department of Urology is located at ground floor of the hospital. It provides clinical services both on OPD and IPD basis involving latest treatment strategies for diseases of the male and female urinary tract and the male reproductive organs.

The department deals with the management of surgical problems of kidneys, ureter, bladder, prostate, and other genital organs like the testicles and penis in the males. In the females it also deals with surgical problems of urinary incontinence, the urinary fistula like the ureterovaginal and vesicovaginal communications.

The department focuses on non-invasive and minimally invasive treatments to give the best possible results with the minimum amount of discomfort.

It deals with both medical and surgical treatment.

PLANNING:

The planning of this department shall depend on following factors (work load);

1. What will be the OPD working hours and days?
2. Many urodynamic studies are envisaged.
3. One OPD chamber shall be provided (120 to 180 square feet, if work load envisaged is not much.
4. Reception and waiting area shall be common for all OPDs.
5. One room for Urodynamic studies.
6. One area for ESWL.

AIM, VISION AND MISSION:

1. To make treatment standards comparable to international and national standards.
2. To create research material and publications of research results in various journals.
3. To organize international and national level conferences, seminars and guest lectures.
4. To provide the most modern services in various fields of urology to patients at affordable cost.
5. To provide all types of services in urology under one roof.
6. To provide high quality holistic care based on Best Practice Principles (BPP)

Vision:

1. To achieve excellence in patient care in urology.

Mission:

1. To provide best possible urological care to all patients with compassion.
2. To impart highest standard of training to subordinate staff.
3. To achieve academic excellence in all fields of urology.

INFRASTRUCTURE/EQUIPMENT:

1. Dedicated Urology Surgery Theatre.
2. Uroflow meter (Urodynamic Machine)
3. ESWL (Lithotripsy Machine)
4. Holium Laser
5. Endoscopes and Endo Urology Instruments: Cystoscopes, TUR set, etc
6. Da Vinci Robot
7. C-Arm

A. **PCNL Set:**
   1. Nephroscope
   2. IP Needle two Piece
   3. Fascial Dilator Set- 8 Fr, 10 Fr, 12 Fr, 14 Fr, 16 Fr
   4. Alken Dilators with Central Rod
   5. Stone Holding Forceps
   6. Clot Holding Forceps
B. **TURP Set:**
   1. Resectoscope Sheath, 26 Fr
   2. Working Element – Passive
   3. High Frequency Cable
   4. Visual Obturator
   5. OTIS Urethrotome
   6. Ellic's Evacuator
C. **Accessories:**
   1. Guide wire: Straight – 0.035 and 0.025 "
Angle tip
   2. Ureteric Catheter – 5 Fr and 6 Fr
   3. DJ Stents- 6/26 Fr, 5/24 Fr, 4/20 Fr
   4. TURP Loops
   5. Three Way Foleys Catheter – 20 and 22 Fr
   6. TUR Irrigation Set

STAFFING:

1. Urologists
2. Urology Technicians
3. Urology Nurses
4. GDAs and Housekeepers.

DUTIES & RESPONSIBILITIES:

A. Duties of a Urologist Doctor:

Urologists diagnose and treat diseases of the urinary tract in both men and women. They also diagnose and treat anything involving the reproductive tract in men.

1. He is overall in-charge of the Urology Department,
2. To conducts Urology OPD with his subordinate staff on specified day and time regularly,
3. To ensure quality performance in the department,
4. Will be 'on call' in all emergency cases,
5. Will be an in-house consultant for all urological emergency situations encountered in the hospital,
6. To diagnose and treat patients' disorders related to the genitourinary organs,
7. Taking daily rounds of his admitted patients,
8. In scheduling of cases and coordinating the department activities,
9. To co-ordinate the Inter and Intra-departmental activities,

10. Documenting and reviewing patients' histories, examination and medication etc,
11. To examine patients and assess their medical condition,
12. To ensure that medications prescribed by him is administered to patients,
13. To perform different medical procedures and treatments using available resources,
14. Ordering, performing, and interpreting diagnostic tests,
15. To prescribe appropriate medications,
16. To advise other physicians whenever asked for,
17. Refer patients to other specialists, when necessary,
18. Adhere to hospital rules and regulations,
19. Supervise all nursing/paramedical & non-medical staff of the department to maintain discipline and high standard of medical care at the department as per standard operating procedure,
20. Interaction with patient attendants to brief them about current status, anticipated recovery and any other specific issues or problems,
21. To ensure compliance with hospital policies about Infection control and biomedical waste management.

B. Duties of a Urology Nurse:

Urology nurses care for patients with urinary tract issues and conditions. They assist with surgeries, assess and order tests for patients, maintain health records, and administer medication and 'Plan of Care'.

1. Educating patient and family members
2. Administering medication
3. Maintaining patient records
4. Assisting with surgeries, procedures, and examinations.
5. Working as per 'Plan of Care' developed by the urologist.

C. Urology Technician:

1. Instructing the patients to undergo proper medication,
2. Managing work schedules,
3. Keeping track of patient records,
4. Maintaining equipment and checking inventory,
5. Performs urodynamic testing on urology patients referred to the urodynamic lab by the Urologist,
6. Performs difficult and routine catheterizations on patients referred from the emergency department, operating room, ICU etc,
7. Must be conversant with use of guide-wires and uretic catheter, etc,
8. Recording of vital signs and history including all medications,
9. Guides patients regarding catheter care, self-catheterization, kegel exercises,
10. Prepares and assists with all procedures performed by Urologists,

SERVICES OFFERED:

1. Daily OPD Services from 9.00 am to 5.00 pm.
2. Daily Operations.
   A. Open Surgery,
   B. Endo Urology,
   C. Oncology Surgeries.

D. Simple Laparoscopic Procedures,
E. Nephrectomy,
F. Ureterlithotomy,
G. Endoscopic Surgeries
H. ESWL
I. Urodynamics Facilities
J. Reconstructive Surgery

FACILITIES AVAILABLE:

1. Lower Urinary Tract Endoscopy:
   a. Cystoscopy,
   b. Visual Internal Urethrotomy (V.I.U),
   c. Cystoscopic management of Vesical calculi (Cystolithotripsy, Cystolithitrity),
   d. Transurethral Resection of Prostate and Bladder tumours & Laser Prostatectomy)
2. Upper Urinary Tract Endoscopy:
   a. Per-cutaneous Nephro-Lithotomy (P.C.N.L)
   b. & Ureterorenoscopy (Rigid & Flexible)
3. Laparoscopic Urology Surgery.
4. Extra Corporeal Shock wave Lithotripsy. (E.S.W.L)
5. Uroflowmetry & Complete Urodynamic Study.
6. Andrology Lab – Ultrasound Penile Doppler Study & Rigiscan.
7. Abdominal & Trans rectal Ultrasound & TRUS guided biopsy of prostate.
8. Holmium Laser
9. Open Urological Surgery.
10. Renal Transplantation
11. Da-Vinci Xi Robot Assisted Urological Surgery.

Facilities may be grouped as under;

A. **Diagnostic Facilities:**
   1. TURS
   2. Digital Ultrasound
   3. Penile Doppler Studies
   4. Uroflowmetry
   5. CECT
   6. MRI
B. **Therapeutic Facilities:**
   1. TURP
   2. PCNL
   3. Uetero Renoscopy
   4. Radical Nephroureterectomy
   5. Radical Cystectomy
   6. Endopyelotomy
   7. Pyeloplasty
   8. Internal Uretherotomy

9. Nephrectomy
10. RPLND
11. Orchidopexy
12. Hypospadias repair
13. Reimplantation of Ureter
14. Ablation
15. Urethroplasty
16. Infertile Surgery
17. Endoscopic Teflon Injection Posterior Urethral Valve

SOME OF DISEASES TREATED IN THIS HOSPITAL:

A. In men:
   1. Cancers of the bladder, kidneys, penis, testicles, and adrenal and prostate glands
   2. Prostate gland enlargement
   3. Erectile dysfunction, or trouble getting or keeping an erection
   4. Infertility
   5. Interstitial cystitis, also called painful bladder syndrome
   6. Kidney stones
   7. Urinary tract infections (UTIs)
   8. Varicoceles, or enlarged veins in the scrotum

B. In women:
   1. Bladder prolapse, or the dropping of the bladder into the vagina
   2. Cancers of the bladder, kidneys, and adrenal glands
   3. Interstitial cystitis
   4. Kidney stones
   5. Overactive bladder
   6. UTIs
   7. Urinary incontinence

C. In children:
   1. Bed-wetting
   2. Blockages and other problems with the urinary tract structure
   3. Un-descended testicles

SPECIALISED CLINICS:

1. Male Infertility Clinic
2. Paediatric Urology: deals with
   a. Stone problem in children
   b. PUJ obstruction
   c. Vesico ureteric reflux (VUR)
   d. Posterior Urethral Valves (PUV)
   e. Ureterocoele
   f. Hypospadias repair
   g. Un-descended testis

SURGICAL PROCEDURES PERFORMED:

1. Pyelolithotomy
2. Nephrolithotomy
3. Simple Nephrostomy
4. Implantation of ureters
5. Vesico-vaginal fistula
6. Nephrectomy
7. Uretrolithotomy
8. Open Prostectomy
9. Closure of Uretheral Fistula
10. Cystolithotomy Suprapubic
11. Dilatation of stricture urethra under GA
12. Dilatation of stricture urethra without anaesthesia
13. Meatotomy
14. Testicular Biopsy
15. Trocar Cystostomy

A. For Children:
   1. Hydronephrosis
   2. Urinary Tract Injuries
   3. (PUV)/Posterior Urethral Valve
   4. Cystic Kidney
   5. Urinary Obstruction
   6. Undescended Testis
   7. Hypospadias and Epispadias
   8. Mega Ureter
   9. Extrophy
   10. Tumours - Urinary Tact

B. For Adults:
   1. All above and
   2. Stricture Urethra
   3. Stone Diseases
   4. Cancer - Urinary and Genital Tract
   5. Trauma Urinary Tact
   6. Genito Urinary TB

C. For Old Age Patients:
   1. Prostate Enlargement and Urinary Retention
   2. Stricture Urethra
   3. Stone
   4. Cancer
   5. (Kidney, Bladder, Prostate, Testis, Penis and Urethra)
   6. Trauma Urinary Tract

FUTURE PLANS:

Future plans include starting DNB training in Urology in the department.

To upgrade facilities to offer renal transplant surgeries in this department.

GUIDELINES FOR PATIENTS:

1. Stay hydrated
2. Drink cranberry juice to help prevent urinary tract infections (UTIs)
3. Limit the amount of salt and caffeine
4. Stay within a healthy weight range
5. Choose a smoke-free lifestyle
6. Strengthen the muscles of the pelvic area with Kegel exercises
7. Encourage children to urinate immediately before bed
8. Limit fluid intake in the night time hours
9. Instruct young girls that they should use a front-to-back motion to wipe the genital area after going to the washroom

STANDARD OPERATING PROCEDURES (SOP)

A. Urology OPD

1. Same system as that of any speciality OPD will be followed.
2. The OPD will function all six days of the week.
3. Timings are as per other OPDs and will be displayed at the front desk.
4. Patients will be escorted to OPD after proper registration on first come first serve basis.
5. Only consultants will be authorised to admit patients.
6. All clinical records will be maintained as per hospital protocol.

B. Urology IPD:

1. Same system as that of any speciality discipline patient will be followed.
2. All admitted patients will be assessed by consultant and medical officers. Assessment will be carried out on daily basis.
3. The case file will be completed by the doctor on duty.
4. Referrals to other departments will be given on written orders of the attending consultant only.
5. Procedures will be governed by SOP for any Surgical Procedure.
6. Documentation will be complete in all respect and as per NABH guidelines.

GENERAL PROTOCOL FOR UROLOGY DEPARTMENT:

1. To provide high quality care based on Best Practice Principles.
2. To use the departmental/hospital resources effectively and efficiently.
3. To provide a safe and comfortable environment to patients and visitors.

4. To provide in-house training to junior staff.
5. To take care of ethical issues.
6. To examine female patients only in the presence of a female attendant.
7. The department should have safe and easy access to support services.
8. Always keep record of various quality indicators to assess the quality of care being provided in this department, and to upgrade the services/make corrections whenever required.

KEY PERFORMANCE INDICATORS:

Much are same as that of an OPD and operation room (Surgical Department).

1. Percentage of emergency readmissions within 30 days for patients following male bladder surgery.
2. The average number of days between diagnosis of urinary retention and surgery for male patients
3. Percentage of emergency readmissions within 30 days for patients following TURBT
4. Percentage of emergency admissions with urinary tract stone that have a stent inserted as a primary procedure during the emergency admission.
5. Percentage of emergency admissions with urinary tract stone that have reteroscopy/ESWL procedure done.
6. Percentage of patients referred to other hospitals.
7. Average length of stay for percutaneous nephrolithotomy (PCNL)

Note: Similarly, some more KPIs may be developed depending on procedures undertaken in the hospital.

Following are common Indicators useful for the Department of Urology:

1. Urinary Tract Infection Rate due to urinary catheter.
2. Surgical Site Infection Rate.

HOSPITAL POLICIES FOR THIS DEPARTMENT:

1. Maximise the use of non-operative procedures where appropriate.
2. Maximise the use of day case surgery
3. Ensure enhanced recovery.

BIBLIOGRAPHY, REFERENCES & ACKNOWLEDGMENTS:

1. "Standard Operating Procedures SOP For Hospitals 2nd Edition" by Dr. Arun K. Agarwal
2. "Duties & Responsibilities of Hospital Staff" by Dr. Arun Kumar
3. "Checklists for Hospitals" by Dr. Arun K. Agarwal
4. Standard Operating Procedures (SOP) For Hospitals In India: Complete with Stationery Formats Used in Various Departments in a Hospital– 19 July 2022 by Arun K. Agarwal
5. https://www.betterteam.com/urologist-job-description

www.ingramcontent.com/pod-product-compliance
Lightning Source LLC
LaVergne TN
LVHW080550160826
845677LV00010B/1793
9798890269461